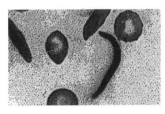

Dying in the City of the Blues

STUDIES IN

SOCIAL MEDICINE

Allan M. Brandt &

Larry R. Churchill,

editors

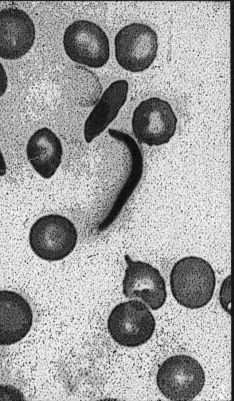

Dying in the City of the Blues

Sickle Cell Anemia and the Politics of Race and Health

Keith Wailoo

The

University of

© 2001

The University of North Carolina Press

All rights reserved

Set in Carter Cone Galliard

by Keystone Typesetting, Inc.

Manufactured in the United States of America

The paper in this book meets the guidelines for permanence and durability of the Committee on Production Guidelines for Book Longevity of the Council on Library Resources.

Library of Congress
Cataloging-in-Publication Data

Wailoo, Keith.

Dying in the city of the blues: sickle cell anemia and the politics of race and health / Keith Wailoo.

   p. cm. — (Studies in social medicine)

Includes bibliographical references and index.

ISBN 0-8078-2584-0 (cloth: alk. paper) —

ISBN 0-8078-4896-4 (pbk.: alk. paper)

   1. Sickle cell anemia — Tennessee — Memphis — History. I. Title. II. Series.

RA645.S53 W35   2001

362.1′961527′00976819 — dc21   00-062865

05 04 03 02 01   5 4 3 2 1

Contents

A section of illustrations follows page 128.

Acknowledgments

I must begin with a word of thanks to the late Dr. Lemuel Diggs — a University of Tennessee pathologist who figured prominently in the history of sickle cell disease and in the story of race and health in Memphis. In 1992 I came across Diggs's corpus of writings on sickle cell disease dating back to the 1920s. I remember inquiring at the University of Tennessee archives about the availability of Dr. Diggs's papers and being quite surprised to hear the archivist say that Diggs (at ninety-two years old) still came in to do research from time to time. During the following years I was able to visit the engaging and lucid Lemuel Diggs and to interview him about his long-standing interest in sickle cell disease. I learned that he had followed the disorder where it took him, from its years of obscurity in the 1920s through its rise to scientific significance in the 1950s and its increasing social and political significance in the 1970s, 1980s, and into the 1990s. His reminiscences and scrapbooks prompted me to begin a broad exploration of the ways in which this singular malady opened a window on the history of race relations, health care, and scientific medicine in Memphis, the South, and America. That exploration has resulted in this volume. Dr. Diggs, who died in 1995, might not have agreed with all that I say in these pages, but I owe him special thanks for starting me on the journey that has resulted in this book.

Along the way, many people have heard me present aspects of this project, and their comments have helped me to sharpen and strengthen the work. My colleagues in the Department of Social Medicine at the University of North Carolina at Chapel Hill have enriched the project in ways too numerous to detail. Also, I must thank the faculties in history departments where this work was presented: at Florida International University, the University of Alabama at Birmingham, Rutgers University, the University of Miami, and Carnegie Mellon University. I received thoughtful feedback from the faculty and students in the Departments of History of Science and of Afro-American Studies at Harvard University where I spent a year as visiting professor in 1998–99. This volume is also much improved thanks to audiences at the College of Physicians of Philadelphia, the Sickle Cell Disease Association of America, the American Association for the History of Medicine, the American Public Health Association, Massachusetts Institute of Technology, the Institute for Health, Health Care Policy, and Aging Research at Rutgers University, and the schools of medicine of Case Western Reserve University, the University of California–San Francisco, the University of Pittsburgh, and the University of Virginia.

Many individuals must be singled out for their critical engagement and helpful suggestions in these and other settings: Caroline Acker, Bridie Andrews, Kwame Anthony Appiah, David Barnes, John Beatty, Suzanne Blier, Charlotte Borst, Robert Brain, Jeffrey Brosco, N. David Cook, Alan Cross, Colin Davis, Jim Edmonson, Jonathan Erlen, Sue Estroff, Judith Farquhar, Peter Galison, Henry Louis Gates Jr., Evelyn Hammonds, Anne Harrington, Gail Henderson, Tera Hunter, John Kasson, Daniel Kevles, Nancy King, Bill Lachicotte, Jane Maienschein, Kenneth Manning, Harry Marks, J. Lorand Matory, Everett Mendelsohn, Robert Murray, Jonathan Oberlander, Robert Olby, James Pittman, Jack Pressman, Kendrick Prewitt, David Ransahoff, Don Reid, Charles Rosenberg, Barbara Rosenkrantz, Des Runyan, Jonathan Sandelowski, Barry Saunders, Todd Savitt, Steven Schlossman, Joyce Seltzer, Lynne Snyder, Donald Spivey, Joe Trotter, Convery Bolton Valencius, Cornel West, and William Julius Wilson. My deepest gratitude goes to those who commented on the entire manuscript, specific chapters, and early outlines. This group includes Chris Feudtner, Nick King, Kenneth Ludmerer, Don Madison, Michael McVaugh, Katherine Park, Reggie Pearson, Stephen Pemberton, David Rosner, Molly Sutphen, Elizabeth Toon, Rachel Watkins, series editors Allan Brandt and Larry Churchill, reader Alex Lichtenstein, and editor Sian Hunter at the University of North Carolina Press. Finally, thanks to Patricia LaPointe of the Memphis and Shelby County Room of the Memphis and Shelby County Public Library, Ed Frank of the Mississippi Valley Collection at the University of Memphis, and various archivists at the Memphis and Shelby County Archives at the Cossitt Branch Library in Memphis, the National Archives and Records Administration in College Park, Maryland, the National Library of Medicine, the Tennessee State Library and Archives in Nashville, and the Library of Congress.

This book could not have been completed without the generous support of several organizations, foundations, and funding agencies. The University Research Council of the University of North Carolina at Chapel Hill provided a small grant that enabled me to begin this study. Later, financial assistance for research came from the Burroughs-Wellcome Fund, from the Ethical, Legal, and Social Issues Program of the National Center for Human Genome Research, and, most recently, from the James S. McDonnell Foundation's Centennial Fellowship. I am extremely grateful to all of these organizations and their selection committees for this encouragement and support.

Finally, I must thank my wife and historian, Alison Isenberg, for her valuable ideas and vital comments from the start through all of the other important phases of this project. Thanks also to my parents, Bert and Lynette, and to my brother, Christopher, for your support, and to little Elliot for being so cooperative, happy, and understanding over the last year. I could not have completed this work without you all.

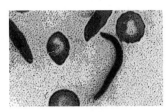

Dying in
the City of
the Blues

Introduction
Pain and Suffering in Memphis

Throughout history, numerous diseases have been used to draw attention to the African American body and to represent particular aspects of the "African-American condition." In the 1850s southern physician Samuel Cartwright invented "dyaesthesia Aethiopis," a disorder that he claimed caused "obtuse sensibility of the body" and insensitivity "to pain when subjected to punishment" in slaves. The "disease" was a convenient invention, for it could be used to highlight just how different enslaved blacks were from their white owners. Biological difference could be used to excuse plantation whippings and to explain the excessive brutality of slavery.[1] Throughout the nineteenth and twentieth centuries many other conditions, syndromes, and pathologies among blacks — from tuberculosis to venereal disease — have been used similarly to moralize about African American status, sexuality, intelligence, education, or economic condition. Whether these discussions focused on what we term "real" pathologies or invented ones, the discourse of "Negro disease" has always reflected deeper moral quandaries in society. Were black people degraded by or biologically suited to slavery? Was black sexuality a danger to whites and to society? Were black people sicker because they were innately different, or because they were kept socially unequal in America? The stories of particular maladies have been mined and interpreted throughout history because they appear to provide the answers to such questions.

The discourse of black disease has often been stigmatizing and controversial, but occasionally narratives of black pathology have also been uplifting. In 1930, for example, a blues guitarist with the stage name of Memphis Minnie brought an obscure disorder into public light, seeking to sow the seeds not of fear or revulsion but of compassion toward ailing African Americans. In her "Memphis Minnie-jitis Blues," the artist Lizzie Douglas sang:

My head and neck was painin' me
Feel like my back would break in two
My head and neck was painin' me
Feel like my back would break in two
Lord I had such a mood that mornin'
I didn't know what else there was to do.[2]

In the lyrics that followed, Douglas sang of the excruciating pain of meningitis, the diagnostic confusion of the doctor, and the enduring faith of her companion. The lyrics dramatized a common, often epidemic, disorder in the South, asking the listeners for sympathy and understanding.

Depending on the time, the context, and the interpreter, the performance of pathology could point in many different directions. The conception of "racial diseases" has provided physicians, patients, and performers ample, ever-changing material for debating race relations in America. From tuberculosis to venereal disease to meningitis to AIDS, the ways in which diseases are defined, characterized, and dramatized provide a window on social relations and social values.

The lyrics of the "Memphis Minnie-jitis Blues" created a drama around a prevalent early-twentieth-century malady, a disorder that affected African Americans in the Mid-South disproportionately. But Douglas's stage performance reflects much about how society had changed since the days of Cartwright's "dyaesthesia Aethiopis." As Douglas sang of her pain on stage, her words portrayed the travail of a woman desperately seeking help from her Lord, from her doctor, and from her companion. In Douglas's time, the blues personalized the obscure, anonymous crises of southern African Americans, attracting ever-wider audiences. Through the blues one woman's experience took shape, gained authenticity and power, and attracted sympathy. Memphis Minnie's was a new voice from Algiers, Louisiana, traveling up through the Mississippi Delta to Memphis, on its way to Chicago. Through the new musical genre, the possibility emerged that African Americans might gain increased understanding for the pain they suffered. Like the blues, Douglas gained visibility and renown on Memphis's Beale Street, and from there her songs of the plight of southern blacks radiated outward via railway, radio, and record player to distant listeners in St. Louis, Chicago, New York, Cleveland, and beyond.

Some 120 years after the rise and fall of "dyaesthesia Aethiopis" and some forty years after the "Memphis Minnie-jitis Blues" had receded from the spotlight, another obscure and painful disorder named "sickle cell anemia" would emerge to exemplify the African American condition. This "new malady" highlighted yet again — but in another political register — painful, hidden, racial experiences. In the turbulent decades of the 1960s and 1970s, and, indeed, through the close of the century, sickle cell anemia — an inherited malady characterized by many symptoms, including repetitive painful "crises" — seemed to embody the problem of unrecognized pain in the African American community. At the same time, it continued to draw attention to the existence of fundamental biological differences between blacks and whites. The interpretation and meaning of sickle cell disease became a potent public issue. The disorder would follow a very different path from its predecessor "race diseases."

The history and transformation of sickle cell disease — from early-twentieth-century invisibility to intense late-twentieth-century politicization — is the subject of this book. This historical study draws attention to the forces that brought the disease to public light, the nature of its dramatization, its evolving symbolism, and the consequences of its high profile as an authentic "black disease." The history of sickle cell disease is presented here as a window on medicine, race, and American society. The story is a narrative of individuals whose ailments were invisible before 1900. Only gradually — in the period from 1910 through the 1930s and 1940s (when Memphis Minnie herself began singing the "Minnie-jitis Blues") — did their ordeal achieve a measure of clinical visibility and scientific significance. In the 1950s came social prominence for "sicklers" (a common colloquial term for sickle cell patients), followed in the 1970s by striking political importance.

The following pages examine the slow process by which invisible suffering has been made visible. Set in Memphis, the story examines how this once-invisible disorder acquired an identity and symbolic significance, and how the malady became a key part of African American identity and a kind of political and cultural currency. The study explores not only the history of the pathology itself, but also the relationship between disease, African American identity, medicine, and American society.

How did sickle cells and the pain associated with the disease acquire this magnitude in the late twentieth century? The disease's transformation resulted from a complex, historically significant reinterpretation of specific signs and symptoms. The transformation reveals changes in the meaning of racial experience, as well as changes in medicine as an economic and political system.[3] Viewing the historical evolution of sickle cell anemia, we witness a series of shifts in which clinicians and scientists, patients and communities, politicians and movie actors, and society at large came to reinterpret and give fresh meanings to pain, blood cells, and disease experience. These various players saw the disease from different viewpoints, connecting the vital symptoms with their own particular scientific, clinical, social, and political agendas. In combination, they shaped an awareness of this single disorder, and through the disease they also informed broader understandings of disease experience, chronic illness, and disease politics in America.

Conventional histories of disease tend to follow only the professional scientists and physicians who, it is assumed, played key roles in shaping the lives of the infirm. Thus the traditional narrative for sickle cell disease dwells on the search for scientific understanding, beginning in 1910 when Chicago physician James Bryan Herrick first reported "peculiar elongated and sickleshaped red blood corpuscles" in one of his patients—a young African American dentistry student from the West Indies (see illustrations).[4] On the basis of this finding, Herrick speculated that the young man was afflicted with a new disease that had never before been seen in the world. Soon afterward other clinicians noted its prevalence among black Americans and speculated that people of African descent were the preferred victims of this mysterious ailment that was characterized by leg ulcers, recurrent joint and abdominal pains, and the telltale sickle blood cells. But just as a river's course is influenced by many factors—topography, climate, and human constructions—so too the history of the infirm has been guided by many factors. For people with sickle cell disease, *three* issues—scientific medicine in friction with race relations and health care politics—have been key factors in their lives throughout the twentieth century.

To date, most conventional histories have focused on scientific medicine and features of the *disease* itself and not on the patient's changing *experience* of the disease. Thus for decades Herrick's clinical recognition of the malady stood as a crucial discovery, for it symbolized the power of Western medicine's laboratory orientation that brought microscopic analysis to bear on clinical problems, making the invisible now visible. But in the 1970s and 1980s, an era shaped by increasing awareness of the patient's perspective as well as of African American culture and identity, some scholars began to weave new discovery narratives—acknowledging, for example, that long before Herrick's "discovery," African cultures must have been aware of sickle cell disease.[5] One Ghanaian-born medical researcher, Felix Konotey-Ahulu, recalled that "unlearned men and women of my own tribe could give accurate descriptions of the symptomatology."[6] Indeed, he noted, well-established tribal names for the disorder revealed a persistent historical concern not with sickled cells per se, but for the intense, agonizing, chronic pain of the disease. In Africa, disease names reflected concern for the illness *as experienced*. "The Ga *Chwechweechwe*, the Fante *Nwiiwii*, the Ewe *Nuiduidui*, the Akan *Ahotutuo* all reflect the onomatopoeia of the repetitive gnawing pains characteristic of sickle cell crisis," wrote Konotey-Ahulu, and this contrasted with Western biomedicine's fascination with cellular morphology.

In the 1970s and 1980s, as attention turned to the patients' experience and to medicine as a cultural force, once-simple questions of discovery, naming, and disease definition became more complex.[7] The questions of who "discovered" sickle cell anemia and how it was named reflected, in microcosm, deeper problems of race relations and cultural difference. They pointed to key divergences between black and white Americans in historical experience. Such issues of how the disease discourse has reflected social relations — from the era of James Herrick through the time of Konotey-Ahulu — are key themes in this book's narrative.

Historians speak of 1949 as another important year in the modern scientific understanding and naming of sickle cell anemia. In that year, physical chemist Linus Pauling suggested that the sickling phenomenon of red blood cells occurred because of a flaw in the molecular composition of the hemoglobin (the oxygen-carrying component of the blood) inside the cells. Sickle cell anemia became, in the parlance of molecular biology, a "molecular disease." Indeed, because of the foundational status of Pauling's research for the emergent discipline of molecular biology, sickle cell anemia was quickly labeled the "first" molecular disease.[8] A subtle error at one point in the vast molecular structure of hemoglobin, it was said, caused the molecules to cluster together, bending the red blood cells they inhabited and thereby creating sickle-shaped corpuscles. It was assumed that the joint and abdominal pains and the variety of clinical problems known as sickle cell disease could be traced back to the subtle molecular error. For scientists such as Pauling, who came to see the disorder through the lens of molecular analysis, the disease became significant in the 1950s and 1960s not because of the pain of its sufferers, but because it served as a case in point of the extraordinary relevance of molecular biology to post–World War II medicine. In the decades after Pauling's work, sickle cell disease was distinguished as the first disorder in which it could be argued that the clinical problems stemmed from a single amino acid mis-substitution on hemoglobin. Molecular biologists comprised a young discipline constructing their legitimacy. By proposing a specifically "molecular" name for the disorder, Pauling's insight closely linked the fate of the then-obscure disease to the vaunting ambitions and ideals of molecular medicine.[9]

This generation of molecular biologists, in conjunction with medical geneticists, shone a spotlight on sickle cell disease, in turn raising many new questions — about the inheritance of this hemoglobinopathy in black people, about its evolution through centuries in Africa, and about whether the disease's continued prevalence among black people was assisted, paradoxically, by its value in fighting malaria on the African continent. People with sickle cell disease became case studies for emerging questions in fields such as evolutionary biology, population genetics, and physical anthropology. In each of these fields, the model disease became rapidly more visible and noteworthy, a test case for establishing the plausibility of novel theories of biological inheritance, adaptation, and evolutionary change. One new theory suggested, for example, that the sickle cell trait began as a beneficial evolutionary protection against malaria.[10] People with the trait (known in the language of biology as "heterozygotes" and in popular parlance as "carriers") showed no sign of ill health. Indeed, the argument went, they were well adapted to survive in malarial surroundings. But when this beneficial trait was passed to children from *both* parents in a "double dose" (one "dose" from each carrier parent), the result was sickle cell anemia, the often-fatal childhood disease. Considered over many generations, the ecological balancing act between malaria, sickle cell trait, and sickle cell disease defined what biologists called a "balanced polymorphism." As such theories emerged in the 1950s and 1960s, the lives of sicklers became more relevant to professional scientific discourse and more widely discussed.

The lives of sicklers as portrayed in these theories also became germane to moral concerns in American society. Had American blacks inherited a "good" gene or a "bad" gene from their forebears in malaria-prone West and Central Africa? Or was sickle cell trait only a "bad" gene when removed from the indigenous context that made it beneficial? Such discussions rendered African American character problematic in the specialized, coded language of science. Would the causative gene and the disease disappear with migration, with intermarriage of Africans among other peoples over time, or with a change in context? Could this disease discussion be applied to debates about the inheritance of other controversial "traits" in American blacks (such as intelligence)? How might the evolutionary understanding of the disease be translated into reproductive policy or the prevention of new sicklers from being born in America?

In the 1950s and 1960s public and professional discourse bound the lives of people with sickle cell disease and their parents to controversial issues ranging from the black diaspora to assimilation to population control. With their increasing visibility in evolutionary biology and clinical medicine, persons with sickle cell disease became more central than ever to Americans' understanding of the complexities of disease experience, to Americans' growing appreciation of the power of scientific medicine, and to sweeping debates over the nature of African American identity.

It was at this moment in the 1960s that the history of sickle cell disease also intersected with the national politics of race, inequality, and health care in America. If discovery and new scientific theories were important in the disease's trajectory, then health care politics — in its local, regional, and national manifestations — became a third crucial force shaping the lives of sicklers. In the late 1960s and early 1970s, as sickle cell anemia was caught up in the torrent of U.S. congressional and presidential politics, the malady became widely characterized as a "neglected disease," a disease of a people whose "pain and suffering" had been ignored for too long, and a disease finally achieving its moment of national recognition. As part of the struggle of black Americans for equal rights and justice, the typical disease experience (repetitive painful episodes) fit neatly with the politics of consciousness-raising. To invoke the pain and suffering of the sickle cell patient was to dramatize the long-ignored social condition of black Americans and to give impetus to social activism. The malady propelled reform in health care and society. For white Americans, embracing the disease and acknowledging the legitimate pain of its sufferers could be an act of symbolic redemption. In the wake of legislative debates about a national health insurance plan, and amidst cuts in biomedical research funding, even Republican president Richard Nixon was compelled to acknowledge the "neglected disease," signing into law the Democratic Congress's Sickle Cell Anemia Control Act in May 1972.

With this legislation came federal funds for medical research, community clinics, and genetic counseling programs. But with national attention also came controversy. As legislation gave recognition to the disorder — splashing its name across television, in newspapers, and through popular media — the intense visibility also nurtured fear, misunderstanding, and resentment. Cautious observers feared that widespread talk of eradicating the "hereditary disease" and the practice of counseling carriers not to have children fostered stigma and discrimination. Enthusiasts, however, promoted mandatory testing for sickle cell trait as an effective method of disease prevention, hoping that the knowledge of their status would lead carriers to make informed reproductive choices about whether to bring a child with sickle cell disease into the world. At the same time, some people resented the "special attention" this disease had gained over other equally prevalent and similarly tragic disorders. Others simply resented the fact that political pressure from African Americans and liberal politicians had influenced the direction of National Institutes of Health (NIH) research dollars.

Indeed, state and national legislation stirred up many fresh controversies. Some states embraced mandatory screening of African American schoolchildren without parental consent. In the name of military preparedness, the U.S. Air Force restricted personnel with sickle cell trait from flying, based on a much-debated theory that their red blood cells would sickle at high altitude and they would descend into painful crisis.[11] To many African Americans, these instances of employment restrictions, coercive testing, and directive counseling about reproduction seemed little more than heavy-handed social control and discrimination. By the mid-1970s, national legislation and increased disease visibility had inspired several backlashes, including defenses of reproductive rights and parental consent and objections to directive genetic counseling.

Sicklers had traveled a long and tortuous road, emerging from clinical and social obscurity to become, in turn, patients with a model "molecular disease," evolutionarily interesting people, part of a powerful social and political cause, and people whose disorder reflected increasingly widespread controversies in the application of genetics to public health. Their disease's clinical, scientific, and political transformation in the twentieth century paralleled the ways in which other hereditary diseases (such as cystic fibrosis and Tay-Sachs disease) emerged from obscurity into prominence, embraced by scientists and by ethnic groups and politicized by patients' advocates and health care activists at century's end. The case of sickle cell disease foreshadowed the rising power of patient advocacy in the 1980s and 1990s (as with AIDS and breast cancer) in shaping biomedical research agendas and popular attitudes about illness and identity.

In writing the history of diseases, scholars often follow these singular currents — clinical discovery, scientific theorizing, and political transformation — as if they were separate events, without attention to how these streams flow together.[12] As we shall see, the disease's twentieth-century transformation can be more fully appreciated if we understand it as a commodity whose value for patients' rights advocates, molecular biologists, and clinical specialists increased rapidly as the economy of biomedical science itself changed and as the politics of illness experience shifted. To call attention to disease as "commodity" is merely to emphasize its place in a network of exchange relationships, where — much like any object — the *disease concept* and the *illness experience* acquired value and could leverage resources, money, or social concessions. Sickle cell disease's trajectory as a commodity reveals, in microcosm, the general trajectory of American health care and medical research in the twentieth century. This way of viewing the history of disease will draw our attention to the ways in which disease discourse meshed with other political and economic developments in health care, including the rise of national institutions like the NIH, the appearance of genetic counseling, the emergence of disease activism, the growing cultural power of illness, the advent of managed care, and the changing political economy of health care in America.

Disease and the Politics of Place

On one level, this study chronicles a national transformation. In every city where sicklers have lived, national trends in politics and biomedicine aided the increasing clinical visibility of their illness. Another national trend — the decline of acute diseases that often masked the very existence of sickle cell disease — also contributed to the rising prominence of the malady. In the 1950s, for example, the disease's rising profile in hospitals across the nation was materially aided by the use of new antibiotics to treat acute infectious disease. To be sure, in large part national clinical visibility drove the malady's social visibility. At the same time, however, the nationwide struggle over racial segregation and civil rights also drove its social visibility, as did the expansion of federally funded biomedical research. Certainly by the 1970s, 1980s, and 1990s it was national activism that made the story of sickle cell anemia a poignant one on televisions and in newspapers across America.

Yet the national history of sickle cell anemia can obscure as much as it illuminates about individual and local experiences. The disease manifests itself in children in their infancy, where it causes its highest mortality. But the experience of the illness varies greatly from one person to the next. In some, pain and infection are overwhelming and recurrent, and in others such symptoms are barely discernible. The illness has always gained significance first as individual bodily experience, and then in the context of families and local communities. As medical anthropologist Arthur Kleinman has noted, "Local cultural orientations . . . organize our conventional common sense about how to understand and treat illness."[13] For most of this century, sickle cell anemia would have been experienced by its sufferers as mysterious, recurrent episodes of severe pain coursing through the abdomen, joints, or bones. Proneness to infection would have stalked many of these sufferers throughout their lives. Children might earn the label of "sickly" and would require constant family care. Many would die early of infectious disease, their deaths attributed to whatever malady prevailed in the community—whether tuberculosis, pneumonia, typhoid, diphtheria, or something else. Rarely recognized as a discrete ailment and never uniform in its effects, sickle cell anemia would not have been perceived by that name. So a child in the early twentieth century might grow to adulthood learning to live with painful episodes and bouts of infection, relying on whatever system of diagnosis or of home or clinical therapy best answered the family's needs. In some places, depending on local diagnostic custom, the ailment might earn the name "spells" or "rheumatism." But for most people who experienced it, the malady would remain nameless and indistinct and yet impossible to ignore. Records of mortality among its sufferers, especially by midcentury, would be scattered widely throughout medical and public health inventories as cases of pneumonia, tuberculosis, rheumatism, or some other ailment, lost amidst the local toll of infant death and infectious diseases.

As we move to the local level, then, the story of disease becomes necessarily more varied, gaining in cultural and geographic complexity. In what follows, we examine the full picture of the disease through the lens of one southern city—Memphis, Tennessee. In this city on the Mississippi River—known for economic and racial conservatism, cotton-oriented business culture, Beale Street blues, fundamentalist religious leanings, and, perhaps surprisingly, one of the nation's first sickle cell anemia clinics—one begins to see the ways in which local values defined the visibility and political significance of the disease long before it became nationally significant. At times civic culture in this "capital city of the Delta" stymied clinical discovery, social recognition, and scientific awareness. But at other times this culture magnified recognition and visibility—indeed, at some historical junctures Memphis could even be portrayed as the exemplary city with a special understanding of the disease. It is only with attention to local culture and the local meanings of disease that we can fully appreciate why sickle cell anemia became a socially meaningful disorder, and how it eventually infiltrated our national politics.

Located in the southwest corner of Tennessee near some of the poorest rural counties of Mississippi and Arkansas, the city of Memphis—self-styled as "America's Distribution Center" — has become a distinctive cross-roads metropolis in the heart of the South. It is a city marked by a checkered heritage — the birthplace of the blues and a center of music tourism along fabled Beale Street, the home of Elvis Presley's Graceland mansion and of St. Jude Hospital (a national landmark in the fight against childhood cancer), as well as the site of Martin Luther King Jr.'s assassination in 1968. The city has come to see itself as an amalgam of characteristically southern urban traits, where close proximity to rural culture bred innovative cultural expression and also fomented vicious racial tensions, where the influences of the rural Delta still mix uncomfortably with cosmopolitan ideals.[14] In the words of a recent historical profile, "Memphis stood where cultures, rich and poor, black and white, urban and rural, did not so much converge as collide."[15] The story of sickle cell anemia in Memphis reveals the impact of this collision on local health attitudes.

Throughout much of the nineteenth and twentieth centuries, Memphis's citizens often blamed the city's poor health record on the constant stream of "indigent outsiders" from the surrounding rural countryside. But try as they might to keep disease at arm's length and to distinguish their own metropolitan health standards from the city's rural surroundings, Memphians drew their identity from those very surroundings. Cotton commerce along the Mississippi River built Memphis, yet the city regarded the influx of people who worked the cotton fields as bad for the civic image, bad for business, and bad for health. The same fact of location that made Memphis a prosperous cotton marketplace thus made it a reluctant center for regional health care; this ambivalence was a key feature of health politics throughout the early and mid-twentieth century.

By the post–World War II decades, however, the city's economy, its relationship to indigent outsiders, and its dependence upon cotton had been thoroughly transformed.[16] Something akin to an inversion of economic values had begun to occur. Cotton was now associated with a single-minded agricultural backwardness and with the region's failure to diversify. Illness, by contrast, once a regional burden, had become a significant economic boon — a new source of income, a commodity in a growing service sector. By the 1950s, in Memphis and other American cities, health care was becoming a booming industry in itself. Post–World War II federal legislation promoting hospital construction and medical research, as well as the passage of Medicare and Medicaid in the mid-1960s, further enhanced the income in city hospitals and transformed the city's view of indigent care. Service to the region's poor could now be used to attract growing amounts of federal health care and research dollars. Private health insurance enrollment had also skyrocketed in the 1950s, further boosting local health care consumption. Such economic developments may seem tangential to the story of sickle cell anemia, yet it is precisely in these postwar years that the malady gained a new measure of local visibility. The question thus emerges, how did local economic transformations underwrite the rising visibility of the disease?

Viewed in this local aspect, the story of disease transformation involves people, institutions, and forces often hidden from the national spotlight. The history of sickle cell anemia involves not only physicians like James Herrick, scientists like Linus Pauling, and national politicians like Richard Nixon, but also mayors and congressmen, countless patients, and local philanthropists. In Memphis local lay healers, from mystical conjure doctors to urban midwives, were as much a part of the disease's history as university researchers, newspaper writers, and ministers. These same people would later become part of the national movement that included television and movie actors, athletes, federal bureaucrats, and scientists. But decades before the national politicization of sickle cell disease, this local economy with its diverse systems of knowledge and belief shaped a particular recognition of the distinctive pain and suffering of the disorder. Through the local lens, we begin to discern how and why individuals and small communities took an interest in this disease, and how their efforts influenced its trajectory on the national stage.

By looking closely at Memphis, we also discern the fine grain of human relationships and the ways in which the worlds of science, medicine, urban politics, race relations, and health belief conjoin in twentieth-century America. Investigating this local dimension of disease requires, of course, sensitivity to society and politics in the South, particularly to the significance of African Americans in the history of the region. It also requires attention to the complex histories of medicine, biomedical research, and public health. In addition, any study of African American pain and suffering in the South must be informed by the history of blues music, the history of regional labor, and the economic history of the region. Accordingly, this study uses a wide range of sources — local newspaper accounts of health crises and controversies, regional musical lyrics, sermons, imaginative fiction, cartoons and popular images, the papers of local congressmen and mayors, the writings of other local Memphians, and the professional writings of the city's physicians and scientists. It also analyzes state and federal government records, including presidential papers, as well as reports from national scientific journals, mainstream media, and medical journals. This range of sources helps us to visualize the history of African American experience and the cultural history of an important disease in America.

Studies of other diseases could yield, and have yielded, similar insights. The history of syphilis, especially in the notorious U.S. Public Health Service (USPHS) study of untreated syphilis in Macon County, Alabama, from 1932 to 1972 (known as the "Tuskegee Syphilis Experiment") has long served as an important reference point — perhaps even an archetype — for understanding region, race, and health care.[17] Such studies of black health in the region have tended to focus on themes such as the history of neglect, the prevalence of racial stereotyping in medicine and public health, the isolation of poor southern blacks and their health conditions from mainstream influences, and the abuses of the segregation system. As James Jones's history of the USPHS study shows, the research project fed into potent regional stereotypes about African American sexual behavior. The perception of syphilis as typical and widespread among southern blacks, and of Macon County's black population as hopelessly ignorant and carefree, played an important role in the USPHS's decision to observe the disease's progress in black men while withholding treatment.[18] The infamous forty-year study was also nurtured in the isolation of rural Alabama, and it was prolonged by the desire of researchers to gather data, despite the deterioration of the bodies of these syphilitic black men and the difficulty of keeping them in ignorance of their condition even after effective therapies became available.

This study of sickle cell disease in Memphis examines similar themes: the driving force of medical research agendas, the potency of racial stereotypes, and the power of social circumstances to dictate patterns of diagnosis and treatment. But different themes also emerge. Black life in Memphis was quite different from life in Macon County, Alabama. Nor was sickle cell disease in the early twentieth century anything like syphilis in its cultural symbolism, in its apparent prevalence, or in its clinical, social, or moral aspects. The history of sickle cell anemia as it unfolded in Memphis was not exclusively a tale of neglect and victimization, and so this is not a story of research scandal. But like the story of "bad blood" in Macon County, the sickle cell story is a narrative of the invisibility of pain and of the long struggle for recognition and political power. It examines the devaluation of black people in the American health care system, but it also explores how, why, and under what circumstances the system has granted visibility and assigned value to the ailments of black people. Unlike the high profile, sexually explosive image of black syphilis, sickle cell anemia offers a portrait of a slowly emerging, chronic experience whose gradual emergence revealed the features of a new society.

The Cultural Meaning of Disease

Assessing the "value" of health and sickness has involved a complex calculus in the South — and therefore the region's history provides an important backdrop for any study of black health. The southern agricultural economy has always relied upon the wellness of black men, women, and children as healthy laborers — the backbone of the region's agricultural prosperity through slavery.[19] Emancipation brought a shift in this calculus. Freedom from slavery offered unprecedented opportunities for former slaves, but as historian Eric Foner and others have noted, it also brought a crisis of health.[20] The high incidence of tuberculosis, cholera, venereal disease, and other epidemic diseases among newly freed people seemed to suggest that emancipation and mobility were double-edged developments. Public health experts predicted the eventual demise of American blacks, unshackled from the supposedly benevolent protection of southern masters, compelled to inhabit squalid shantytowns, and forced to compete in a laissez-faire world for their own food and clothing. Discussions of "racial health" in the late nineteenth century were inseparable from postemancipation politics, particularly since southern apologists saw rising mortality rates as an indictment of emancipation and of the federal Reconstruction agenda. Disease among black people, these apologists insisted, was a sad commentary on the slow demise of the freed slave in America. But all agreed that the health of black Americans entered a period of instability and crisis with the death of the slave system.

At the same time that Herrick noted the possible existence of a new sickled cell disease, discussions of racial disease differences continued to reflect these lingering cultural anxieties. To southern physician Thomas Murrell, for example, syphilis sent a compelling political message to northerners. "If Negro health is a political menace," he wrote in 1910 in the *Journal of the American Medical Association*, "then the diseased one is doubly a social menace, and the invasion of the South by the North forty years ago has brought about an invasion of the North, and that by the man they freed."[21] Although the predicted postemancipation extinction of black Americans had not occurred, analysts such as Murrell continued to interpret disease statistics as if they told a moral tale about emancipation, about the flight of African Americans from rural plantations, and about the dangers awaiting them in urban America. Disease patterns revealed the face of changing social relations and economic arrangements, and in this context, disease discourse carried moral weight, warning Americans about the fallout from migration, urbanization, and the rise of the northern ghetto.

Such debates about black health were inevitably intertwined with political debates about race relations in the South and in America.[22] White southerners, now fearful of losing black labor in the exodus known as the "Great Migration," continued to champion the benefits of the plantation system for the mental, physical, and even spiritual well-being of African Americans. Some, like Murrell, believed that the demise of planter paternalism would only bring an increase in pain and suffering. For others, however, the "backward," rural, and "peasant-like" customs of southern black people — in an age embracing germ theory and the "new public health" — were to blame for black-white health disparities. There were also those who insisted that economic deprivation among black people — dating back to slavery — was responsible for the high rates of death and disease. But for many it was enough simply to state in blanket fashion, as did one southern public health official, that "tuberculosis . . . is today almost a synonym for the word 'Negro.'"[23] Everyone was aware of the ways that factors such as "human nature," diet, morality, innate biology, historical deprivation, or poverty could be invoked as causes of disease, and of how these explanations might serve political ends.

Thus the southern discourse on black health — as well as white health — was linked to regional historical sensibilities, to deeply ingrained notions of white paternalism, and to the question of labor in an agricultural economy.[24] Healthy African American people meant hardy workers, which in turn augured well for economic prosperity.[25] As historian Ulrich Phillips observed in 1915, slave ownership brought with it the responsibility to provide food, shelter, and clothing, and the slave "might also be given medical attention in time of need and perhaps some occasional reward as an incentive. All this was required for the sake of the master's prosperity, if from no other consideration."[26] Though willing to cause pain and suffering in order to punish, subdue, or coerce their human property, plantation owners were often concerned that disease be treated promptly, especially when illness (whether "real" or "feigned") intruded upon the slave's ability to work the crop and thereby bring prosperity to the land, the landlord, and the region.

This moral economy of pain and suffering on the plantation was extinguished for some black southerners as they migrated toward northern and southern cities after freedom. But the paternalistic plantation system remained unaltered for many who continued to work the cotton, tobacco, rice, and sugarcane fields. In the 1880s one Mississippi sheriff could opine that planters wanted "to see cotton grow too well to let Mr. Nigger suffer."[27] As historian James Cobb has noted, "Complain as they might about the fines and medical bills they had to pay for their tenants, few planters appeared to let the economic costs of supporting and retaining labor cut into their profits."[28] Well after slavery had ended, plantation owners' paternalistic interests still dominated regional health concerns wherever traditional plantation labor relations thrived.

By the early decades of the twentieth century, planter paternalism was no longer the primary force influencing black health. A new municipal economy distinct from that of the rural hinterlands began to emerge with the "rise of a new, segregated, urban geography" of cities like Memphis.[29] The federal government's freedmen's hospitals intruded, if briefly, into the traditional southern system, elevating the health of emancipated slaves to a national concern.[30] In addition, by the 1890s small medical schools and hospitals organized by entrepreneurial black southerners had sprung up throughout the region.[31] Simultaneously, the "laboratory revolution in medicine" promised to reshape both individual and public health in the cities.[32] Thus, when Miles Vandahurst Lynk's medical college for black physicians opened just outside Memphis in the 1890s, he envisioned the school as a distant relative of Booker T. Washington's uplifting, self-sufficient, and race-proud Tuskegee Institute.[33] In cities like Memphis, black and white religious congregations pooled funds to build their own hospitals, thereby promoting physical as well as spiritual well-being. Philanthropic organizations supported ventures such as Nashville's Meharry Medical College at an unprecedented rate.[34] Health had become a more complex social and cultural issue, a different kind of concern than it had been on the plantation. Certainly health was still an economic and labor issue for planters, but it was also part of greater public goals of uplift, moral advancement, and urban reform.[35]

Health care, accordingly, became an increasingly significant municipal concern, and a modern (if rudimentary) health care "system" began to emerge.[36] A department of public health was formed in Memphis in the face of the yellow fever epidemics of the 1870s and 1880s; it fell out of use in the 1890s, only to be reconstituted in the early twentieth century in the wake of typhoid epidemics. The city constructed sewer systems and occasionally launched health campaigns (for pure milk and against tuberculosis, for example), but even so, mortality rates increased. By 1910 the city offered an even larger variety of health services, among them a large municipal hospital providing charity care to the poor, a number of modestly equipped hospitals built by Baptist and Methodist congregations, new pharmacies, and a small public health infrastructure struggling to be something more than an office of political patronage. Still, death from infectious disease remained ever present and the burial business thrived. The existence of even this small amount of public health activity in Memphis represented a regional novelty that stood out in sharp relief against the absence of such work in the surrounding rural counties.

In the southern city, the illness as well as the health of black people would become valued in new — and sometimes perverse — ways. Consider, for example, the world of medical education, where "disease" had always held a peculiar appeal to teachers and researchers. In 1924 the University of Tennessee pursued an affiliation with Memphis's ever-expanding municipal hospital in order to gain access to sick patients for educational purposes. The agreement between the school and the municipality reflected much about the new urban economy, for here the dense accumulation of the poor and the diseased actually constituted a net economic gain for teachers and students. The school's dean saw affiliation with the charity hospital as a "golden opportunity for the university. The almost limitless wealth of clinical material afforded by the General Hospital . . . brought [students] into intimate contact with practically all the diseases that they will be called upon to treat."[37] In this urban confluence of teaching with charity health care, sick bodies were valuable educational commodities.[38] The dean's comments were an index of economic and medical change in the city, signaling how the academy itself was expanding and altering ideas about the value of disease. Over the next four decades, the school and the municipal hospital would become the centerpiece of Memphis's growing health care system, constantly introducing new and unconventional notions about disease into civic discourse. Later, as the growth of clinical research added even more "value" to sickness, this new health care system would become one of the most important forces defining disease and black health in the city. The tensions that arose between the declining plantation complex and its way of placing value on health, on the one hand, and this emerging health care / research enterprise and its values, on the other, are central conflicts in the story of sickle cell disease in the urban South.

The transformation of the meaning of disease thus reflected the convergence of many factors — the expansion of medical education, the growth of biomedical research, and the embrace of disease as a worthy social cause by government and social groups. Indeed, the commodification of health and illness is one of the most important and understudied developments in twentieth-century society. Where early-twentieth-century public health promoters spoke of health as a "purchasable commodity," we now see this style of thinking as only one part of a larger commodification of illness and disease in this century.[39] Marx, of course, highlighted such processes of commodification as key aspects of capitalist development. Anthropologists and historians have extended Marx's insights to any number of developments, although rarely have they examined commodification in the realm of health and disease.[40] For their part, historians of consumer culture have explored the processes by which "commodities appear in virtually every space twentieth-century American culture affords," but, again, only occasionally have such scholars touched upon health and disease as new commodities.[41] In using "commodification" in the context of medical history, I mean to draw attention to the processes by which bodily experiences such as pain are assigned value (monetary and otherwise) by physicians, patients, insurance companies, and others. "Commodification" also turns our attention to the ways in which ambiguous collections of experiences are named, take on conceptual coherence, and are subsumed under the title "disease," in such a way that they can be called upon by professionals, laypersons, and politicians in bargaining for rights, power, status, or economic position. It is this profound transformation in disease — from the early twentieth century through the age of AIDS — that the story of sickle cell disease chronicles.

Finally, this transformation gives us insight into the rise of chronic disease in the twentieth century. Acute infectious childhood diseases declined sharply in significance, and as populations aged, chronic diseases rose gradually in importance.[42] Writing in 1940, physician Ernst Boas could observe that "we escape the invasions of microorganisms to succumb at a more advanced age to diseases obscure in origin and chronic in character."[43] Sickle cell anemia stood amidst this spectrum of "obscure" diseases that became more visible in the wake of the decline of infectious disease. By the time of sickle cell disease's emergence in the post–World War II years, the very notion of "disease" had taken on many new connotations, becoming not only a burden but a long-term lived experience and a new kind of economic boon for hospitals and growing research-oriented medical complexes. The story of sickle cell anemia in the Mid-South is not, therefore, merely an isolated narrative of race and health in one region. It is fundamentally a story of the changing meaning of health and disease in America.

Understanding Memphis

The city of Memphis offers particular insight into these transformations. Its civic culture evolved as a tense compromise between urban ideals and rural traditions. The hot, moist climate of the low-lying West Tennessee region reached an extreme in Memphis, distinguishing the city from its home state in climate and in culture and wedding it more intimately to the climate, culture, life, and economy of the Mississippi Delta.[44] As James H. Robinson noted in the 1920s, "Memphis bears a relationship to the eastern part of Arkansas, the western and northern parts of Mississippi, as well as to West Tennessee, that is more vital and immediate . . . than its relation to East and Middle Tennessee."[45]

According to H. L. Mencken, Memphis was — and arguably still is — a "rural-minded city," its economic, cultural, and political concerns dominated by migrants from the vast Mississippi River region, the Delta, and the "Black Belt" of Alabama, Mississippi, Louisiana, and Arkansas.[46] In the words of a regional author, Memphis was the "metropolis of the Delta . . . its financial, social, and cultural capital."[47] Yet the city also strove to distance itself from the rural cultures from which it grew. If Mississippi in the early twentieth century was a rural "closed society," then Memphis was one of the few doorways opening from the Deep South onto a metropolitan world.[48] Rural influences continued to filter into the city in many forms, however. They were visible in the efforts of the regional Ku Klux Klan (and later the white Citizens' Council) to control city hall, in the performance of the Delta blues on Beale Street, in the practice of "conjure doctors" and lay midwives in the city, and in the influx of thousands of refugees who sought relief whenever the Mississippi River flooded. As their city expanded in the early twentieth century, Memphians knew that their enclave could, in the blink of an eye, be reclaimed by the surrounding elements. Chief among those defining rural elements was the traffic in cotton, for everyone in the city knew that the cotton market defined the city's priorities, its prosperity, and its identity.[49] As Clarence Poe wrote in 1904, "When cotton prices drop, every man feels the blow."[50]

Any Memphian in the early twentieth century would also know that the city was run by Edward "Boss" Crump, a Mississippi native with strong ties to cotton and to the insurance business. Crump was an enigma in the region, a Democratic Party boss who blended southern paternalism and humor with brutality toward those who disagreed with him. The juxtaposition of rural and urban cultures gave rise to a particular kind of politics, which helps us to understand the delicate political compromises that surrounded black health.

The blues was an integral part of that distinctive Memphis politics; indeed, in its aesthetics and its lyrics, the blues evokes much about this civic culture, its politics of compromise, and the prevailing paternalism.[51] As novelist Richard Wright once noted, "The blues could be called the spirituals of the city," the songs of a people "whose life has been caught up in and brutalized by the inflexible logic of modern industrial existence."[52] The musical form, while part of a new urban, African American economy on Beale Street, also reflected a political paradox. A popular music born in the Delta region and thriving in the city, the blues celebrated the difficulties and vagaries of African American life throughout the region.[53] Memphian W. C. Handy's 1909 song "Memphis Blues" gave rise to the urban art form. As Memphis writer George W. Lee described it, the song's style and composition "carried the same backward over-and-over wailing that characterized the sorrow songs of those people farthest down . . . though with a slightly different arrangement."[54] Handy's music combined elements of field work songs with an urban message suggesting, at least on its surface, that black people found true freedom and frankness of expression in the city. African Americans rallied around Handy when he sang, "Mr. Crump don't 'low no easy riders here. / I don't care what Mr. Crump don't 'low, / I'm gonna bar'-house anyhow."[55] The lyrics suggested a certain disdain for Crump's rules, and the existence of freedoms that were unknown on the plantation. But these were limited freedoms. In fact, "Memphis Blues" also carried the title "Mr. Crump," for Handy had composed it for the mayoral campaign of E. H. Crump himself. Men from the crowds around Handy were soon ushered by Crump's supporters to the polls, where their poll taxes were paid and where they might receive other rewards in exchange for voting for Crump (or, in later years, for his preferred candidate). To a large extent, this was the style of black voting in Memphis throughout the first half of the century. The freedom that Handy sang about served Boss Crump, architect of a political machine that would rule the city from the 1920s through the late 1940s.[56] Such cultural negotiations in the birth of the "Memphis Blues" foreshadowed the ways in which African Americans were compelled to negotiate — for a voice, for freedom, for political power, and for health — in the city of the blues.

Chapters 1 and 2 of this study provide portraits of disease and health in Boss Crump's Memphis. They examine the conceptual framework that Memphians used in thinking about health care and provide insight into the invisibility of sickle cell anemia and its gradual emergence as a social force in the 1940s and 1950s. In this setting, one lone white Memphis pathologist named Lemuel Diggs took an unusual interest in the obscure sickle cell disease, seeking to promote its wider awareness, but he had little success. In time, the expansion of urban, segregated institutions like Diggs's University of Tennessee Medical Center fostered a new interest in such odd maladies.[57] In exploring these years of invisibility, Chapters 1 and 2 examine the ways in which Memphis — with its diverse ideas about race, region, and health — maintained a rural-mindedness while also separating itself gradually from plantation culture. It is against this backdrop that we must understand local problems such as infant mortality or the local meanings of the painful crises of black children with sickle cell disease.

Chapters 3 and 4 explore the unraveling of the health care system that had taken shape in the early twentieth century. The World War II era had a transforming effect, ushering in the medical and research-based economy of the 1940s and 1950s and a new faith in science and medicine that transcended regionalism and set the stage for civic health activism in Memphis and other American cities. The new health politics brought chronic childhood diseases like leukemia and sickle cell anemia into the public spotlight for the first time, and for some Memphians these diseases became symbolic of the city's maturation. As Diggs proclaimed after the creation of the St. Jude Research Hospital for leukemia-stricken children, "There is no reason to think that all of the superior mental chromosomes of the country are localized in Boston, New York, and Baltimore . . . and that no scientific good can come from Memphis."[58]

The aftermath of World War II brought challenges for Jim Crow, and the struggles over segregation in schools and hospitals heightened local awareness of sickle cell disease.[59] One beneficiary of these trends was Diggs, who emerged as a leading researcher on the obscure disease that was itself rising in importance. The social visibility of doctor, disease, research, and community activism led to the creation of one of the nation's first sickle cell clinics in 1958, signaling that the city had indeed undergone an important transformation since 1910. The new health politics in Memphis revealed a brief flirtation with liberalism, and Chapters 3 and 4 explore the ways in which sickle cell anemia's civic prominence reflected both the political coalition between liberal whites and blacks that appeared with the demise of the Crump political order and the workings of the booming research and health care economy of the 1950s that changed discussions about health. The national crisis over integration and segregation would soon fragment this liberal coalition, but by then sickle cell disease had already achieved visibility and legitimacy.

Chapter 5 examines the ways in which the black protest movement would seize upon this now-visible disease as a symbol of the hardships endured by the black community. The disease became much more than a rallying point for polite local civic groups. It was remade into a national — and even an international — symbol of pain, social suffering, social inequality, and even the forceful uprooting of African Americans and the black diaspora.[60] In this atmosphere, the pain and suffering of sickle cell anemia victims became nationally politicized, used by many black Americans — from college sororities to women's auxiliaries to the Black Panther Party — to raise consciousness about their long-ignored social condition and their civil right to health equality. The disease gained ever-wider renown among scholars and social policymakers. It became a centerpiece of new research programs in molecular biology, and evolutionary biologists began to link sickle cell anemia to the history of African people and to malaria. In short, the disease had become a cultural commodity — a crucial force in the pursuit of social equality and justice, a vital reference point in debates about African inheritance and identity, and an expression of the patient-centered activism that was reshaping American medicine.

In the aftermath of this new era in health care and racial politics the disease's political visibility reached a peak, and it became a foil for many competing political agendas, both in Memphis and in America. The personal testimony of victims gave drama and vitality to the malady as a lived experience, as a series of painful trials to be weathered day by day. At the same time, the disease became integrated into militant liberal as well as conservative political campaigns. Chapter 6 explores how the disease became a crucial part of national health care politics and of the southern politics of racial realignment. In 1971 and 1972 the malady became one of Washington's three or four most important health care and research concerns, moving into the political spotlight alongside Nixon's "War on Cancer" and the Tuskegee syphilis scandal. Speaking on sickle cell disease,

President Nixon told Americans, "We cannot change the history of neglect, but we can do much to alleviate the pain and suffering."[61] Sickle cell anemia also became a double-edged political tool for the Nixon administration and for Memphis's Republican congressman — and strong Nixon supporter — Dan Kuykendall. Fighting for reelection in a district with a growing black population, the congressman saw the disease as a means of "reaching out" to now-enfranchised African Americans while also emphasizing the dangers of drug addiction and using the prominence of sickle cell anemia in his region as a vehicle for ensuring that federal dollars would continue to flow to his city. It is not surprising that Memphis's African American communities saw the disease quite differently and used it to pursue their own political ends.

Chapter 7 explores the therapeutic promises that came out of this political activity, as well as a disturbing new portrait of the disease that has emerged since the 1970s. The health care politics surrounding the disease in the 1990s differed starkly from that of the early 1970s. In that earlier era, mainstream Americans accepted the authenticity of pain and suffering and embraced a complex agenda for its prevention, care, and alleviation. By contrast, in the 1990s the authenticity of the very experience came into question in the clinic and in society. Some people insisted that pain relief in sickle cell anemia rewards "drug-seeking" and came to see sicklers as a variant of the inner city drug addict stereotype. In an era of cost cutting, others began to scrutinize the high costs of the liberal protocols for disease and pain alleviation. Debates over the morality and economics of pain management in sickle cell anemia took on new significance with the national expansion of managed care, anxieties about health care costs, and fears about inner city pathology. If this disease became a symbol of increasing compassion and awareness of black health in America in the 1970s, then Chapter 7 examines what its subsequent displacement from the celebrity spotlight reveals about civic activism, race relations, and consciousness-raising in the 1990s. What does the recent history of celebrated and hyped "cures" tell us about the alleviation of African American pain and suffering or the promise of molecular medicine? What does the rise of managed care and free market medicine portend for the visibility of sickle cell disease and for race and health policy?

Although this book examines a wide range of black health concerns in the nineteenth and twentieth centuries, sickle cell anemia, with its early invisibility, changing symbolism, and rising clinical, social, and political prominence, provides the central thematic thread. The question of *clinical and scientific visibility* prompts an examination of one kind of social/ conceptual issue: the ways in which a disease could gain meaning for medical practitioners and scientific disciplines, its changing meaning from generation to generation, and its gaining or losing utility as a model in clinical and scientific discourses. As suggested earlier, questions of clinical and scientific visibility have always been linked to economic, intellectual, and professional goals. *Social visibility* speaks to another kind of issue: the ways in which people experiencing illness have been labeled by physicians and scientists, and how they and others have folded their plight into larger social causes. Social visibility also highlights how these groups themselves, especially in recent decades of patient activism, have embraced their "disease" label publicly, proudly, and with a measure of political defiance. In dramatizing their appeal for recognition, they have taken on new forms of identity that can intersect with a larger body politic.[62] These questions of disease visibility point us toward the wide range of processes by which illness, syndromes, disease, poor health, and symptoms like pain have become the sites of negotiations about power, governance, justice, and social order.

1 Conjurors of Health in the New South

Just take her 'round to the city hospital
Jus' as quick, quick as you possible can
Take her 'round to the city hospital
Jus' as quick, quick as you possible can
Because of the condition she's in now,
You will never go home live again.
— Lizzie Douglas, "Memphis Minnie-jitis Blues"

In order to understand the health care system for African Americans that emerged in Memphis in the early twentieth century, we must first understand the city itself. Who were the people that built and maintained the system? What kinds of political machinations shaped their institutions? How did their economic interests and their racial agendas inform their perceptions of health and disease?

When Joseph Edison Walker arrived in Memphis in 1916 from Indianola, Mississippi, he was part of a steady stream of black southerners coming into town. Neither farmer nor field hand nor domestic servant, Walker was a professional — a physician fleeing oppressive small-town southern life. What was true in 1916 about the small-town South remained true for decades; as sociologist John Dollard later observed, "There is not much money [in Indianola, and] . . . this situation has a tendency to force the Negro professionals out . . . into more lucrative opportunities."[1] In migrating to the city, Walker left behind a restrictive rural world where black professionals often inspired jealousy and resentment in local whites.[2] By contrast, the rising Memphis skyline evoked promises of economic prosperity. In the heart of the Bible Belt, the city was a place where "even the church spires were dwarfed by a number of imposing skyscrapers."[3] Soon after Walker arrived in Memphis, he dedicated himself to the insurance business.

Turning away from medical practice per se, he became one among several prosperous black businessmen and a spokesman for business as a means of racial uplift and advancement.[4] His success suggests that Memphis, unlike Indianola, provided fertile ground for the aspirations of such men.

Some years before Walker arrived, Thomas O. Fuller (see illustrations) had fled Durham, North Carolina, for Memphis. He too had made the Mid-South city his haven and his pulpit. After a term as senator in the North Carolina legislature, Fuller's brief political career had come to an abrupt end in 1898, when North Carolina whites began to employ the poll tax and use coercive measures to prevent African Americans from exercising the vote.[5] As Jim Crow restrictions in voting and public accommodations swept across the region, Fuller headed for the high ground of Memphis, some 700 miles to the west. Memphis was a beacon in a region undergoing dramatic urbanization. In the South it was second only to New Orleans in overall population, and it had a large black population — 48 percent of the total.

Widely known as a transportation gateway to the North and West, the city symbolized escape, possibility, and rebirth for many southern African Americans.[6] Traveling through Tennessee to its westernmost point at Memphis, Fuller would have witnessed the harsh aftermath of the Supreme Court's 1896 *Plessy v. Ferguson* ruling — the creation, state by state, of formal, separate racial worlds in transportation, education, and health care. But at the end of his journey, the city of Memphis seemed to stand above this tide. Black Memphians had held onto some of their voting rights, surviving the regional floods that swallowed the African American vote primarily because their ballots served the interests of the local Democratic political machine. But with his arrival in Memphis, Fuller, like Walker, had already transformed himself. He had lost his taste for party politics and now embraced less overtly political interests, seeking new ways to promote the health and political well-being of his people. He was ready to accommodate himself to Memphis's political culture.

As Baptist minister Blair Hunt recalled, Fuller "was quite a politician out there in North Carolina." But in Memphis he assumed a role consistent with the city's cautious black leadership — the ministry. "They worshipped in a little frame building there on Beale Street called Zion Hall," Hunt recalled. In shifting his vocation, Fuller joined a large group of black preachers who had created their own sacred spaces in a city whose landscape was dotted by such enterprises.[7] From the pulpits of Zion Hall and other small churches, ministers like Fuller and Hunt preached what historian David

Tucker has called "a healing, soothing ministry." Their sermons eschewed formal politics, even as the tide of lynching and segregation pressed upon their people. Their careers represented a compromise with the emerging "New South" social order — a recognition that segregation had arrived and that the goal was to survive amidst this new order.[8] In time Fuller became, in Tucker's view, "the most prominent local black pastor during the age of accommodation . . . [elevating] racial adjustment to a major ministerial art."[9] In Memphis the North Carolina outcast politician had found a pulpit, a religious following, and a home.

Both Fuller and Walker settled in a city seen by many African Americans as a sanctuary within the increasingly hostile and racist South. As these men knew, Memphis was far from a welcoming city to reformers, black or white.[10] Accommodation was the local watchword. Moderation, many believed, had allowed Memphis to avoid the urban race riots that bloodied East St. Louis, New Orleans, Knoxville, Chicago, Springfield, and other regional cities in these decades.[11] One minister cut from the same cloth as Fuller reflected that "this was what they called a preacher's town. They said in those days stay in your place. . . . If you could stay in your place as a negro preacher here, why you could have it very fine, very good. That is, don't bother with no politics, don't bother with no status quo, just preach and shout the folks."[12] In Memphis many like-minded, ambitious black men with a gift for preaching eschewed activism for this politics of the pulpit.

Memphis's status as an economic promised land for black businessmen was confirmed by the regional fame of real estate magnate Robert Church, builder of Beale Street and reputed to be among the wealthiest black men in the nation.[13] The luster of Church's accomplishment shone across the region, drawing others to Memphis. Physician and educator Miles Vandahurst Lynk (see illustrations) saw similarly grand possibilities in the Bluff City in 1912, when he moved his West Tennessee Medical School — one of eight existing African American medical schools in the country — eighty miles from Jackson, Tennessee, to Memphis.[14] For businessmen and preachers, the Memphis of Lynk, Fuller, Walker, and Church was a city of promise. It was a city bustling with streetcar traffic and cotton commerce, a place where black men might prosper and black institutions could flourish — as long as they adjusted themselves to the politics, economics, and ideologies of the region.[15]

The vast majority of Memphis's energetic African American newcomers in the 1920s, 1930s, and 1940s were not professional men but agricultural laborers — men, women, and children — whose interests, aspirations, and trajectories diverged from those of the professionals. But it was these working-class people who made the ideals of men like Walker and Fuller attainable, for these were the people who provided the clientele for the professionals in a segregated society. Their arrival meant that Memphis's black population would climb steadily from some 50,000 in 1900 to over 120,000 in 1940 and ensured that African Americans would consistently comprise around 40 percent of the city's population. Some of these new-comers continued to work in the fields of northern Mississippi and western Arkansas by day, returning to Memphis to live and rest at sundown. But others reinvented themselves as domestic servants, laundresses, carpenters, draymen, masons, clergymen, schoolteachers, musicians, and nurses.[16] Some enterprising people opened saloons, lunchrooms, retail groceries, barbershops, and beauty shops. Because of their numbers, their rural roots, and their working-class concerns, the city that emerged was more rural than cosmopolitan in character. Half or more of its residents at any time hailed from small towns in the surrounding territories. By their presence and spirit they contributed a contentious, rustic, and small-town aspect to Memphis's civic life.[17]

Rural black southerners moved into Memphis neighborhoods north, south, and southeast of the downtown and Beale Street.[18] Poverty haunted many of the African American neighborhoods, which observers character-ized as blighted "darktowns," filled with one- and two-room shanties.[19] Still, there was nothing in Memphis resembling New York's Harlem or Chicago's South Side, where one could find congested and unhealthy tene-ments.[20] As some black people prospered, a certain measure of economic, residential, and labor differentiation emerged through these decades. By 1930 over 20,000 black Memphians worked in domestic labor; only 1,500 became professionals.[21] Black North Memphis neighborhoods became more affluent than black neighborhoods to the south.[22] Yet, despite these signs of diversification and economic disparities, economic interdepen-dence continued to define the relationship between black professionals and the black working class in the segregated society.

The reality of economic and social interdependence was but one of the factors defining the character of the health care system for African Ameri-cans and for white Memphians in these years. Memphis's system, like the city itself, was a delicate compromise — between urban and rural cultures, between black and white citizens, between insiders and outsiders, and be-tween professional and working-class concerns. This system was composed of a changing set of actors: midwives moving in and out of the city, street-corner conjure doctors practicing with roots, herbs, and charms, an aging charity hospital, a medical college with a few university-trained physicians, and a wide range of other practitioners. Their coexistence reflected the balance of urban and rural healing cultures; as the city itself changed, some of its healers would be incorporated into mainstream health institutions while others would become discredited and marginal.

Like any health care system, Memphis health care reflected the local political economy. A system evolved, shaped by Memphis-style politics, regional economics, and Mid-South race relations. Also, like any health care system, Memphis's arrangement of institutions determined which patients had access to which kind of health care, which patients were seen and how they were diagnosed, and which among the many ailing people of the region remained invisible. The evolving system determined which disorders attracted great attention, which health crises made local headlines, and which were suffered in the solitude of home and the privacy of family.[23]

Three features of this early-twentieth-century health care system warrant closer attention. First, health educators (ranging from black physicians like Miles Vandahurst Lynk to the physicians at the University of Tennessee medical school) were a relatively minor force in the city. For these educators, the sickness of indigent African Americans began to take on a particular economic value. That is, health educators realized the utility of sickness, and the fact that their enterprises would not prosper without the presence of concentrated pools of people as patients and teaching material. Second, this system evolved with the growing political power of Edward "Boss" Crump and the Tennessee Democratic Party. Thus the shape of health care institutions in Memphis inevitably depended upon negotiations with the Crump regime. Third, the need to preserve racial segregation and white supremacy also dictated the shape of the Memphis health care system. These factors — economic, political, and ideological — drove the system not in one direction, but along many trajectories, creating numerous conflicts in the early twentieth-century city over what the system should look like and whose interests it should serve.

When we speak of a health care "system" today, we think of the conjunction of large academic medical centers, massive health insurance corporations, and huge federal programs like Medicare catering to millions of people. We also think of expansive public health programs and multibillion-dollar pharmaceutical companies and research institutions — all of which interact with one another, shape access to health services, and influence our perceptions of disease and mortality. As we shall see in the story of

Memphis, however, small, local institutions defined urban health care and shaped perceptions of disease early in the century. City government played a much greater role than state or federal government. Boss politics was a more formidable force than the university, the research institutions, or the insurance companies. Written into the character of "the system" was the city's culture — its ambivalent relationship to its rural surroundings, the changing relations between the city, the university, and the neighborhoods, the power of the Democratic Party, and long-established, ingrained regional attitudes about race, paternalism, and social order. The interplay of race, politics, and economics in Memphis produced a conflicted municipal health care system that was born of compromise. It was also a system that proved resistant to outside influences, whether from philanthropists or federal officials.

In such localities, diseases — whether we mean the personal experience of illness, clinical symptoms and syndromes, or the scientific understanding of pathological mechanisms — evolved in a context. Disease perceptions were shaped by social and political negotiations and by racial ideologies. For example, radical segregationists might argue that the high rate of tuberculosis among black people proved that separation was justified, and that blacks posed a constant danger to whites. Yet white moderates might answer that the presence of African Americans as servants in white households showed that some racial interaction was economically valuable, and that this interaction required at least modest attention to black health.[24] This logic was agreeable to many surrounding plantation owners and overseers, who depended upon healthy workers for their own economic prosperity. This chapter describes the tensions among such ideologies and the system of health care that emerged in the Memphis of Lynk, Walker, Fuller, and Church.

Conjuring Health on Beale Street

A panoply of institutions sold, marketed, promoted, and conjured health in early-twentieth-century Memphis. Building viable and secure institutions was never as important in America as in the decades around 1900. Urban institutions gained special significance for black Americans in the wake of emancipation and their migration toward cities. "In the cities," wrote historian Eric Foner, "many blacks believed 'freedom was freer.' Here were schools, churches, and fraternal societies . . . offering protection from the violence so pervasive in much of the rural South."[25] Such institutions created a sense of social order and community for black Americans and other ethnic groups, as urban in-migration fueled new churches, schools, hospitals, civic clubs, labor unions, and professional organizations.[26] Accordingly, American cities saw a large increase in hospitals, many of them built as extensions of the missions of churches.[27] These institutions symbolized communal security to those being uprooted by migration or being tossed about in the tumultuous waves of ethnic and racial intolerance.[28] A key question confronting Memphians was which of these institutions would survive the economically and politically tumultuous 1910s and 1920s — an era when, in order to survive, institutions were forced to expand, affiliate, and incorporate.

For black Americans, the church assumed a central role in the organization of civic life and exercised a sweeping influence over matters of public health and individual hygiene.[29] "Up until 25 years ago," wrote T. O. Fuller in 1938, "the Churches used one or two glasses in passing the wine. . . . Since that time the large Churches of the more intelligent groups adopted the individual glasses. . . . This facilitated the services and was also more sanitary."[30] The process of sanitizing religious ritual, however, could also foment division in black communities. Even though some members of Fuller's congregation embraced the new ritual of individual communion glasses, others regarded sharing wine from a common cup as a valued expression of mutuality, solidarity, and faith. Fuller noted that "the older people felt that it exhibited a lack of faith in God to use individual cups."[31] In Fuller's view, the role of the church included uplifting the people into an informed, sanitary individualism. Implicit in his comments was a criticism of the traditional beliefs of many southern blacks, who bought the services of conjurers to cast spells and work magic to heal ailments, tied charmed pouches around the necks of babies to ward off disease, and persisted in the belief that sharing cups was an index of their faith in God.[32] As historian Nancy Tomes has argued, such disagreement over the wine ritual suggests the subtle ways in which a wide array of institutions promoted the modern "gospel of germs" and how this new gospel could conflict with older, established faith.[33]

In the South, the rise of segregation reinforced the significance of institutions such as churches, hospitals, and schools, for they assumed an even more crucial role in the formation of modern identity.[34] But even as they promoted health and sought to alleviate the effects of a violent, Jim Crow social order, segregated institutions also accommodated black people to the new order of things.[35]

In traveling from countryside to the city, men and women left behind a paternalistic plantation system and entered a commercial world of bankers, cotton merchants and brokers, and hospitals and insurance companies selling health services. In Memphis an embryonic, consumer-oriented health care system was developing in the early twentieth century, including pharmacies, religious hospitals, university clinics, doctors' offices, and urban midwives. The city achieved a solid reputation as a health care marketplace with modern practitioners, novel hygienic practices, and up-to-date treatments for ailments like malaria (one of the region's most endemic problems). The General Hospital—providing care to thousands of indigent patients a year—was perhaps the most distinctive health care facility in the city, even if it was not the most modern or best regarded. Memphis was fast becoming a regional clearinghouse for health care and medicinal information. Writing to a Memphis pharmacist in 1928, one woman from Widener, Arkansas, could request, "Please send me something that you know will kill malaria. I have bought drugs from you for 27 yrs and know you are capable and reliable."[36] Despite these developments in health care, however, it was not medical services or drugs that dominated the city's booming commercial and economic system, but "King Cotton."[37] In the planter-dominated world around Memphis, moreover, medical care was still regarded as a labor issue, a necessary expense to maintain workers' productivity.

Through the 1910s, church, hospital, and municipal government struggled to define their roles in civic health. Municipal officials remained reluctant reformers, pushed into action only by population growth or by one health crisis after another. Their battles against tuberculosis and typhoid epidemics, high infant mortality, and hospital deterioration were always constrained by what one observer called "the retarding influence of political indifference," and by the power of local businessmen wary of taxes and expanding government services.[38] In a campaign to fend off bovine tuberculosis by restricting infected cattle from city markets in 1910 and 1911, for example, health officials found themselves locked in battle against local farmers wary of health inspections of their cows. Health regulations, it seemed, encroached upon commercial interest.[39] In 1919 "a sudden gross pollution of the city water supply with human fecal matter, the result of a broken sewer main," pushed Memphis to the top of a national list of cities in typhoid deaths. Yet administrators remained reluctant to renovate the sewer system.[40] Even in the face of such typical urban crises, many citizens believed that the city's major disease problems were not homegrown but had their roots in rural in-migration. Moreover, the public health department was staffed with part-time, political appointments, and it was often left to the private hospitals, university clinics, and the churches to address the health problems that came with urban growth.[41] By the 1920s, these diverse and separate institutions were being more closely knit into an inter-related network that defined a southern health care "system."[42]

One defining feature of this system was racial segregation. In health care as in schooling, housing, and transportation, Jim Crow was both codified by laws and established through fear and terror campaigns. Jim Crow struc-tured black deference to white authority along the streets, in public places, and in workplaces throughout the city. Jim Crow in medicine was a com-plex affair. It meant the exclusions of black people as patients and physi-cians from white-only hospitals. However, it did not mean their exclusion from work crews building these hospitals, nor did it mean their absence as low-level laborers within such institutions. The exclusion of patients from white-only hospitals opened up opportunities for black businesses, for it meant that enterprising people like T. O. Fuller and J. E. Walker were able to build thriving institutions for African American patients and consumers. Additionally, in an era of expanding public health initiatives in states throughout the region, segregation also meant the creation of separate and unequal neighborhood clinics, maternal health programs, and nursing ser-vices.[43] Structured paternalism and selective exclusion, rather than any ab-solute separation of blacks and whites, defined Jim Crow medicine as it evolved from the 1910s through the 1950s.

Even as the segregation system offered opportunities, it also placed boundaries on the economic ambitions of such men as Lynk, Fuller, and Walker.[44] In his 1910 report on medical education in North America, Abra-ham Flexner had indicated that segregation created clear roles for black pa-tients as consumers and for black physicians as providers. To Flexner, "the physical well-being of the negro is not only of moment to the negro himself. Ten million of them live in close contact with sixty million whites."[45] In Flexner's estimation, this white anxiety defined the subordinate, second-class role (and limited the aspirations) of black physicians. He noted that "the medical care of the negro race will never be wholly left to negro physicians . . . [but at the same time] the practice of the negro physician will be limited to his own race."[46] As professionals like J. E. Walker left the small-town South, they must have seen clearly that any health care system would enforce this white paternalism and this separate but unequal relationship with their clientele.[47]

Walker's Universal Life Insurance business appealed to a segregated mar-ket: black consumers who were searching for security against the prospect of crises, distress, or death. In general, such insurance firms grew rapidly in the 1910s, as companies like Prudential Life Insurance and Metropolitan Life generally denied coverage to African Americans.[48] Insurance coverage was summarily denied because the actuarial linkage of high mortality and race labeled all African Americans as "high risk."[49] Insurance stood, then, as one among numerous modern commodities beyond the reach of many black consumers. In this segregated context, Walker's business and other black insurance companies thrived. Such enterprises promised sickness benefits, made payments to families in case of loss of life, and even covered the cost of burial. Like the black church, such institutions catered to community health and well-being. Even as they alleviated the injustice of segregation, they also became profitable companies.[50] In the 1910s and 1920s Walker's firm was one among many such health institutions on Beale Street, which itself had grown into a vibrant business corridor and a nationally recognized center of black commerce and culture.

As Flexner's words indicated, white businessmen also saw profit in catering to the well-being of Memphis's black citizens. Pharmacist Abe Plough, for example, opened a small pharmacy near Beale Street in 1908. Over the next decade he did a steady business among both black and white Memphians, making enough money to build a manufacturing plant to produce his own best-selling Plough's Antiseptic Oil.[51] Also serving Memphis's growing black population was a small but growing group of white physicians, along with the black physicians, numerous midwives, many root and herb doctors, and many conjure healers—who invoked spirits or supernatural forces in the name of healing. The almost entirely white world of scientific medicine was also slowly developing an interest in the black patient, and this spectrum of business interests defined the system of medicine in the Bluff City.

In the 1910s several new hospitals appeared, some of them seeking to address the needs of black citizens. These hospitals reflected the coalescence of religious values and economic trends. The two largest white hospitals — organized by Methodist and Baptist congregations — expanded rapidly in these years, but they did not admit African American patients. Answering with hospitals of their own, African American Baptist and Colored Methodist Episcopal (CME) congregations gathered funds not only from the city's faithful but also from regional churches and built two modest infirmaries in Memphis. Their actions highlighted not only the strength of black Baptist and Methodist networks throughout the region, but also the city's particular significance as a cultural and demographic magnet for black people in eastern Arkansas, northern Mississippi, western Tennessee, and parts of Missouri. The Baptists' Terrell Infirmary opened in 1909, and one year later the CME's Collins Chapel Hospital opened its doors.[52] By 1920, Collins Chapel offered seventy-five beds and twelve private wards for paying and charity patients from the tri-state region. It was equipped well below the standards of other private hospitals of the day, with only a modest array of technical facilities. Moreover, while large urban hospitals increasingly divided the tasks of physicians, clerks, nurses, laboratory staff, and others, Collins Chapel's doctor, W. S. Martin, and his wife served as medical attendants, orderlies, and administrators. The pooled funds from regional congregations to finance the venture were part of the CME pastors' "alliance for mutual helpfulness."[53] Pursuing a similar regional mission, the Terrell Infirmary also expanded in the 1910s from a facility equipped for ten patients into the renamed Terrell Memorial Hospital, offering nearly 100 beds by the late 1920s.

Regional religious commitments and the growing demand for hospitals drove these developments. The Terrell and Collins infirmaries sought to maximize their appeal by declaring themselves to be "open to all reputable physicians, white and colored." All physicians could thereby bring their own paying black patients into the wards.[54] Black physicians and patients enjoyed no such privileges in white institutions.[55] The Terrell and Collins Chapel hospitals exemplified self-help and mutuality, the same ideals that sustained black-run insurance companies, African American banks, and other institutions in the segregated community. The hospitals identified themselves as regional centers, and their moral obligations extended well beyond the boundaries of the city.[56] Built by the "good works" of black worshipers throughout the Mid-South, these institutions ignored state and city lines, catered to paying as well as charity patients, and established healing and relief within the pale of the church's mission.[57]

In the 1920s, however, even as prosperity came to institutions like Terrell and Collins, economic collapse came to others like Miles Vandahurst Lynk's West Tennessee Medical School. The difference reveals how the health care economy and medical education economy moved along different economic trajectories. In 1920s America, even while rising patient demand ensured a place for the new infirmaries, the production of black physicians in small proprietary schools became increasingly difficult. Flexner's 1910 report had stated that "of the seven medical schools for negroes in the United States, five [including Lynk's] are at this moment in no position to make any contribution of value." Furthermore, Flexner had written, "they are wasting small sums annually and sending out undisciplined men, whose lack of real training is covered up by the imposing M.D. degree."[58] Lynk's college (then located at Jackson) was designated one of these five "wasteful" and "undisciplined" institutions. In the wake of the criticism, Lynk had moved to Memphis in 1912 in an effort to build closer connections with Memphis physicians and their new hospitals.[59] But the operating costs of medical education were spiraling upward, particularly in the 1920s, an era where "rising standards" became the watchword and where colleges needed expensive laboratories, regular access to hospital patients, and full-time faculty to keep up with the competition.[60]

The same economic trends that were redefining American business — the need for new technical facilities and horizontal integration between institutions — were also crippling Lynk's enterprise. The Flexner report forecast and also hastened the demise of such small-scale, fee-dependent, proprietary medical colleges founded by lone entrepreneurs like Lynk.[61] Even established medical schools found that generous endowments, posthumous bequests, and philanthropic donations were increasingly crucial to the task of building hospitals and laboratories. Lynk's school attracted none of this financial support. Indeed, philanthropists who were interesting in supporting black medical schools took their cue from Flexner's report, aiming funds selectively farther east to Meharry in Nashville and Howard in Washington, D.C., deemed more promising by Flexner. By the mid-1920s, the doors of Lynk's school closed for good. Minister Blair Hunt eulogized the school for doing "a great work in its day, but," he added, "they didn't have any hospital facilities, or anything like that."[62]

Ironically, the hospital — a repository for the sick, the disparate, and the vulnerable — was becoming a key to economic survival for medical colleges. Another of Memphis's schools — the University of Tennessee medical school — came very close to a similar demise, but it was a fortuitous hospital affiliation that allowed the school to avoid collapse. Flexner had labeled the college a "showy, but quite mercenary concern at Memphis [that should] be liquidated."[63] No philanthropic bequests appeared on the horizon that might rescue the school from extinction. But college leaders maneuvered to link the school to the Memphis General Hospital (MGH), hoping that affiliation with another ailing institution would save it. The city hospital had also drawn Flexner's criticism for being "divided between two schools, though [it does] not supply enough material for one."[64] By "material" Flexner meant, of course, "clinical material," a common professional euphemism for patients — a crucial commodity in the turbulent economy of medical education. By the early 1920s, the medical college was maneuvering adeptly to sign a contract with the city to staff the MGH. In return, university physicians gained exclusive control of MGH's "material," and this access would become a key to the school's survival. The integration of teaching with health care at the city hospital was consistent with the economic trends of the 1920s.[65] As one key educator noted, "The almost limitless wealth of clinical material afforded by the General hospital . . . places the medical department in some parity with the non-state [private] medical colleges."[66] Even as Lynk's school became a victim of these trends, many Memphians looked at the university-staffed MGH as a promising and progressive development.

With this merger, an important shift in the valuation of poor patients in Memphis had occurred. The general hospital, with its imposing brick façade, its several hundred beds, and its central location, had long reflected the city's own charitable self-image.[67] Built in 1829 and remodeled several times through the century, the hospital housed many of the "diseased, destitute, and friendless persons . . . cast upon the charity of the citizens of Memphis."[68] By 1910, the hospital could claim to provide free care for several thousand residents and nonresidents alike, about 60 percent of them African Americans.[69] One national survey of the hospital noted that this was a "good hospital and doing good work, even though the patients are charity and not of the high type, as ordinarily found in private institutions."[70]

But charity aside, a utilitarian calculus also explained the hospital's existence, for the control of infectious disease among the urban poor (who were disproportionately black) was widely portrayed as a vital concern for white people themselves, especially since many black people worked as domestic laborers in white homes. To some southerners, the municipal hospital represented a public health insurance policy as well as a charitable act. It was built and sustained as an act of white "self-preservation."[71] To look at the Memphis General Hospital (the largest for hundreds of miles around) was to see the face of regional poverty as well as the visage of white anxiety. The 1920s affiliation with the medical college merely extended this economic calculus. In the process of merging, the value of the old and decaying hospital and of the ailing patients within its walls was realized. This arrangement also meant a shift in the clinical visibility of disease.[72] Poor patients became more visible to students, to educators, and to the few research-minded teachers who constituted a tiny minority of the college's teaching staff. In the wake of affiliation some of the college's teachers, seeking to distinguish themselves among their peers, wrote of interesting cases encountered in the MGH's clinic. Case reports based on these observations of patients at MGH began to appear more and more frequently, for example, in the *Memphis Medical Journal*.[73]

Expanding their reach farther, university physicians also built closer ties to the city's department of public health in these years, and here too black Memphians found themselves incorporated into new roles. In 1923, for example, the city's health department, the university, and the general hospital organized a segregated corps of thirty-nine nurses (thirteen of whom were African American) to work in the clinic and the communities. Their purpose was to provide prenatal examinations, give home education, and also "to assist in home deliveries."[74] The corps was created in response to crisis — specifically, Memphis's continually dismal infant and maternal mortality rates. But it was also created as a concession to political necessity, for it was built in the wake of women's suffrage and amidst increasing political sensitivity to maternal and child health in the 1920s.[75] The nursing corps further developed the relationship of city government and the university, extending the reach of the university-hospital complex into neighborhoods. Dispatching nurses into previously unmonitored Memphis neighborhoods, the corps sought to ensure that the sick might be assisted at home and that patients would find their way to the MGH.[76] Nurses collected health data on tuberculosis, diphtheria, and other ills, and they promoted hygienic practices.

But the corps also pitted educated middle-class black nurses against the less formally educated urban black midwives. The public health nurses were agents of the university-hospital system, a crucial part of a strategy to redefine urban health, and their practice reflected the university's economic agenda as well as the continuing urban-rural struggle over Memphis's civic identity.[77] From its inception, the corps was assigned a specific task: to monitor the midwives, who represented, especially in the minds of many physicians, an unwelcome rural presence and a nuisance among the city's poor. "In 1920," recalled one university obstetrician, "there were 75 midwives practicing in this city, and at present [1932] there remain only 16."[78] Such specialists saw the nursing corps — black and white — as integral to driving out the midwives, for "in communities where physicians are not available . . . intelligent nurses, with special training, will solve the problem."[79] Another observer commented that "the practice of the health department is to control the work of the old midwives and to restrict the number of new permits issued to younger women."[80] The black nurses were key to the strategy, holding monthly meetings with "midwives, at which a colored nurse gives instructions, with occasional assistance from a white nurse." The nurses were also encouraged to go beyond education and instruction, to inspect midwives' bags and to investigate their homes.[81]

Symbolizing science advancing against outmoded rural beliefs, these nurses were also part of the economic strategy of an emerging health care system bent on incorporating would-be consumer/patients as hospital clients. "We have almost eradicated the ignorant midwife, who has so markedly affected our colored population," one obstetrician noted in 1932. "[This trend] has sent [black patients] to private physicians and to our [university] clinic."[82] With the battle against midwives launched, "colored patients who are able to pay are seeking white and colored physicians."[83] Such authors also believed—without much evidence to support them— that the decline of the still high infant mortality rate was a result of this assault on the midwives, and a by-product of the expansion of their urban health care system.[84]

The system that began to emerge in Memphis, therefore, spoke in diverse ways to the problems of black health and sickness. It marginalized some practitioners—like Lynk and the urban midwives—while it integrated public health nurses into the battle against rural influences. The system fomented the rise of those black institutions that were consistent with local culture. Yet it also proved responsive to national trends in medical education, women's health, and indigent care. The developments of the 1920s created new, if circumscribed, roles for black citizens—as nurses, as maligned midwives, or as valued patients in the teaching hospital.

In the prosperous Roaring Twenties, these and many other practitioners who capitalized on the health and well-being of Memphis's black population could be found near Beale Street, "home to one of the largest Negro enterprises in the country, the Universal Life Insurance Company . . . [a street where] small shops and saloons gave way to banking establishments and large stores. Negro doctors, dentists, financiers, lawyers, politicians, writers, real-estate promoters, and insurance men flocked to the area."[85] Beale Street's sidewalks were also home to those who trafficked in rural cures, where "barkers entreat passers-by to stop and inspect bargains [and] conjure doctors sell good luck bags, love powders, and graveyard dust charms."[86] At the confluence of magical healing, conjure and mysticism, and scientific medicine, Beale Street sustained a brisk health care business. Along comparable streets in New York's Harlem (much farther removed from the countryside), black doctors waged fierce campaigns against sidewalk "magic doctors" with their "Obiah," "voodoo," and "magic dust."[87]

But in Memphis the sellers of roots, herbs, grape leaves, rabbit's feet, and wine and whiskey concoctions maintained a steady, interested clientele. Those who invoked spirits to relieve one's rheumatism or to subdue one's enemies would not be driven easily from the Bluff City.[88] Even in the mid-1930s, one source could note that the work of public health nurses and the growth of the university had not eradicated rural traditions of healing, for "midwives still practice here, despite the county's million dollar hospitals and its learned members of the medical profession."[89]

As Memphis's health care system emerged, spiritualism, religious faith, and nonmedical notions of healing remained overarching factors in its shaping. Church hymns and blues music swayed audiences, in different ways, with songs about loss, suffering, salvation, and healing.[90] Noted one contemporary, "A spiritual is a matter of a choral treatment; a blues is a one-man affair."[91] But both spoke, in their distinctive registers, of suffering and healing. Existential pain and human suffering figured prominently in church services as well as in sidewalk and saloon performances.[92] At the same time that blues performer Lizzie "Memphis Minnie" Douglas sang plaintively about the devastating effects of meningitis — moaning about her failing health and telling listeners of her flight to the city hospital — choral groups in small churches were singing of salvation and the alleviation of pain.[93] "Long ago," wrote minister T. O. Fuller, "the people of the South learned that religion had a quieting and soothing effect upon the mind of the Negro."[94] Fuller believed that the church could modernize the message, spread the gospel of health, soothe congregations, and accommodate them to the norms of the new segregated system. But even Fuller encountered resistance to these modernizing trends. Though he preached of ventilation and drinking from separate communion cups and sought to make his church an exponent of the new public health beliefs, he observed that "unfortunately, Negroes have the idea that when at Church, the laws of health are suspended."[95] Indeed, even as their institutions tried to accommodate them to the cultural and economic currents as patients, practitioners, and modern believers, many black Memphians refused to abide by the new laws and resisted being incorporated into the new system.

Boss Crump's Political Economy

If this health care system was shaped by new economics and old faiths, it was also defined by the paternalistic political interests of Boss Crump. E. H. Crump was the closest thing to a plantation master Memphis had. His police force, business associates, and political machine controlled the city from the 1910s through the 1940s. His men harassed union organizers, out-muscled political adversaries who challenged his control, frustrated reform-minded newspaper journalists and editors, doled out patronage jobs to loyal cronies, and gained enormous leverage over Democratic Party and West Tennessee politics.[96] Officially, Crump served only one term as mayor and one as U.S. congressman, but he controlled these and many other elected posts for decades. He ran the party, personally selected candidates, and determined the outcome of elections.

Crump's attitude toward black Memphians was shaped both by the paternalism that pervaded the region and by his desire to maintain political power. As historian William Miller noted, after Crump's mayoral election in 1910 "periodic roundups of transients and vagrants were made, and for a while every Negro found on the street after midnight was taken to the station house."[97] Crump maintained power and popularity precisely because of these actions—battling vagrants and poor blacks. He also maintained his popularity, especially in the early days, by openly campaigning for the common citizen against the domineering corporate interests of the day—the railroad companies, the gas and electric utilities, and other big business interests that threatened to take over his city.[98] But collaboration with some black Memphians was also key to his control. According to historians and contemporaries, at election time the Crump machine "made use of policemen in the black wards to shepherd Negroes in wagons and on foot to registration places, many of which were saloons. The saloonkeepers cooperated, with the expectancy of special favors from the Crump regime."[99] Business leaders paid the poll taxes of these "independent" voters, prompting some to muse that black vagrants were transformed on election day from eyesores to respected citizens. Several of the city's black ministers also assisted in getting voters to the polls for Crump. In return for their support, Crump encouraged the construction of parks, swimming pools, schools, and health facilities to serve Memphis's black citizens. Through these moves, and occasionally more violent tactics, Crump consolidated his hold on the city in the 1920s and strengthened it through the 1940s.[100]

Throughout Crump's reign, public health was widely treated as just another aspect of party patronage. One U.S. Public Health Service inspector noted that "the expansion of public health activities in Memphis has been influenced to a considerable degree by political conditions. Many of the personnel 'put on the pay roll' of the health department have received their appointments . . . because of certain political considerations and not because of . . . special experience and training or other qualifications."[101]

From the standpoint of such outside experts, Memphis represented a backwater of cronyism and political influence where innovations in health, sanitation, and hygiene would be closely scrutinized for their fit with the needs of the political order.

During these years the Crump regime proved to be responsive, however, to small changes in the political power and visibility of black citizens. The 1920s, for example, saw Memphis's black businessmen resisting Crump's influence and criticizing his use of black ministers and saloonkeepers to "get out the vote." The wealthy and independent-minded Robert Church became a symbol of this resistance, taking control of the weak Republican Party apparatus of the region. Church had successfully mobilized numerous black voters to support the 1920 Republican presidential ticket, and the success of Warren Harding's campaign — particularly his ability to carry Tennessee, which was Republican in the east but strongly Democratic elsewhere — earned Church modest influence in Republican circles and in making federal appointments. From his now-elevated position as Memphis's leading black businessman, active citizen, and successful Republican, Church pushed with other businessmen against the paternalistic despotism of Crump.[102] Men like J. E. Walker and George Lee, proponents of Booker T. Washington's self-help philosophy of economic advancement, also aligned themselves against those black leaders who supported the Democratic machine. Church and his backers preached self-help and praised the "thrifty intelligent group of Negroes [who would] by their own shoulder straps . . . lift themselves to the highest plane of self-determination."[103] Their wives belonged to the city Federation of Colored Women's Clubs, whose motto was "Lifting as We Climb."[104] These women and men, most of them living in the better-off North Memphis neighborhoods, styled themselves as enlightened alternatives to the liquor-dispensing saloonkeepers and soothing ministers who, they insisted, helped to keep Crump's exploitative regime in power.

If the vigor of black business in the 1920s posed problems for Crump's control, so too did the advent of woman suffrage. A wide range of observers, from *New York Age* writer James Weldon Johnson to Crump himself, saw the coming of woman suffrage to the South as a significant turning point in race relations. Heading into the 1920 elections, Johnson had predicted that "the colored women will be less easily intimidated and kept out of voting than the colored men have been. This has been realized all along by the opponents of suffrage especially in the South."[105] In the aftermath of Harding's unexpected success in Tennessee, Crump too realized that the combination of Church's influence and the women's vote had delivered the state to the Republicans. He noted to one colleague that "women not having to pay poll tax [had permitted] so many of them in East Tennessee and negro women in other sections of the state, to vote without cost, [that it] carried Tennessee into the Harding column."[106] Concerned that these national and statewide trends would have ripple effects later at his local level, Crump lobbied with the state legislature to do more for local blacks, pushing for the building of a state Vocational School for Negro Girls in Memphis. Crump's concerns were real and his strategy was preemptive, for he was convinced that "if the negro women should exercise their prerogative, the Republicans would receive a large and dangerous vote down this way."[107] Some contemporaries viewed such political calculations as evidence of African American progress in the South, since they revealed that black Memphians had "made a breach in the white party system." Others, however, insisted that Crump would always maneuver to make African Americans merely the pawns of his machine.[108] Indeed, both observations were essentially correct. These double roles for black citizens — as pawns as well as political forces in the urban power struggle — made Memphis a distinctive city in the region.[109]

Crump's occasional concessions to African Americans aside, Memphis health politics remained unyieldingly segregated. In New York City in the 1920s, by contrast, the admission of black physicians to staff positions in the white-controlled Harlem Hospital became the focus of loud debate. Local medical boards lobbied at City Hall, and newspapers weighed in heavily on the matter.[110] In New York and Chicago segregation was openly debated both within black medical circles and among reform-minded white politicians, and in both cities subtle changes in hospital policy followed. But no such discussions were possible in Memphis.[111] Most urban southerners accepted the obstinate reality of segregation. They debated only the ways in which it could be made less paternalistic, more humane, and more economically rewarding.

Crump worked occasionally with the black clergy to improve the health care system for African Americans, earning a continued faithful following among such leaders.[112] Minister T. O. Fuller, disagreeing with Church, characterized Crump as a well-meaning "bridger of racial chasms." He praised the boss for supporting projects like the hospital for crippled African American children and portrayed Crump as sympathetic, respectful, and father-like in his regard for Memphis's hardworking black people.[113] Crump's opponents insisted that his sympathy was insincere and that the only hard work he truly respected came on election day.[114] Black businessmen condemned the saloonkeepers and ministers for helping exploit those "with an imagination that easily conceive[s] the wonders of the other world when things become too hard in this."[115] While his critics fumed that the machine was using "ignorant, fraudulent, Negro voters . . . herded to the polls by dive-keepers and political bosses," his supporters insisted that in exchange for support from blacks, Crump had improved their living conditions, doing particular "yeoman service for Negro health by creating twelve free hospital wards and some neighborhood clinics."[116]

If economic possibility defined Memphis, so too did the constraints of the Crump political order. African American migrants coming to Memphis from small-town Mississippi or Arkansas in the 1920s would have encountered a complex economic and political world. As they ventured into the city, they left behind an exploitative plantation credit system that systematically deprived many tenant farmers of their full pay for work, keeping them tied to the land by the accumulation of debt.[117] But as these newcomers would have known, this older system was in transition, for the boll weevil was devastating the cotton crop. At the same time, sharecropping and wage labor — including the availability of day laborers from Memphis — had begun to undermine the older labor system. The end of a nineteenth-century system of obligations and dependency seemed to be at hand.[118] For newcomers, Memphis was where African American men like Robert Church had accumulated vast wealth, where others had found reliable wage labor, where some attained a measure of cultural visibility in the church or on stage, and where others exercised limited political influence.[119]

Newcomers would have also encountered an expanding Terrell Memorial Baptist Hospital, now with two operating rooms and a small training school for nurses. They could venture past the newly created Royal Circle charity hospital, sponsored by one of the numerous black fraternal societies.[120] These societies, like the churches, were one of the many symbols of mutuality in the African American community. Newcomers could buy burial insurance from J. E. Walker's company, and they might worship in T. O. Fuller's congregation. They would also see black women dressed in white, the public health nurses representing the university/hospital/public health department reaching out into their neighborhoods and homes, and policing the midwives.[121] Crump's police would be ever vigilant, keeping watch over such casual strollers and "foreign elements" and preventing them from gaining too much visibility in the city except on Beale Street. In Crump's view, black men and women were most valuable for the city when they were supervised — as domestic servants, as field hands, as industrial laborers, or as compliant "voters" on election day. In exchange for their accommodation to his rules, Crump ensured African Americans space and visibility in segregated municipal parks, in vocational schools, and in small clinics.

Outsiders Looking In: Feds, Philanthropists, and the MGH

In these very decades, federal and state health agencies were tentatively expanding their presence in cities like Memphis throughout the South. But in confronting Memphis's formidable political economy, these agencies stood outside the local system cautiously looking in. This wariness was evident in numerous controversies, particularly in the restructuring of the Memphis General Hospital in the 1930s, as we shall see. The cautious stance of federal agencies and philanthropists in the South in the 1920s was in reaction to a strong suspicion among southerners of northern "do-gooders" and "carpetbaggers." Such suspicions were deeply etched into the regional psyche from antebellum assaults on slavery, from Civil War scars, and from the failed attempt to create a biracial democracy in the Reconstruction era.[122] Even with the rise of a new, prosperous, and self-consciously progressive Memphis in the 1910s and 1920s, antagonisms toward outsiders were still evident, albeit in new forms and revolving around new issues like health care.

Since before the Civil War, the federal government had regarded Memphis as a vital military post overlooking the Mississippi River. But after the failure of Reconstruction policies and the resurgence of regional autonomy in the late nineteenth century, the federal government remained a weak force in the city. The early 1900s, however, brought a new Washington-based activism in matters of health. State and federal agencies promoted the application of the new science of bacteriology to public health surveillance, national legislation urged oversight of purity in food and drug products, and the rise of the hospital as a popular consumer institution provoked these governments to ensure new standards in food packaging, hospital care, and individual consumption. States and cities also created new regulatory agencies and gradually enlarged their role in monitoring public health. Thus the federal government's decision to expand the Veterans Hospital in Memphis in 1919 would not have been greeted with local alarm. Rather, this move would have been seen as the fulfillment of a national obligation to veterans, a welcomed development especially in an era of booming hospital construction. The expanded Veterans Hospital was a benign but significant federal presence, a sign of continuing government interests in urban health care.[123]

With this presence came the possibility of increasing federal oversight over the Memphis health care system, and the likelihood — however small — that local conflicts in health care might receive a sympathetic national hearing. In 1921, for example, one black World War I veteran in Memphis appealed to federal authorities for justice and equality in health care. He did so as a patient as well as a U.S. citizen. In his mind, his treatment at the hands of local white nurses reduced him to a lowly status, incommensurate with what he believed he had earned through military service. Writing to the army's adjutant general, the soldier (designated "3462.27") described the hospital as a "ward of Humalation of Black negro from some of the nurses."[124] Patients, though ill, were forced to scrub toilets and tubs, and they were compelled to act as their own orderlies. The black soldier wanted, he said, only to be "treated and spoken to as citicines of this Civil America, who showed loyaliness, on the field, and will repeat the same should it need be."[125] The soldier's appeal as a U.S. citizen to federal authorities does not appear to have provoked a response from the adjutant general, however. Federal agencies remained cautious, ineffectual investigators of such local controversies. Soldier "3462.27" remained anonymous, his plight — save for the letter — more or less invisible.

By contrast, the Veterans Hospital at Tuskegee, Alabama, became the site of a high-profile struggle over race, government, and health care that would send ripples throughout the region. In 1923 debate erupted over whether black doctors and nurses would be allowed to staff this new facility, created at the site of Booker T. Washington's famous Tuskegee Institute. The debate exposed complaints about respect and status similar to those of patient "3462.27." But the fight in Tuskegee, because of the national profile of the Institute, attracted the interest of black professionals across the country. At Tuskegee, already a national symbol of black self-help, the question of how to structure health care in its Veterans Hospital also reflected the conflict between regional white supremacy and federal power.

The debate pitted President Warren Harding and the Veterans Bureau against Tuskegee's white citizens. Many Alabama whites objected to the idea that the hospital might be staffed with African American physicians. This made it, in their eyes, a nearly autonomous black institution accountable only to the federal agency. To many whites in Alabama, this was federal interference with a regional way of life. They called for supervision of any black staff and patients by white physicians and administrators. The resurgent Ku Klux Klan sounded the most vehement criticism of the federal plan, arguing that "if our government wanted negroes to manage this hospital, they should have located it in the north and if they now want northern negroes to manage it, for God's sake, let them move it quickly."[126] Yet Harding (a Republican with little to lose by taking a firm stand in the Democratic South) upheld the plan. He pledged to give the "colored race [this] opportunity to show its capacity for service," even as white Tuskegeeans warned that "violence and bloodshed" would surely follow if a black administrator was named to head the hospital staff.[127]

The Tuskegee dispute raised the possibility of strong federal intervention in race and health care, and it unearthed some of the complexities of segregated medicine. As historian Pete Daniel has noted, whites were essentially calling for an extension of their paternalism rather than segregation per se. They wanted white involvement and oversight. The arrangement championed by some Alabama's white citizens called for complex divisions of labor in which, "most humiliating to the blacks, the white nurses, who were forbidden by Alabama law to touch the black patients, would have black maids to do the actual work."[128] But other white Alabamans questioned whether such an arrangement did not, in fact, undermine the principle of racial segregation. Why, they wondered, would any white person (and particularly white women) *want* to work in such a facility?[129] Ironically, their commitment to pure segregation and the "honor" of white southern women supported the position of Harding, the Veterans Bureau, and black professionals. The dispute thus highlighted the ways in which the interests of black physicians reinforced institutional segregation. It also showed that although federal agents were outsiders looking in, they could nevertheless leave a lasting imprint on institutions in the South.[130]

As with the Veterans Bureau in Tuskegee, some agencies could be aggressive and outspoken in the South. U.S. Public Health Service workers regularly came through the region (sometimes at the request of civic officials), investigating public health crises, commenting on the hospital situation, and comparing one city's health statistics to another's, all while avoiding direct confrontation on matters of race and hierarchy.[131] In Memphis, for example, inspectors rushed to the city in the wake of a typhoid outbreak in 1919, in the aftermath of the Mississippi River floods of 1927, and after a dramatic climb in infant death rates in the mid-1930s (see Chapter 2).[132] In the first case, inspector Paul Preble concluded in frank language that local politics were an impediment to public health: "The conditions responsible for high morbidity and mortality rates . . . are very largely the result of an unorganized health administration. . . . The influences of pernicious politics must be credited with most of the responsibility for such a condition of affairs."[133] Such outsider surveys shone a critical spotlight on the city, and while some of the criticisms led to calls for reform, the calls often went unheeded.[134] Generally, federal agencies remained circumspect in their language about civic politics and regional health, so as not to offend local sensibilities. It would take a staggering rise of poverty, particularly during the Depression, to begin altering this equation.

Philanthropists were another group of outsiders looking at Memphis's health care system, and the work of the Rockefeller, Rosenwald, Carnegie, and other foundations provoked considerable concern among southerners. Perhaps the first high-profile model of philanthropic involvement in regional health was the Rockefeller-financed campaign against hookworm, the so-called germ of laziness.[135] The hookworm campaigns exposed "a hidden feature of Southern life": an endemic, parasite-borne disorder causing anemia and lethargy.[136] The disorder gained widespread attention as a new and highly visible disease because it was easily identified using the novel tools of bacteriology, it was easily treated with thymol, and it was preventable by reforming sanitary norms in the South — that is, by distributing shoes and building privies. In short, its visibility reflected the rising power and interest of corporate philanthropy, bent upon demonstrating the superiority of private rather than government initiatives in spreading the gospel of public health. But the hookworm campaigns also spotlighted southern poverty for the nation to see. "Germ of Laziness Found," proclaimed one northern newspaper, establishing a stereotypical portrait of this "disease of the cracker" and of supposedly lethargic African Americans.[137] Even as private philanthropy spearheaded such a regional health campaign, the outsider initiatives also fomented stereotypes and fed anxieties.

Together, private philanthropies and federal agencies comprised a formidable force for change in the region — for good and for ill. In the late 1920s, for example, the U.S. Public Health Service received extensive support from the Julius Rosenwald Fund to begin studies of syphilis in Macon County, Alabama — a research project that would later become known as the Tuskegee Syphilis Experiment. The project, based in Tuskegee, began as a simple health survey and gradually evolved into a long-term study of untreated syphilis in African American men.[138] The Chicago-based Rosenwald Fund paid the costs of the study during the early survey phase, only to withdraw in 1932. At that point, the USPHS made the decision to begin systematically observing the advance of the disease process in these men. Writing in 1934, and reflecting on the survey phase, black sociologist Charles Spurgeon Johnson saw the study as a positive model, one of the notable attempts by philanthropies to seriously chronicle disease among African Americans in the region.[139] In his view, the study shed light on the kindness of philanthropy to patients, the absence of coercion, and the respect of southern blacks for paternalistic authority: "The greatest kindliness was shown the patients, and the invitations were in no sense supported by force, either direct or implied."[140] Johnson noted that the "tradition of dependence and obedience to the orders of authority, whether these were mandatory or not, helps to explain the questionless response to the invitation to examination and treatment."[141] He believed that the success of such campaigns depended in no small part on the malleability of the people.

In cities like Memphis, Rosenwald money rebuilt many African American public schools.[142] But Rosenwald dollars were no match for the city's contentious health care politics. As Memphis's George Lee recalled, when the fund sought to aid the construction of black hospitals, it encountered local rivalries and political obstacles. "Julius Rosenwald decided to build five hospitals in the black belt of the southland," wrote Lee in 1934, "[and] Dr. L. A. West, former president of the National Medical Association, made application for one of the hospitals to be built in Memphis."[143] West convinced Rosenwald that Memphis was "the gateway to the midsouth" and "that Memphis, serving three hundred thousand Negroes in three states as a hospital center, was a good location for further hospital development, and that Beale Street had a sufficiently large number of Negro physicians to staff such a hospital."[144] The foundation dispatched an investigator to the city, making it clear that any plan's success depended upon the "unanimous endorsement by the colored physicians together with a pledge of cooperation on the part of the city officials."[145] As Lee recalled, the plan fell apart in the face of factionalism and rivalries among the black physicians.[146] Yet, he noted, a second significant obstacle was the city's resistance to the plan, and a third was the fund's concession to local white prejudices against a hospital staffed with black physicians. The mayor wished to build a facility modeled on the city hospital. "Though Negro patients were admitted to the city hospital of Memphis," noted Lee, "Negro physicians were denied admission, and hence cut off from the chance to elevate their medical standards by such practice."[147] The leaders of the small black hospitals (W. S. Martin at Collins Chapel and C. A. Terrell at Terrell Baptist Hospital) "objected to the plan for a hospital, that would have a white consulting staff, and when their opposition was made known to the Rosenwald Foundation that hospital program failed to materialize."[148] Foundation money flowed instead to causes like the Tuskegee Institute, Atlanta's black educational institutions, and Nashville's Meharry Medical College.[149] Indeed, in the state of Tennessee, Nashville rather than Memphis was perceived as the center for the production of physicians and nurses.[150] The Bluff City had no such renowned institution around which philanthropic interests could be mobilized.[151] Memphis's small black hospitals, which had grown and prospered in the expansive 1920s, were now struggling in the 1930s. Its black college, LeMoyne College, possessed nothing like the national reputation of Meharry, Tuskegee, Howard, or Fisk.

Even locally generated philanthropy, which had also become a force for altering health arrangements in cities across America, proved ineffective in Memphis. Certainly Memphis had no industrial giants or commercial magnates of the stature of Rockefeller, Carnegie, or Rosenwald, and it had no George Eastman to create the University of Rochester or James Buchanan Duke to reinvent the college and medical school bearing his name.[152] Memphis did produce John Gaston, who, with his wife, Teresa Gaston Mann, promoted a modest vision of health care reform. However, the effort to create Gaston Hospital revealed, yet again, the wary political and economic conservatism of the Memphis civic establishment.

After amassing wealth and building one of Memphis's leading hotels, John Gaston had given generously to the city in 1900, donating five acres of land for a public park and playground.[153] The well-regarded Gaston died in 1912, leaving his estate in the hands of his wife. When Teresa Mann died in 1929, her will stipulated that some $300,000 to $400,000 would be left to the city for the construction of a new municipal hospital bearing her husband's name.[154] The bequest supported charity care, but one crucial and controversial stipulation attached to the gift dictated that the charity ward of the Gaston Hospital would be open not only to Memphis residents, but also to the citizens of Mississippi and Arkansas. In Mann's view, the new hospital would serve the region.[155] This stipulation cut against the grain of local culture. Like the Rosenwald proposal, it provoked internal rivalries about the control of the hospital, but it also exposed Memphis's prejudices about its place in the region.[156] Civic officials feared that Teresa Mann's bequest would be an open invitation to area vagrants, the rural poor, and the diseased of neighboring states. Even as the old hospital facility deteriorated, the Gaston/Mann bequest remained politically suspended. Into the early years of the Depression, the generous grant sat in escrow. Without success, Memphis officials negotiated with the executors to amend the terms of the will to limit outsider access to the planned hospital.

Local interest in the Gaston-Mann endowment was revived with the continuing decline of the economy, with journalistic exposés on the appalling condition of the General Hospital, and, most important, by the availability of new matching funds for hospital construction from the federal government's Depression-era Public Works Administration (PWA). The patient burden at Memphis General had increased dramatically with rural migration away from the economically ravaged countryside. The question looming over Memphis was this: Would philanthropic generosity combined with federal funds alter the landscape of urban health care? Civic pragmatism compelled city leaders to apply for PWA construction dollars and to take up again the challenge of the Mann bequest.[157] At the same time that Memphians were reading about rats and frightened patients inside Memphis General Hospital, a PWA loan office opened in May 1934.[158] Mann's bequest was suddenly pushed back into the headlines by reform-minded journalists. But city officials held firm in their reluctance to open the hospital to the citizens of nearby states, taking their case to the courts. After a series of hearings, the city of Memphis ultimately won the right in the state supreme court in June 1934 to amend the five-year-old will.[159] Four days later, a PWA loan for hospital reconstruction was approved. The city's xenophobic and fiscally anxious concerns had triumphed over Mann's broad-minded regionalism. Construction on the new John Gaston Hospital began later that year. While the *Memphis Press-Scimitar* claimed credit for pressuring Crump's machine through "a series of news articles and [having] urged this action editorially," the victory in many ways was the city's. Civic officials had proved adept at leveraging funds from local philanthropy and from the federal agency, but on their own terms.[160]

These new Depression-era relationships created a civic awareness that the strategy of making "regional need" visible, however painful and embarrassing to the city, could attract dollars to the struggling metropolis — even if, ironically, those dollars would serve the needs of only Memphians.[161] The hospital represented a new economy and a compromise among ideals in the 1930s. It represented a new stage in the growth of an integrated health care system with economic ties and debatable moral obligations outside the city itself. Already staffed with University of Tennessee medical school faculty, but now financed by the Mann/Gaston bequest, by PWA funds, and by an additional sale of $170,000 in city bonds, the facility symbolized the confluence of multiple agendas revolving around health care for the poor.[162]

The Depression had tipped the balance of health patronage decidedly toward the federal government, yet this shift had not fundamentally altered the city's view of its regional responsibilities or changed race relations.[163] The flow of federal dollars into the city matched the influx of migrants, resulting in one new facility after another: a new maternity ward at the Gaston Hospital, new public housing, new dormitories at the medical school, and improvements to public schools, parks, bridges, and sewers. From the PWA alone, the city obtained some $8 million.[164] If such programs did not challenge the existing political order, they did reshape familiar institutions and compel subtle changes in the political economy of health care.[165]

The Value of Bodies and Disease

By the early 1930s, the economic crisis and its political and demographic fallout had increased the visibility of pain and suffering in Crump's Memphis, particularly as institutions like the John Gaston Hospital took form. Yet the eyes of merchants and politicians remained fixed on declining cotton prices and on the struggling economies of the cotton-producing states.[166] The dwindling value of the crop led cotton farmers themselves to accept generous federal subsidies, linking the fate of "King Cotton" itself to federal largesse.[167] In an ironic development, the newly created Agricultural Adjustment Administration began a policy of paying farmers *not* to produce, laying the foundation for the withdrawal of thousands of acres from cotton cultivation and for the eviction of thousands of tenant farmers. Released from the land, agricultural laborers headed for cities like Memphis where New Deal agencies were also creating jobs and financing urban development.[168] In the early 1930s, cities like Memphis stood out even more sharply as havens from rural blight than they had for T. O. Fuller, J. E. Walker, and Miles Vandahurst Lynk in the 1910s. The city's health care facilities had become all the more attractive for the uprooted, the ailing, and the infirm of the region. As early as 1931, a Rosenwald-funded survey found that "a considerable proportion of the beds for Negroes in Memphis are occupied by residents of neighboring states."[169] Tennessee cities, noted one Memphis physician in 1932, already had "24 percent of the population and 44 percent of the physicians."[170]

The Depression era provoked Memphians to rethink familiar truisms about cotton, their health care system, and their role in the regional economy.[171] The material basis of plantation paternalism was eroding. Just as African Americans had been valued as laborers in the cotton economy, in Memphis they had become crucial to the domestic economy as workers in white homes, and sick and indigent Memphians (many of them African Americans) were slowly becoming valuable in the city's health care economy. Not only were they recognized as useful "clinical material" by the expanding university; from the city's perspective, African Americans also defined a demographic group whose presence could attract dollars to re-build civic infrastructure. Institutions such as Universal Life Insurance Company, for example, sprang up and thrived in Memphis precisely be-cause they served distressed African Americans in the city and throughout the region.[172]

Economic crisis and dislocation attracted attention not only to the city in the South, but also to the rural surroundings. Fisk University's Charles Spurgeon Johnson observed, for example, that out on the farms of Mis-sissippi and Arkansas where African American tenant farmers, sharecrop-pers, and day laborers performed backbreaking work, the landlord still could "determine the kind and amount of schooling for the children, [and] even . . . the relief they receive in the extremity of distress."[173] Health problems, he pointed out, were "a part of the very culture of tenancy."[174] In Johnson's view of African American life on the plantation, "startling inbreeding . . . violent eruptions of nutritional disorders, and the rapid contagion of infectious disease [were] intricately bound up with their iso-lation."[175] Other observers spoke of "the neglected Negroes in the rural communities . . . embalmed in their ignorance of the laws of health."[176] "That they carry germs is known here and there," historian Carter Woodson suggested, "but the thought with them is still a theory. Most diseases result in the natural course of things, or come as the vengeance of God to afflict the wicked. Of course, the 'conjure doctor' there is still active."[177]

In the 1930s, mobility and escape from the cotton-obsessed rural South into the city were still on the minds of many black southerners, just as they had been for J. E. Walker when he left Indianola, Mississippi, in the 1910s. In the 1930s, however, Memphis projected a somewhat different image. The city, with its complex institutions and array of services, was now seen as a healthful place.[178] For observers like Charles Spurgeon Johnson, cities like Memphis held the possibility of improvement through "definite cultural penetration through the medium of the school, the church, the influence of persons educated outside the community, the exposure to demonstrations in health and agriculture, and through returned migration."[179] Yet civic officials remained wary of the burden of migration and ambivalent about the city's role as a regional health care center, even as they now vigorously used Memphis's centrality to promote economic growth.

Memphis represented a haven and a stage where the invisible might emerge into the light, a place where nascent economies generated new regional sensibilities and new perceptions of health. Consider the early career of blues musician Lizzie Douglas. Born in 1897 in Algiers, Louisiana, near New Orleans, she moved with her family to a small town in Mississippi in 1904. By 1917 Douglas had left for Memphis, where she was already well known as a Beale Street guitarist. Taking the name "Memphis Minnie," Douglas played with jug bands through the 1920s before recording her first songs in 1929. By 1933 she had migrated to Chicago. The trajectory of her career symbolized much about upward and outward mobility in the region, as well as about the growing commercialization and national visibility of the region's culture via the popularization of the blues. When Douglas performed the plight of the ailing on a blues stage, it was at once an expression of the new economy and an index of the rising visibility of regional culture and health.[180] Among Douglas's songs, "Hoodoo Lady" celebrated the power of the conjuror to transform water into wine, old into new. In "Memphis Minnie-jitis Blues," Douglas bemoaned the epidemic disease that took a woman away from her lover, the inability of the doctor to diagnose the malady, and what seemed to be her final trek to the city hospital.[181]

In the 1930s many such individuals were positioned to see the value of disease as a centerpiece of an expanding health care system.[182] When most Memphians sought to shun the sick, labeling them as social and financial burdens, the city's academic physicians, like Douglas, seized upon sickness as an opportunity for teaching and illumination. For the academic physicians, to visualize disease was a way to build a professional name, to claim distinctive insights, and to boost public confidence in medical care.[183] To be sure, however, some physicians and many civic leaders (particularly those we shall encounter in the following chapter) continued to echo the disdain felt by fellow Memphians for the infirm, particularly if they were outsiders.

Certainly many black southerners came to Memphis to flee the oversight and paternalism of the plantation system.[184] Many newcomers, like Lizzie Douglas, came to the city to work within the emerging social system — to *gain* visibility, to find opportunity, to create a new identity, and thereby to rise in stature and prominence. Memphis was a city where, for many different reasons, the obscure, unseen, and hidden pathologies of the rural South could be revealed and dramatized. The city was an urban stage, an evolving political and economic culture, where various kinds of conjurors might give value and visibility to disease.

2 Race Pathologies, Apparent and Unseen

My companion take me to the doctor
"Doctor please tell me my wife's complaint"
My companion take me to the doctor
"Doctor please tell me my wife's complaint"
That doctor look down, shook his head
Said "I wouldn't mind tellin' you son, but I can't"
— Lizzie Douglas, "Memphis Minnie-jitis Blues"

How is it that a disease that today is widely noted for its distinctive, recurrent, and singularly painful episodes could have been so obscure in early-twentieth-century America? The obscurity of sickle cell disease — a disorder characterized by lethargy, repeated infections, frequent joint and abdominal pains, and high childhood mortality — was due to many factors. One factor, as we have seen already in Chapter 1, was that local health care systems allowed for the visibility of some disorders and not of others, giving selective meaning to African American pain, distress, and disease. Another factor shaping disease visibility was the landscape of prevailing diseases, the local diagnostic preoccupations, and the attitudes about race and disease that pressed upon Memphis's collective mind-set.

Memphians and practitioners in the South focused their attention on the overwhelming acute infectious diseases and on the heavy burden of child mortality throughout their region. Diphtheria, pneumonia, tuberculosis, and typhoid fever claimed the lives of many of their children, commanded much attention, and left little-known ailments like sickle cell anemia in their shadow. Malaria, in particular, mimicked the pain and other common symptoms of sickle cell anemia, obscuring it even further from clinical and public health view. But another reason for the obscurity of sickle cell disease relates to the local habit of mind, that is, to the prevailing attitudes toward the maladies and deaths of black infants. Early in the century, black infant mortality was widely perceived as an all-too-common, expected, and unsurprising regional experience. In the thinking of many whites, "negro ignorance" itself explained many of these deaths.

Considering these overlapping factors, then, the invisibility of sickle cell anemia must be examined in relation to the existing landscape of perceptions. To the extent that perceptions about death and disease were rooted in time, place, and cultural context, sickle cell disease's invisibility presents a complex puzzle. This chapter seeks to examine that invisibility and thereby to sort out the pieces of that puzzle. Through this exploration, we learn not only about the disease per se, but also about the region, about the reconfiguration of disease perception, and about the roles of medicine, science, and politics in redefining black health in the South and in America.[1]

Looming over all problems of black health in early-twentieth-century America was one overwhelming, widely accepted image: that of a naturally diseased people. The stereotypic "Negro" portrayed in news accounts and by health professionals was a social menace whose superstitions, ignorance, and carefree demeanor stood as a stubborn affront to modern notions of hygiene and advancing scientific understanding. Mindless tradition and "ignorance" posed great dangers to blacks and whites alike. Stereotypes of these spreaders of disease — the syphilitic black man, the tubercular black woman, and the black child harboring infectious disease — were variations upon old racial themes, updated to fit with new twentieth-century anxieties. In the language of modern bacteriology — which had only recently discovered the "asymptomatic carrier" — black people were like Typhoid Mary, carrying disease maliciously and unwittingly. Such views were becoming increasingly prevalent in public health discourse in the early twentieth century.[2] It was this image of "the Negro" as "carrier and vector" that physicians (both black and white) invoked time after time, either to stress the importance of education and behavioral reform or to highlight the virtues of segregation for public health. One typical southern physician argued that "the safeguarding of the health of the Negro . . . [was] anything but an easy task, for the fight is not against disease, but against physical, mental, and moral inferiority, against ignorance and superstition, against poverty and filth."[3] For health professionals, contending with such unruly, lawless individuals constituted a significant challenge. Determining their actual impact on mortality rates was a central problem in cities like Memphis and throughout the Mid-South, as in much of America in the first decades of the twentieth century. The heavy burden of tuberculosis, syphilis, and other infectious diseases among African Americans (or, as some contemporaries simplified it, "negro disease") seemed only to confirm the correctness of the stereotype.[4]

Writing in the 1930s, African American sociologist Charles Johnson added another dimension to the portrait. For him, ignorance, folk superstition, and fatalism combined to weave a deadly web of misinformation among black southerners. "That child there," he quoted one black Alabama woman, "has spells since she was a little baby. Jest one right after another from eight to four o'clock every day for two years. I dosed her with calomel and I sent to Montgomery and got some worm powder and got nineteen worms from her in one day. But she can't learn nothing in school now. She jest sets with her mouth open . . . most of the time."[5] In his portrait, the vague diagnosis of mysterious "spells" only confirmed the appalling lack of education among poor blacks in the region, and the continuing dangers of folk medicine. There were no hospitals for this woman and her child. Medication consisted only of home remedies and sending away to the nearby city for "worm powder." Such women represented, in Johnson's view, not the virtues of tradition and self-reliance, but an unfortunate isolation and the persistence of dangerous attitudes. Her words emphasized the fundamental separation of rural folk from centers of knowledge and commerce in Montgomery, Atlanta, Nashville, and Memphis. These mysterious "spells," along with malaria, stillbirths, influenza, tuberculosis, and pellagra, were the leading causes of death in the region. In Johnson's opinion, the tragedy of the region was that folk beliefs impeded good health while modern medicine in unreachable urban centers had the capacity to recognize and remedy these ailments.

Johnson believed that illness left unrecognized in the isolation of rural poverty destroyed the capacity to thrive. The Alabama woman's complaints evoked the general situation of black women and children living in the shadow of the plantation. Their clinging to "folk knowledge of disease" was an indicator of their hopelessness and isolation. It was, Johnson concluded, "the heavy fall of death [that] prompts [them] to reliance upon both herbs and something akin to magic, in the attempt to bring about cures." A pervasive resignation reigned in the region, where "children die in great numbers and mothers accept their death with a dull and uninquiring fatalism." That women spoke in matter-of-fact tones about the deaths of multiple children, showing no deep mourning, no social outrage, and no pervasive grief, suggested the presence of a "casual and uninformed" disposition.[6] Modern diagnosis and treatment remained particularly difficult where such poverty, isolation, and folk practices prevailed. By contrast, the city seemed to be one of the true agents of progress.

But what Johnson and others failed to understand was that modern urban medicine's concepts of disease were themselves problematic and evolving, defined by local cultures and contexts. In the burgeoning American metropolis as in the rural countryside, cultural values shaped access to care, diagnosis, disease recognition, and attitudes toward death. In Memphis and other cities, an emerging health care system with its own diagnostic habits left many complaints unrecognized. Here too infant death was intertwined with the fabric of cultural perception, regional belief, and particularized knowledge. The obscurity of sickle cell anemia and its emergence as a discrete recognized disorder proves the point. For here in the story of one disease is a portrait of a city's cultural and intellectual transformation, a narrative illuminating the ways in which medical thought, scientific insight, and politics informed one another.

With the rise of laboratory methods of diagnosis in the early twentieth century, new diseases like sickle cell anemia emerged into medical and public health consciousness. In 1910 Chicago physician James Bryan Herrick had embraced the use of microscopic blood examination for disease detection and noted the existence of the peculiar elongated sickle-shaped red blood cells. He perceived these cells as the signature of a possible new disease, and in the next decade a handful of other urban practitioners—in New York, St. Louis, Chicago, and Memphis—took an interest in this peculiar new pathology, seeking to determine its prevalence in the population and its racial character. But in every context where medical scientists sought to establish the meaning of the disease, local factors shaped their diagnostic practices and their interpretation of these peculiar red cells. In an age when the tools of the laboratory were being widely applied, the recognition of disease depended upon a subtle negotiation between these experts and established diagnostic customs.[7] This was true in all regions and contexts—whether in the rural hinterlands, in the intellectual backwaters, or in the emerging American metropolis. Specifically, in cities like Memphis and elsewhere in the Midwest, the malaria diagnosis took precedence in the minds of the public, physicians, and public health workers. As we shall see, this malady's very prominence—and the way in which its own "shakes" and "spells" were perceived—was one aspect of local diagnostic custom in Memphis that obscured recognition of sickle cell anemia as an independent entity.

This chapter focuses on the relationship between the *visible* pathologies of the region and the *invisible* pathology, sickle cell disease. The burden of malaria highlighted the city's ambivalent rural-urban identity and its tense relationship with its rural surroundings. By contrast, sickle cell anemia attracted little professional concern and no popular attention. The story of its emergence from invisibility draws our attention to the ways in which public attitudes, professional practices, and civic discourses evolved at the local level.[8]

From today's medical perspective, it is clear that the disease we call sickle cell anemia would have manifested itself in various kinds of infant death. Examining the historical invisibility of sickle cell anemia leads, then, not only to an investigation of the malaria diagnosis, but also to a study of infant death. Even as the disorder was emerging into clinical view in the 1920s, 1930s, and 1940s, physicians called it the "great masquerader" because its sufferers often fell victim to pneumonia, tuberculosis, and other infectious diseases, and many of its symptoms appeared to clinicians to be some other disease.[9] Deaths from the disease would simply have faded into the background of general, undifferentiated infant mortality. Anywhere that repetitive aches, overwhelming infections, or lethargy in children appeared, or wherever mysterious deaths occurred, one might suspect that authentic cases of sickle cell anemia lay hidden. One might be tempted to reinterpret even the Alabama woman's home diagnosis of "spells" as, potentially, a case of sickle cell disease. But where some historians have striven to uncover such "real" and "misdiagnosed" cases from the sparse records of the past, I have taken on a different interpretive challenge.[10] In what follows, I have sought to understand how the deaths and ailments of these black infants were perceived at the time, why they were so perceived, and what these perceptions tell us about southern culture and race politics.

Indeed, a crucial turning point in the story of disease perception was the politicization of infant mortality in Memphis, particularly after a 1934 infant death crisis brought federal officials from the U.S. Children's Bureau into the city. Such events highlighted the ways in which the contested meanings of shakes, spells, and infant death in the city itself were part of a deeper struggle among Memphians to define a civic identity as well as to define their relationships to rural migrants and to the nation at large.

Interpreting Pain and Pathology

Regional mortality figures in the early-twentieth-century South told a grim tale of infectious diseases, and observers often saw high mortality as a natural result of regional poverty.[11] Urbanization, it seemed, merely fed the rising death toll. A familiar range of diseases shaped local memory—pellagra, tuberculosis, and typhoid among them. Any Memphian could tell stories about the devastating yellow fever epidemics of the 1870s in which thousands died, even more fled, and regional commerce was destroyed.[12] But diseases like malaria lingered long after yellow fever had passed, leaving a very different kind of mark on regional consciousness. Elbridge Sibley, a Fisk University statistician, believed that "plausibly, malaria may be endemic among Negroes living in certain urban areas" of Tennessee. Mortality rates from the disease remained quite low—between 15 and 20 deaths per 100,000. But its endemic nature and its intimate association with Mississippi River communities were as noteworthy in 1930 as they were one hundred years earlier.[13] Malaria was one of the "natural" diseases clinging to the river valleys, etched onto Memphis's local landscape.

Into the early twentieth century, endemic malaria had specific cultural meanings. Writing about the Mississippi Valley, historian Erwin Ackerknecht noted that the rising and falling incidence of the disease in the nineteenth century was explained by a variety of factors—transportation, agricultural development, and popular as well as diagnostic perception.[14] Into the 1920s, state health departments confirmed by statistics what every Tennessee doctor knew from experience: "The malaria death rate varies almost inversely as the distance from the Mississippi River, with a minor increase as one approaches the Tennessee River."[15] The shakes and fevers associated with malaria were commonplace occurrences in the lives of Mississippi River cultures, and the anemic appearance of people along the river valley was regarded by visitors and locals as a natural feature of the land, not much more noteworthy than the river itself. It was common, for example, to hear people say, "He ain't sick, he's only got the ager."[16]

The meaning that was assigned to symptoms like the shakes, pain, disease, or even death was shaped by regional culture, by local tradition, and by social institutions.[17] Religion, of course, played an important part in the discourse of illness and healing throughout the nineteenth century and would continue to do so into the twentieth century.[18] Even popular music expressed regional attitudes toward pain, suffering, and death. As Memphis Minnie sang of the "Minnie-jitis Blues," for Robert Johnson the blues was nothing but "a low down shakin' chill"—a phrase resonating with meaning in the malaria-prone river valley. The character of *any* new pathology involving shakes, spells, episodic pain, or lethargy would have to be carefully distinguished from this background of spells, shakes, fevers, and periodic pain if it were to achieve an identity of its own.[19]

Southern cities created their own stories of pathology, and these inter-sected with regional politics and urban anxieties. Public health officials and editorial cartoonists in Atlanta, for example, graphically depicted black women domestic workers mingling with flies and insects, all of them por-trayed as carriers of tuberculosis, and then flying over the defenses of aver-age white homes, transmitting the disease as they went. Racialized images of disease, from hookworm to pellagra (and, later, to sickle cell anemia), were commonplace.[20] Disease — for the public and the professional alike — acquired a definite social character and stood as a poignant commentary on the new social and political relations associated with urban growth.

In their civic discourse, Memphians emphasized the dangers posed *by* blacks in their town, much more than the dangers posed *to* black citizens. Progressive-minded citizens championed pure milk campaigns, carried out typhoid and malaria warnings, and endorsed the eradication of venereal disease in the black population.[21] In Memphis as throughout America, public health discourse drew heavily on bacteriological metaphors. The "Negro health problem" was thus frequently portrayed as a close relative of the hookworm nematode infection, the boll weevil parasite's invasion of cotton patches, and the spread of the syphilis organism. All of these motifs represented invading organisms bringing blight where health and pros-perity might otherwise reign. This style of thinking about animal vectors, parasites, and infections appealed to the local agricultural mind — and to those in a world dominated by the cotton planter, the cotton merchants, and financiers.[22] By the 1910s, religious leaders, elected officials (including the public health leaders), physicians, businessmen, and the popular citi-zenry had become accustomed to using these motifs in shaping the regional understanding of black health.

Accordingly, the first case of sickle cell disease reported in Memphis at the Veteran's Hospital in 1926 posed a local interpretive challenge. J. F. Hamilton, a doctor stationed at the hospital, reported the plight of a thirty-three-year-old farmer: "Married . . . has [four children] living and in good health . . . but [three deceased children] . . . three of his half-brothers died . . . in infancy." At the age of twenty-one, the farmer "had recurrent attacks of pain in the back, muscles, and joints of extremities and stomach, that did not cause him to stop work, but left him sleepy and drowsy."[23] As a self-employed black farmer, this man would have been something of a regional anomaly.[24] He drew upon home remedies to relieve the pain and returned to farming, for Hamilton noted that a dose of soda and an occa-sional drink of whiskey sometimes brought relief.[25] While serving in the

U.S. Army in 1918, the farmer had an acute attack on the drill field. He "fell out with extreme pain . . . refused gall stone operation . . . and worked as a hospital orderly for the rest of his Army service," where he suffered several more attacks.[26] The scattered references to gallstones, tuberculosis, and other disorders highlights the fact that such patients were at risk not only from the disease, but also from the treatments.

Based on the sickled cells in the blood, Hamilton believed that this farmer presented an authentic case of a relatively new disease — sickle cell anemia. After he presented the case before the doctors of the Memphis Medical Society, discussion revealed the weight of diagnostic custom, particularly the impact of malaria on the local medical mind. One supportive colleague urged Hamilton on, noting that "we are likely to see many others."[27] But another warned against moving too hastily toward these diagnostic novelties. He observed that "sickle cells are sometimes associated with malaria . . . [and such findings] might lead some one to suppose that such cells were due to sickle cell anemia" when in fact the problem was actually malaria.[28] This warning was both a clinical and cultural commentary, an indication of the weight of "rural-mindedness" in the city; the burden of malaria produced a knee-jerk diagnostic conservatism. Only the most adventurous doctors (or perhaps a newcomer to the region unfamiliar with local medical culture) would stray beyond the bounds of diagnostic custom. Those who ventured into novel terrain, like Hamilton, would find it hard to convince their peers that this was a new category of pathological experience.

Local diagnostic custom prevailed, especially where chills, shakes, fevers, and painful episodes were found clumped together in one suffering person. Writing in 1927, the editor of the *Memphis Medical Journal* noted that "every physician is familiar with the 'chills and fevers' that is so common in . . . patients in the locality. And he is likewise familiar with the fact that not one out of fifty . . . has had the diagnosis confirmed by examination of a blood smear."[29] Local practices were such that most physicians did not need to rely upon laboratory observations to spot the telltale malaria organism that invaded blood cells, depending instead on the well-defined, familiar range of physical signs and symptoms. Moreover, the disease was by definition evasive. Lloyd Graves, head of the Memphis Department of Public Health, believed that "malaria is one of the most important health problems in this territory . . . a disease in which accurate statistics are difficult to keep . . . largely due to [its] chronic and relapsing course."[30]

By contrast, typhoid fever — a disease caused by a water-borne pathogen — was perceived as a distinct, and distinctly urban, problem. "Typhoid," wrote Graves in 1929, "is perhaps the best index to the general sanitation of any city."[31] Yet here too, observers drew upon local custom to explain the etiology. Graves attributed this problem (as he did with many Memphis health problems) to two vectors — not microscopic organisms, but easily seen, inwardly migrating ones: nonresidents and blacks. As he and other Memphians saw it, "31.8 percent of the cases and 40.9 percent of the deaths were of non-resident infection. This unusual non-resident element is no doubt due to the large territory which Memphis serves with her splendid hospital facilities and her widely known medical personnel."[32] Graves noted that "the negro population is also an important contributing factor to the high morbidity and mortality rates." For support, he cited statistics showing that almost 50 percent of all typhoid deaths in the city from 1926 to 1929 were in the black population, while "only 35.4 percent of our total population is colored." For health officials like Graves, these numbers did not suggest sympathy for blacks, a group that carried an excessive burden from diseases linked to poor sanitation. Rather, the numbers suggested the need for increasing surveillance and control of inward migration, for without black people and nonresidents, he believed, Memphis would undoubtedly see typhoid rates that were among the nation's lowest.

The battle against malaria and typhoid fever in the city was a battle against population mobility and urban geography. The malaria struggle involved housing reforms such as requiring screens on dwellings to keep the mosquito at bay, and swamp drainage to deprive the insect of a breeding place.[33] Graves argued that here too "non-resident infection and the negro population doubtless affect our rates in this disease more than in typhoid fever."[34] This was especially true when natural disasters (like the floods of 1927 and 1937) forced thousands of people into Memphis from their homes along the Mississippi. Noted Graves, "The 1927 flood with its many refugee camps has no doubt played an important part in disseminating the disease throughout this entire region."[35] But even under normal circumstances, black Memphians and poor whites lived precisely in these undervalued, low-lying areas with poor drainage — ideal circumstances for the proliferation of swamp conditions, mosquitoes, and malaria.[36] To Lloyd Graves and others, slum clearance thus became a necessary method of population control, as well as a centerpiece in malaria and typhoid fever control and public health reform.[37]

For Graves the problem of malaria was as much perception as reality, and he blamed black doctors for falsely increasing the high incidence of the disease. He noted that over the years, the public health department had come to dismiss the malaria diagnosis when it came from black doctors. Graves believed that "much of our decline of malaria mortality is due to not accepting this as a cause of death without proper proof . . . some of the negro doctors . . . were using this as an alibi [that is, to hide their ignorance]. In this connection, I would say that there are about eighty negro doctors in this community whose favorite diagnosis is malaria."[38] In his view, by the late 1920s malaria had become a catchall diagnosis associated with thoughtless custom. Considered alongside Hamilton's case report, Graves's comments indicate that popular and professional assumptions about malaria were well established, and also that this thinking was beginning to change.

When Lemuel W. Diggs, the Johns Hopkins–trained pathologist (see illustrations), arrived in Memphis in 1929, he brought with him a distinctly new, laboratory-oriented perception of disease, and he turned his critical lens on Memphis. His education at Hopkins tied him to a small but fast-growing world of clinical research, to modern tools of analysis, and to the emerging discipline of hematology — a field that took a specialized interest in the blood and in blood diseases like sickle cell anemia. Throughout Diggs's career, these national professional attachments — in addition to local disease patterns and diagnostic customs — would guide his writings on disease. Because of his training, Diggs came to Memphis quite a bit more familiar with obscure new diseases like sickle cell anemia and pernicious anemia than with malaria. Soon, he became the second Memphis author to write about sickle cell anemia as an independent affliction.

He too noted that the diagnostic attachment to malaria played a large role in determining what was seen and unseen in the region. But to Diggs, it was not just the "Negro doctors," as Graves insisted, who overdiagnosed malaria. It was the Memphis medical and public health establishment itself that overestimated its prevalence while ignoring the significance of novel disorders. Diggs found that most health care practitioners concealed sickle cell disease by their embrace of mundane diagnostic procedures. Even where laboratory tools were used, he suggested, the dominant style was to hunt for malaria parasites — and this practice itself hindered recognition of sickle cell anemia. Writing in a local medical journal, Diggs reminded his peers that looking for malarial parasites involved a particular "thick drop" blood analysis, but that looking for sickled cells necessitated another, more refined blood smear technique. Malaria diagnosis was the easier and more common of the two, "because any doctor can make a puddle of blood on a slide, whereas it is the exceptional doctor who is capable under field conditions of making good smears," wrote Diggs. "Moreover," he continued, "the parasites in a thick drop are concentrated and the searching time is greatly reduced."[39] Diagnostic efficiency and the lack of skilled training meant that most local doctors used the thick drop method. This technique, Diggs suggested, actually precluded the diagnosis of sickle cell anemia, making the visible detection of discrete sickled cells almost impossible.

Thus the relationship between the visible malaria and the invisible sickle cell disease was culturally complex, highlighting, in part, a clash of medical cultures. Many cases of sickle cell anemia would certainly have been perceived symptomatically as malaria, and other cases might have been obscured because of the hunt for malaria even where laboratory tools came into play. Still other cases would be diagnosed as some other health problem — appendicitis or gallstones, pneumonia or other infections. Finally, even if it were uniformly accepted as a discrete new disease, sickle cell anemia would have remained a minor complaint compared to these others. As it was, only Diggs and a few others understood sickle cell disease as a rare disorder. Its appearance in medical journals was limited to interesting anecdotes, and it faded into the background of infectious disease in adults and children.[40] Any disorder that included fever, shivering, recurrent pain, or the "shakes" took its meaning from the culture of Memphis medicine. Spells and recurrent painful episodes might easily be interpreted in light of the local disease ecology.[41] Any unconventional interpretations of these symptoms presented locals with a challenge.

Death and the Infant

If the disease rate was high among blacks, it was commonly explained that "the Negro" was little more than an "ignorant" child. Blacks were portrayed as an undifferentiated and superstitious "folk," natural carriers of disease who were responsible for dangerous pathologies streaming into the city. Malaria, tuberculosis, syphilis, and meningitis exemplified the situation, their visibility highlighting the existing racial anxieties of the city.[42] Other health problems, however, like infant mortality, were thrust upon the city's consciousness by national events, forcing civic officials to engage diplomatically with alternative explanations of disease and death.

The 1920s brought a national politicization of the child, framed by the 1921 Sheppard-Towner maternal and child health legislation and by Hoover's 1930 White House Conference on Children. Child health became a subject of national debate and soon constituted a potent political issue. The topic was given force by women's suffrage, but it also carried distinct racial overtones and regional dimensions.[43] Reductions in infant mortality in these years became an index of community progress. In 1920s Memphis, politicians and public health officials gained political mileage from the fact that the infant mortality rate had declined dramatically. Parents' expectations about infant survival were rising year by year, and all were aware that improvements in sanitation, diet, and housing were primarily responsible for children's surviving the early "fatal years."[44]

The South itself, wary of the stereotype of its backwardness, changed in response to the child welfare movement. States became more inclined to enforce school requirements and to move some young children out of the labor force.[45] Legislated paternalism resulted in new protections for women workers and child laborers in the 1910s, and these trends culminated in the Sheppard-Towner Maternity and Infancy Protection Act. As historian Molly Ladd-Taylor has argued, Sheppard-Towner's proponents effectively "turned women's private suffering to political advantage."[46] The act represented an unprecedented national commitment to child health, providing federal matching funds to bolster state programs on maternal health education. Its passage, however, involved political compromise, for the legislation had been opposed by the American Medical Association (AMA), which saw it as a step toward government health care. In 1926 organized medicine mounted another campaign against Sheppard-Towner's renewal, and the 1928 election of Herbert Hoover sealed its demise.[47] But child health had gained both political and cultural significance — for physicians safeguarding their economic interests, for reformers, and for American families.[48]

The existence of black-white differentials in infant mortality had also become a common concern, for they enumerated what most people in the region easily recognized: black children died in higher proportions than white children.[49] In Tennessee these differences spanned all regions and covered a range of diseases. In the writings of African Americans, child death was seen as a tragic consequence of a social system defined by economic inequality and ignorance. Such scholars commonly portrayed infant death as an offshoot of inequalities in economic status or as part of the gap between the "learned" and the "uneducated folk" trapped in a world of superstition and ignorance.[50] Women's clubs seized upon child health as a public extension of maternal responsibilities. As one participant in National Negro Health Week wrote, "The mother is the force which influences and controls the child and . . . the home is the seat of this influence."[51] The target of reform energies was often the ministers, who were frequently charged with fostering backward beliefs. Charles Johnson and George Lee, for example, both saw the church as a repository of superstition and folk practices.[52] Writing in the pages of *Opportunity* in 1926, another author noted condescendingly that churches had no qualms advertising "We believe that all manner of disease can be cured. Jesus is the Doctor. Services on Sunday."[53] Such learned authors and would-be reformers portrayed infant death not as a matter for prayer and charms, but as the by-product of a failed social system.

Where the church stood on the death of children is a more elusive question. Black churches were instrumental in creating a framework for thinking about worldly matters, the afterlife, and the place of people in these worlds. Baptists, Methodists, and other religious traditionalists placed emphasis on *adult* repentance; baptism (the powerful gesture of accepting Jesus Christ and being saved) was a practice reserved for those who consciously chose to believe. "Does any one ask why the Baptist churches condemn infant baptism?" wondered the Reverend M. W. Gilbert, pastor of the First Colored Baptist Church of Nashville, in 1890. The belief among such conventional theologians was that infants could not be baptized because they lacked self-awareness, experience, or demonstrable faith. "John the Baptist preaches repentance before baptism. Surely infants cannot experience repentance . . . where there is no exercise of faith, there is no baptism."[54] Baptism, for Gilbert, was a burial and a rebirth — an immersion in water, a cleansing that no infant could initiate or undergo. In 1937 John Dollard confirmed the point, noting that adolescents were typically the ones baptized, and that "the parents or family of the one being baptized did the most shouting; perhaps they were overjoyed by the certainty of being united with their loved ones beyond the grave."[55] Later Dollard observed members of the congregation "testifying before the church as a proof of a valid conversion."[56] Infants had no place in such rituals, and their status after death remained a matter of faith rather than conversion.

It was not the church, then, but secular, reform-oriented forces that drove these new questions about the meaning of infant death. Social critiques of infant mortality implied that social and economic reforms were necessary to save babies. Moreover, attributing infant death to the presence of particular diseases proved increasingly appealing, for it suggested that perhaps medicine and public health experts would have something to say about infant death. Civic boosters, who were concerned about how infant mortality reflected on the city, actively promoted public health campaigns.

Memphis civic leaders were prepared to perceive the death of children as a civic embarrassment and, as we shall see, as a lingering public relations nightmare.

The promotion of child health took many forms in Memphis, and there was debate about who should properly promote it. In 1932, for example, Memphis physicians objected to one form of promotion, the "baby show" — an effort by one local doctor along with a "vaudeville shyster" to popularize child health by staging a fitness contest in a local department store. "When will our local pediatricians stop, look, and listen before falling for the scheming machinations of the silvery-tongued gentry who invade the sacred precincts of ethical medicine," wondered the editor of the *Memphis Medical Journal*.[57] Local physicians railed with even more intensity against the prominent black midwives, announcing with delight the gradual decline in their numbers in Memphis.[58] These debates highlighted, of course, the physicians' own desire to commandeer the proper promotion of child health. Their rhetoric must be understood as consistent with the rising stature of the specialty of pediatrics and its consolidation of authority in the early 1930s.[59] In Memphis the midwives, charlatans, and traveling "baby show" hucksters thus became favorite targets of pediatricians' venom and medical parody.

In rural parts of Tennessee, other promoters of child health encountered a very different politics, and it became clear to many that in the South the economy itself, organized around cotton, posed a danger to the health of black children. As one worker for the U.S. Children's Bureau noted, it was planter and mill town paternalism — and the desire to get people working in the mills and the cotton fields — that shaped the meaning of child health in these areas. Fieldworker Margaret Koenig described how her group "parked [in a small town] in the pretty young grove adjoining the Baptist church. . . . Soon the local colored chairman appeared, very much distressed, saying she thought we would not have much of a day as most of the mothers were in the field picking cotton."[60] At the close of the day, a wave of mothers finally came in "from the cotton fields" accompanied by their small children. "Thirty-six children, one of school age, and thirty-five of preschool age were examined," Koenig noted. Traveling from town to town, Koenig and the people she visited were never far from cotton — or from the purview of mill managers or plantation overseers. In one town, Koenig described how the mill manager "looked in on us several times during the day."[61] Even in towns just outside Memphis, child health was closely joined to the labor issue. "Much of the correction of physical defects," concluded

Koenig, "will depend upon the outcome of the cotton crop, on which these people depend chiefly for subsistence and even with this the means for obtaining a fair living is seemingly a struggle."[62] As it had been in the nineteenth century, child health remained bound to cotton.

Across southern states, such reformers sought to map and describe these rural and urban facets of child health by defining its relationship to the local economy and encouraging "proper" health practices. State public health officials, increasingly sensitive about child health as an indicator of the state's general condition, began to collect data on infant death in the rural and urban sectors and in both the black and white populations. Memphians too began to focus on these issues in the early 1930s. But in the city, particular political interests circumscribed the civic debate about infant death. In Memphis the attitudes and interests of public health officials, Chamber of Commerce businessmen, the professionalizing physicians, and the elected civic leaders shaped public discussions of child health.[63]

In 1934, when these leaders first learned of a newly published report from the U.S. Public Health Service that drew national attention to infant mortality in their city, their response revealed — as much as any other event — their ingrained, interwoven attitudes about the character of African Americans and the city's place as a regional health care center. The infant death controversy in Memphis can be seen as an important turning point, for it set the stage for new habits of mind and habits of surveillance over obscure pathologies like sickle cell anemia.

Redefining Infant Mortality, 1934–1937

In July 1934, Memphians awoke to read in their newspapers that the U.S. Public Health Service had sullied the image of their city. A report by the federal agency stated that Memphis, when compared to other cities with populations over 150,000, had the highest infant death rate in America.[64] According to the report, in 1933 a stunning 11 percent of its babies died before the age of one. The report cast no blame, pointed no fingers. Yet clearly a pall had been cast over the Bluff City. Who, or what, was responsible?

Over the next three years, business leaders and elected officials, medical and public health workers, and citizens orchestrated a response to the findings. Infant death became far more than an individual or family tragedy; it was now a social drama with obvious implications for the city's self-image. The publication of the national report made it a regional embarrassment for Memphis as well as a political crisis. The report shocked many, and it could not be easily explained away, because Memphians believed that they had been doing better than ever in these areas. More than ever, city leaders faced a crisis about civic progress. As they felt the impact of the national report, they responded defensively, resorting to familiar local diagnostic customs and shifting blame to "strangers" in their midst.

Days after the news had hit the newspapers, the city's doctors and Chamber of Commerce officials conferred with the mayor. They found two reasons for this statistical disaster. As one news account noted, "Because Memphis has a large Negro population, and because it is a medical center for a large area in the tri-states, its infant mortality rate is necessarily higher."[65] Memphis's politicians and civic leaders responded to the report by scapegoating the poor and blacks, portraying infant death as an unavoidable artifact of interstate commerce. The "ignorance of Negroes" was also cited as a powerful explanation.[66] The city's obstetricians and pediatricians were eager to explain away the critical report as a by-product of the city's location, but they also charged that the report was damaging to their reputations as healers.[67] The chief of Memphis's health department drew clear boundaries between deaths of Memphis babies and deaths of babies *in* Memphis, noting that "babies die in Memphis who were not born here and whose parents do not live here. They were never in Memphis in many instances until they were brought here in a dying condition."[68] It seemed to such civic officials that black and white outsiders — all of them poor and of rural origins, and many of them unaware of the most rudimentary principles of hygiene — were responsible for bringing this blight upon the city's image.

In many respects, their response echoed the city's position in the Gaston Hospital controversy (see Chapter 1). Memphis was a city attuned to the movement of people and goods across its borders, a city closely tied to its rural surroundings, yet deeply ambivalent about those ties. It was, officials believed, this traffic from the hinterlands that brought infant mortality to their doorstep and into the center of municipal politics. But the death of babies raised issues quite different from the death of adults because of the national political significance infant health had taken in the previous decade.[69] As Depression-era poverty rose in the South, child health once again became a national political concern.[70] In these years, the U.S. Public Health Service and the U.S. Children's Bureau reified the ideal of saving babies, and such agencies represented a new kind of political player in Memphis's health care arena.[71] The infant mortality findings revealed a city that was caught in a dilemma created by geographical circumstances, by its status as a regional commercial center, and by the rising power of the federal government to address problems in the region.

Into early 1935, as poor statistics continued to embarrass Memphis, civic officials reassured citizens that the mobility of rural residents and their children into the city was the leading contributor to infant mortality. As one newspaper account noted, "Physicians, scientists, and city health officials have tracked infant mortality deluxe in Memphis to its apparent retreat of safety — the Eleventh Ward — [where] many foreign born residents [from adjoining states] and Negroes . . . keep the infant mortality rate up."[72] Finding these pockets of high infant death (and putting the faces of African Americans and outsiders on the pall of death) presumably reassured some white Memphians that the problem was not their own. But blame the Eleventh Ward as he might, Mayor Watkins Overton also saw that as long as the federal government collected data for his city and others, as long as it published comparative reports, and as long as Memphis's rates continued to be high, an "unprejudiced" study by a reputable federal agency was in order.[73]

Mayor Overton turned to the U.S. Children's Bureau, a federal agency with a national image of benevolent concern for children and an established expertise in raising community awareness of infant health. Overton and others were aware of the need for some kind of federal arbitrator to explain the regional problem that the USPHS had uncovered. Their hope was that an unbiased outsider would agree with local wisdom — that this was a statistical aberration born of Memphis's problematic location. The Children's Bureau's 1937 report, *Infant Mortality in Memphis*, ultimately produced a compelling statistical picture of infant death in the city. The report must be understood as an act of diplomacy by federal authorities seeking to address issues of racial stereotyping, interstate commerce and mobility, and sensitivity to regional stigma in the Mid-South. Indeed, the negotiations that led to the 1937 report reveal the ways in which new ideas about child health were being crafted — and also highlight the growing role of federal agencies in the politics of infant death.

From the start, the bureau (an arm of the Department of Labor) saw this study as a kind of diplomatic mission into the Mid-South, a mission requiring carefully chosen language that would avoid bruising Memphians' self-perceptions. Southerners were still smarting from Secretary of Labor Frances Perkins's comment, two years earlier, that, in order to stimulate purchasing power, the South might be regarded as "an untapped market for shoes."[74] When Memphis officials first approached the Children's Bureau in February 1935, federal officials insisted that formal invitations be issued by specific civic organizations before they dispatched an investigator. The bureau's assistant chief, Martha Eliot, explained to bureau chief Katharine Lenroot that "Memphis apparently attracts many sick persons from surrounding territory in Arkansas and Mississippi. The people in Memphis blame much of their high mortality rates to this non-resident group. I do not know how much truth there is in it. I should be glad of your reaction to the whole situation."[75] Lenroot dispatched an experienced investigator, Ella Oppenheimer, to begin an extensive survey. While preparing for her trip, Oppenheimer corresponded with the Chamber of Commerce and other business organizations, physicians' groups, and a few individuals like Memphis's Dr. Edward Clay Mitchell. Most of them made clear the civic and commercial implications of her study—the good image of Memphis seemed to be at stake.

Oppenheimer arrived in Memphis in August 1935, greeted by a curious and receptive local press—including the anti-Crump, reform-oriented *Memphis Press-Scimitar*.[76] Oppenheimer kept her distance from the press, however, concerned that her findings might be used to criticize the Crump regime's public health record. In July 1935, in fact, Martha Eliot assured Edward Mitchell that the bureau's findings would first be discussed with local physicians and civic officials. "At least one or two newspapers have written . . . asking for statements," wrote Eliot, "but I have told [Oppenheimer] that . . . when her report is ready it should be submitted to you and a few other people in Memphis and that releases to the newspaper should come after you have had an opportunity to go over the report. . . . I do not think the report itself should be given to the press without your consent. That is a matter for you and the others in Memphis to decide." The bureau assured such leaders that they alone would control the dissemination and interpretation of the findings. Mitchell agreed: "I think that you are quite right that the detailed report should not go to the press, as many of the reporters have a way of changing the entire complexion of a report to suit their own convenience."[77] Into late 1935, Oppenheimer collected information from the city hospitals, the public health department, and other institutions. In the end, her conclusions would span over 100 pages, with some forty tables and thirty-six graphs and charts.[78]

The Children's Bureau had cultivated this habit of diplomatic caution based upon years of battle with the AMA, local pediatricians, and civic authorities skeptical of its competing with organized medicine. Under siege from established medicine, the bureau remained at once fiercely committed to the goals of child health and, at the same time, fearful that public findings might offend Memphis's doctors and civic leaders. In January 1936 Eliot wrote again to Mitchell to discuss the release of data. "The question," she said, "has arisen as to whether it would be desirable to place some of the material obtained in this study before the medical public at the American Medical Association convention next May in Kansas City in the form of an exhibit" that would include "charts showing some of the phases of the study." Eliot cautiously noted that "I would not even want to consider doing this . . . unless you and the other medical individuals in Memphis interested think that it is wise. Would you mind writing me what you think."[79] Mitchell, now a key spokesperson for the Memphis pediatricians, gave his approval for the exhibit to the "medical public." Even in July 1936, Eliot continued to be cautious. As one staff worker reported, "One day at lunch Dr. Eliot said to me that she did not think we should print the report unless the Memphis people concerned were willing." Indeed, this staffer recalled that when the Kansas City AMA exhibit had first come up in January "the question again arose as to whether this would seem to make Memphis 'the goat.'"[80]

During 1936 Oppenheimer gradually released her preliminary findings to Memphis civic leaders, and through them the picture of infant death slowly became public. Included in Oppenheimer's statements, and especially in the final report, was graphic confirmation that mortality in Memphis for babies in the first month and for the first year was in fact higher than in comparable cities such as Birmingham, Alabama; Jersey City, New Jersey; and Oakland, California. Charts showing the worst cases offered an implicit critique of a group of southern cities that were disproportionately represented on the list: Atlanta and Birmingham to the south, Louisville to the north, and Dallas to the west.

In a section entitled "Residence of Mothers in Relation to Infant Mortality in Memphis," Oppenheimer tackled the delicate issue head-on, concluding that Memphis's fears of nonresidents were unsubstantiated. Although Fisk University social scientists had written in 1930 that "it is unquestionable that the death rates of cities are swelled considerably by numbers of persons who go from surrounding areas to hospitals for treatment,"[81] Oppenheimer decided to poll public health officers in three other cities — Atlanta, Birmingham, and Louisville — for comparable information. But Birmingham was the only city of the three that could furnish the information she sought. John Kennedy of Atlanta responded that his city kept no such information: "I am extremely sorry that our records are not kept so as to give the births of non resident mothers and deaths of infants of non resident mothers."[82] Perhaps emboldened by learning that Memphis's concern was a particular (but not necessarily isolated) anxiety, Oppenheimer concluded that the city's fears were unsupported by the evidence: "The deaths of infants not born in Memphis have obviously had no significant influence on the neonatal mortality rates."[83]

Oppenheimer did find that "in the second to twelfth month mortality . . . [nonresident cases] have exercised a large influence on the rates for white infants and [a small but] apparently increasing influence in recent years on the rates for colored infants."[84] Nevertheless, she played down the significance of these nonresident births since they constituted only about 20 percent of total overall births and therefore could not be seen as solely responsible for the rise in mortality. She suggested that the high death rate might indeed be an outgrowth of urban expansion and, specifically, that the annexation of thirteen outlying wards in 1929 had been a precipitating factor in the rise in infant mortality. Not only had the city incorporated many poor, undeveloped, and unsanitary districts in its pursuit of physical growth and increasing tax revenue, it had also increased its population of the rural poor. But Oppenheimer concluded that even as Memphis pursued these goals of incorporation and expansion, it "did not expand its health services for mothers and babies"; she suggested that Memphis had failed to take on necessary civic responsibilities along with its desire to grow.[85]

There remained, however, a wide disparity between Oppenheimer's findings and the unfolding coverage of the study in the local newspapers. The final report (with its supporting charts, graphs, and findings) was published in 1937, some two years after Oppenheimer's initial visit. But preliminary reports, sent to Mitchell and circulated to the press, established quite a different image of infant death in the mind of Memphians. Indeed, leading Memphians used her preliminary findings to generate their own understanding of infant death. News accounts routinely focused on indigent outsiders as the cause of Memphis's image problem, with headlines like "Infant Death Figure Blamed on Non-Resident Cases—Terms Problem Complex—Urges Cooperation." Some articles suggested a more insidious, hidden reason for the deaths—a "mysterious epidemic" of an unknown pathology at the county hospital, including among the victims numerous "non-resident cases." Other accounts reported that "non-resident deaths and the large territory we annexed [in 1929] are partly responsible."[86] Thus, while some were willing to discuss the role of annexation and urban growth in the crisis, and others might explain the crisis by attributing it to an unknown epidemic, most Memphians clung to the image of the stranger, the outsider, the foreigner, as the primary source of the city's public health and image problems. For a city with a tiny presence of non-Americans, Memphis exhibited a striking degree of xenophobia and immigrant scapegoating — similar to that found in cities with much larger immigrant populations.[87]

Images of "indigent outsiders," graphic representations of "non-resident baby deaths," and portraits of "ignorant Negroes in the Eleventh Ward" filled the newspapers, informing municipal health policy throughout the 1930s. Dots or shaded zones on the civic map represented acute pathology in the city, and these images imposed a kind of conceptual quarantine on the infant death crisis — confining it in the minds of many to specific neighborhoods and wards. From the first recognition of the crisis, through denial, to the invitation of an unbiased study, and to the attribution of blame, the controversy sketched out a moral narrative. It was primarily the stranger (rather than germs, or poverty, or urban expansion per se) that featured as the central actor in the drama. The city leaders of Memphis went to great lengths to place blame with strangers, and thereby to limit this unwanted traffic of "outsiders." Ironically, the Children's Bureau proved valuable in propagating this view, so that despite Oppenheimer's 1937 findings, infant death continued to be widely represented in Memphis and Mid-South professional journals, in local newspapers, and in policy documents as a "foreign" blemish on the city.

What did the death of black children mean in the city, and how might this backdrop ultimately explain the local meaning of sickle cell disease? From the civic booster's perspective, child mortality was an economic disaster, not because it robbed farms of healthy workers but because it was bad for civic prosperity, urban commerce, and public relations. Infant death was no great mystery; it was certainly no medical puzzle warranting deep investigation. It was not particularly satisfying to think of infant death in terms of obscure, mysterious pathologies. To do so would suggest that vague, hidden processes beyond the grasp of customary local thought accounted for these deaths. The answer to why infants died seemed obviously connected with rural to urban mobility, and with slum conditions in the Eleventh Ward.[88] The Chamber of Commerce, Memphis physicians, and the city's dominant business interests perpetuated this belief, voicing the anxieties of an ambivalent, rural-minded metropolis. "Ignorant Negroes," desperate nonresidents, and the waves of undesirable newcomers were to blame for the city's high mortality rates.[89]

Even particular pathologies could fit this compelling local model. Confronted with a rise in meningitis cases in 1930, for example, health officer S. L. Wadley insisted that "in the spring of 1929 . . . we noticed a good many cases coming in here from Arkansas. We had 50 cases in 1929. Forty-one of these were from out of town."[90] In cases of typhoid fever, meningitis, or malaria, health officials again pointed to blacks and indigent outsiders. "You will notice," Wadley went on, "that the number of white cases is relatively small."[91] Referring to a map where the blemishes of disease were represented with small dots, he continued: "This black dot represents a negro picked up by an ambulance and carried to the hospital last week. . . . He came in . . . two weeks ago and stated he had been in Helena, Arkansas." The Eleventh Ward attracted Wadley's attention less than Beale Street, a popular locale for African Americans (resident and nonresident alike). "It seems a lot of cases center around Beale Street. I don't know why, but I suspect it is due to the fact that all negroes some time go down there," Wadley wrote. And, of course, the issue of unregulated mobility also seemed to define meningitis. "I go into the house and find all kinfolks congregated in the house to see the people. They just move about . . . have no homes, sleep five and six in one room with the windows down. . . . No wonder they are suffering from it," he concluded.[92]

Even as Oppenheimer's study began in 1935, the city, seeking to avoid further embarrassment, enacted measures that would result in a new kind of attention to hidden, obscure pathologies in Memphis. Twenty-three new clinics were built, twelve of them located in black neighborhoods, and nine of these staffed with black physicians.[93] An influx of PWA funds not only helped to build the John Gaston Hospital but allowed for a new wing dedicated specifically to maternal and child health. The crisis resulted in closer scrutiny and surveillance of the ailments of Memphis's poor and African American populations. Writing in 1938, physician David Goltman described the careful handling of premature babies in the hospital, their placement in boarding homes if their own homes were deemed unfit, and their subsequent follow-up by nurses. "Since the vast majority of these babies are colored," he noted, "and the colored well baby clinics are in charge of negro physicians a problem file is kept on all these babies and their feeding is supervised by this means."[94] Extensive testing programs began — for syphilis, pneumonia, malnutrition, and numerous other disorders. As another physician noted of Goltman's study, it "brings out clearly that where *patients are properly watched* and *mothers properly instructed* that the death rate among all children can be reduced materially."[95] Scrutiny and surveillance became the watchwords in the battle against infant death. For pediatricians working in the wake of the crisis, a new habit of clinical surveillance emerged, and further incorporation of African American health workers into the system seemed crucial for these surveillance practices to succeed.

The infant mortality controversy gave rise to real physical and cognitive changes in Memphis's health care landscape. As the Eleventh Ward and the outlying districts became linked with high mortality, conceptual connections were established between disease, housing, and slum conditions. The linkage also gave new impetus to a Memphis public health strategy of slum clearance. Indeed, the very maps of infant death that had been generated in 1934 and 1935 became the basis for slum clearance programs funded by the PWA.[96]

But perhaps most important, the infant mortality crisis introduced Memphis to a new economy based on the flow of federal dollars from New Deal programs in public health, housing, and hospital infrastructure. As historian Edward Beardsley has argued, the New Deal constituted a crucial turning point in the "federal rescue of southern health programs."[97] As a major shift in the political economy of southern health, such programs defined a new kind of health care commerce, an alternative economic system for a city still nostalgically clinging to its identity as a cotton trafficking center. At the inception of the infant death controversy, publicity about death and disease had been unquestionably "bad for business." But by the late 1930s, city leaders realized that the pall of infant mortality could be leveraged at the national level to bring funds into Memphis, to build new hospital facilities, and to aid in the expansion of the medical and public health complex. Indeed, the intense poverty of adjacent rural regions could actually benefit Memphis, for the widespread regional poverty only reinforced the city's appeal for federal aid. In this New Deal economy, Memphis's status as a regional health care center could be considered a geographic virtue rather than an embarrassing burden. By the time of the 1937 Mississippi River flood, which sent thousands of devastated lowland refugees streaming into the city, some physicians could see that crisis as "one of the most exciting periods for pediatrics in our city." Such disasters created opportunity in the minds of some enterprising Memphians, reinforcing the centrality of the city as a regional center and further justifying the influx of Red Cross funds and federal aid.[98]

The Great Masquerader: Sickle Cell Anemia

In 1920s and 1930s Memphis, few people would have been concerned with the pain and suffering of sickle cell anemia patients. Such a concern would suggest a level of attention to particularities of experience that simply did not then exist in medicine or in the city's political culture. Tuberculosis, syphilis, and meningitis symbolized the high-visibility problem of black health in this era; sickle cell anemia stood shrouded in the shadows of these threats, emerging here and there in medical discussions as a weak signifier of the African American condition.

The idea that specific diseases embody the condition of black people has had an enduring appeal in America, for every generation discovers different "racial disorders" and endows them with powerful cultural meanings. In the immediate postemancipation era, for example, many southerners believed that the rise in mental illness among freed men and women represented the consequences of freedom and, retrospectively, the health virtues of slavery's paternalism.[99] For much of the early twentieth century, tuberculosis and syphilis symbolized the condition of the new urban African American communities.[100] Such discourses held meaning partly because of the diseases' prevalence, but also because of the ways in which they intersected with politics, culture, and racial anxieties.

In the early twentieth century, innovations in laboratory diagnosis fed new discourses on disease, reshaping popular ideas about race and health. After James Herrick's microscopic detection of sickled cells in the blood of a patient in 1910, for example, a tiny coterie of physicians constructed knowledge about this obscure disease.[101] Their ideas also expressed general attitudes about race. For many of them, the capacity to develop sickled cells was an inherent feature of "Negro blood." As more cases of this peculiar, seemingly rare disease were discovered, hematological specialists scattered around the country came to depend upon a particular test for diagnosing the disease. The diagnostic tool also created a particular image of this disease as a Mendelian dominant trait that could be spread *outward* from the black population into whites through intermarriage. This discourse of sickle cell anemia became well established among a small group of experts in the 1920s and 1930s. These attitudes are considered fundamentally wrong in today's genetics, framed by their concerns about miscegenation and racial purity. However, the wide appeal of hematology and laboratory diagnostics helped to give their discourse contemporary cultural authority, if only for medical insiders.

This specialist interest in Mendelian dominance and the inheritance of sickled cells was not widely followed in medicine or in society at large. Most southerners did not need the example of an obscure pathology to confirm their prejudices about racial mixing, or to sustain their anxieties about the consequences of integration. Common prejudice and the case of tuberculosis, syphilis, and other well-known diseases provided enough evidence for already developed theories about race, blood, and disease. In such discussions, theories about sickle cell anemia remained obscured by the discourse of those familiar diseases.

There was little cause for reformers or liberal-minded experts to call attention to sickle cell anemia. All talk of "hereditary disease" rang with fatalistic implications concerning the possibilities of improving black health. The label implied that neither medicine nor public health nor social reform could change the course of the disorder. Many southern physicians had long asserted that such natural, inherited, biological differences between the races accounted for differences in mortality. Insurance underwriters assumed that African Americans were biologically weaker and hereditarily prone to disease.[102] One Fisk University researcher believed that "it would be unprofitable to speculate about hereditary factors which are beyond our control before investigating to the fullest extent all clues to conditions which may be subject to amelioration by human intelligence."[103] Precisely in order to refute the do-nothing implications of hereditary science, many black physicians "wasted their efforts in disgusted denials" of these assertions.[104] Sickle cell anemia would never have appealed as a special cause for those who sought to improve black health in the 1920s and 1930s, for it fit too neatly into hereditary discourse and reflected too clearly the scientific fatalism they were fighting against.

But the fact that Memphis pathologist Lemuel Diggs's writings in this era reflected none of the prevailing themes contributed to the difficulties of establishing a wider knowledge of this obscure pathology. Diggs arrived in Memphis in 1929, importing a scientist's fascination with the mechanistic puzzle of disease into a place with no significant academic tradition.[105] His interest in sickle cell disease was piqued while he was a student at Johns Hopkins, and he had expanded his knowledge of similar blood disorders during a stint in Rochester, New York. He "had worked previously [at Rochester] on thalassemia, mainly, which is a disease very similar to sickle cell anemia, but affects Italian people." Thus, when he "came across cases of sickle cell anemia in the Old Memphis General Hospital . . . [and] there was no one [who] had any interest in it," Diggs saw this as an opportunity for expanding the knowledge base of pathology.[106]

Diggs's view of "disease" stood out in Memphis for several reasons. Where many saw diseases as local civic burdens, he saw them as interesting puzzles and case studies in general pathology. Furthermore, he had no background or interest in regional problems such as malaria. Finally, because Diggs was a pathology professor and not a full-time medical practitioner, he had the laboratory resources and motivation to develop his insights on the mechanisms of disease. As Diggs himself noted, "I figured [sickle cell anemia] was an important disease, so I began to study it in every way I could possibly do so."[107] To Diggs, however, the disease's importance was determined not by its prevalence among blacks (for it was deemed to be rare), but because it was one of only a few hematological disorders about which little was known, and in which the possibilities of contributing to the national literature was great. It was the *disease* that interested Diggs, not the *patients*, and not their particular complaints. This made Diggs, and his academic view of disease, something of an anomaly in the ecology of local knowledge in 1929 Memphis.

Diggs viewed himself as an innovative teacher and as a student of minute aspects of pathology—and his recollections highlight the ways in which sickle cell anemia was presented to students and faculty as a fascinating locus of academic intrigues. One of Diggs's often-repeated stories was set in the surgical amphitheater full of students in the 1930s, and it highlights the nature of his theoretical concern with disease. A patient from the Memphis General Hospital diagnosed with sickle cell anemia lay on the operating table. A large swelling on the left side of the abdomen indicated the presence of an enlarged spleen that was quite common in such cases. Dr. McGee, the surgeon, was present, as was Dr. McElroy, the chief of medicine, and Diggs. The operation was innovative—one of the first to remove the enlarged spleen of a sickle cell patient in an effort to improve the blood disorder. "All the medical students were assembled to see this historical event," Diggs explained. "Dr. McElroy told them about what they were going to do and what the theory was, and the surgeon, Dr. McGee, began to operate and opened up the abdomen [but] he couldn't find the spleen." Diggs recalled this as a moment of great embarrassment to McGee. "He was all perturbed about that and he wiped the sweat from his brow and resected another rib and called in another resident and he kept fiddling around and couldn't find the spleen with all the medical students there . . . watching him in his failure."[108]

The surgeon's failure, however, gave birth to one of Diggs's new research puzzles: What happened to the spleen in sickle cell anemia? McGee had become so frustrated in his search for the spleen that eventually he stalked out of the amphitheater, claiming that the organ was impossibly small and could not be found. Indeed, as Diggs recalled, McGee left with a dramatic statement: "He said he'd eat it if it weighed as much as ten grams."[109] Diggs's story did not end there, however, for the patient soon died, and the hunt for the missing spleen continued in Diggs's postmortem examination, where he was finally able to locate the minute, shriveled organ: "The patient didn't die soon after that operation, but did die later and came to autopsy." What Diggs found was a spleen that "didn't weigh [even] ten grams." "It weighed seven and a half grams, and [McGee] didn't have to eat it," Diggs laughed. Diggs saw the postmortem as a crucial step in the solution of the puzzle, and he regarded the incident as the birthplace of a research problem. It was "a spark that spurred me on in research because I tried to know why in the world that spleen had disappeared or had gotten so small."[110] His fascination, common for a pathologist, was with disease as a pathological process.

By the mid-1930s, medical and public awareness of sickle cell anemia remained limited to specialists like Lemuel Diggs — a few other pathologists, some surgeons, and some clinicians with puzzle-solving interests. "Early on [other doctors] wouldn't even accept the diagnosis," Diggs claimed. "A professor of pediatrics would say, 'Why, he's got rheumatic fever' or 'He died of pneumonia.'"[111] Indeed, one counterpart to Diggs in Houston, Texas, noted that most of *his* colleagues would perceive a case of sickle cell anemia as simply another case of respiratory infection. "There is nothing remarkable in finding acute respiratory infection in a young Negro woman; however, I am sure all of you who deal with the clinic patients here in Houston have often wondered why the Negro is so susceptible to the acute respiratory infections." For this pathologist, the answer to the puzzle was sickle cell anemia, at least for a small percentage of these cases.[112] But few of his peers embraced this new vision of disease. Indeed, despite the work of such specialists in expanding the national literature on the disease, two 1938 surveys on various anemias by Memphis authors in the local medical journal said nothing about the disorder.[113] In 1941, however, a glimmer of local recognition came when the journal editor drew readers' attention to a small educational conference at Memphis's famous Peabody Hotel. Among the exhibits "of interest and value," he noted, was a presentation by Diggs on sickle cell anemia.[114] The sickle cell exhibit stood near another exhibit on tuberculosis, and it would have been a fitting imitation of clinical reality if the tuberculosis display had stood in front of Diggs's display, obscuring it and drawing more attention from the clinical gathering. Diggs, the editor noted, was encouraging his peers to "obtain a broader medical vision."[115]

Thus one of the key challenges to be met before sickle cell anemia could attain *social visibility* was the struggle for *clinical visibility* in the 1920s and 1930s.[116] Not only did pediatricians and surgeons (and Diggs as well) see the symptoms of sickle cell anemia through the lens of their particular training, but public health workers as well, trained to diagnose malaria or tuberculosis, saw only what they were trained to look for. Despite Diggs's efforts, sickle cell anemia never featured centrally in the micropolitics of clinical diagnosis, and it did not resonate with broader scientific, social, or political debates on black health. However, one trend did make the disease more visible — the negotiation of meaning among experts, the gradual expansion of their academic complex, and their reinterpretations of conventional understanding. Whether they were reinterpreting folk beliefs or conventional academic wisdom, in the 1930s university researchers promoted a distinctive academic culture. At Fisk, sociologist Charles Spurgeon Johnson was reinterpreting "spells" and pains of black southerners as indicators of social relations in the "shadow of the plantation." At the University of Tennessee, Diggs was reinterpreting obscure symptoms. This academic culture gradually but forcefully sought to revise popular notions of disease. For Diggs, this meant educating medical practitioners, students, and the public alike.

The visibility and invisibility of disease can thus be understood as a complex cultural negotiation, a social, political, and intellectual process that can not be taken for granted. The emergence of sickle cell anemia represented the reinterpretation of symptomatology in urban centers like Memphis, Chicago, and Houston — places where academic cultures were struggling to give new meaning to familiar phenomena amidst the city's struggle to define its own identity. But even in these academic settings, recognition was slow in coming. In 1942, for example, physicians in Richmond, Virginia, would agree that sickle cell anemia was still frequently confused with appendicitis, and that "it represents one of those unique problems challenging the profession of the Southern states."[117] Meanwhile, in cities like Memphis the burden of malaria and the politics of infant death also guided local disease perception. For these reasons, the disease would remain obscure.

In the 1950s, 1960s, and 1970s, a new generation of medical scientists would discover that sickle cell disease was a puzzle even more intriguing than Lemuel Diggs had imagined. As the academic cachet of the disease increased, a wide range of specialists would embrace the novelty of this obscure disorder and use it to theorize about large-scale population migrations, disease ecology, and the interrelations of malaria and sickled cells. They would follow the lead of British physician and biochemist A. C. Allison, who suggested that sickle cell trait offered protection against one form of malaria and that persons with the trait survived in areas where the disease was prevalent.[118] Sickle cell anemia would become a centerpiece of modern theories of molecular biology and disease, serving a high-profile function similar to that which tuberculosis, syphilis, and others had served in earlier times. Sickle cell anemia, as a cutting-edge disease, would offer new insights into questions of African American mobility and human biology and be used to legitimate new theories of black identity. But none of this would have been imaginable in xenophobic Memphis in the 1920s and 1930s, when the pall of malaria, infectious disease, and infant death shaped the professional and public understanding of race, region, and health. Such academic interpretations would have been marginal factors in local accounts of race and disease. Only after the political environment had changed and after the clinical visibility of sickle cell anemia was better established — when it had infiltrated the mind-set of doctors and scientists as a "real" disorder — did their theorizing about the disease lead them to construct a new black identity linked to African genetics, environments, and evolution.

3 Remaking Jim Crow Medicine

In the years around World War II, Americans grew profoundly aware of their role in remaking their nation, and they consciously measured how well their institutions met their professed democratic ideals. The war fostered widespread civic involvement; Americans were called upon across ethnicity, gender, religion, and region to sacrifice comfort at home for the greater good. Government marshaled science and technology to accomplish great feats, and these accomplishments reoriented the citizenry to expect a prosperous, technologically sophisticated postwar age. The year 1946 thus brought a new sense of the possibilities of democratic governance and national greatness for Americans, black and white. Medicine embraced science and technology and helped foster these higher expectations. Armed with new "life-saving" therapies like penicillin and blood plasma transfusion, physicians and scientists were poised for a break with the past. They were bolstered by rising public faith in their practice, even as they confronted a changing landscape of disease challenges. But such dramatic changes in society and health care also provoked worries in some places, especially in cities like Memphis where white citizens were already anxious about what these postwar developments augured for Jim Crow medicine.

A variety of segregated institutions that had crystallized during the early decades of the twentieth century seemed suddenly in danger of dissolution. Amidst the institution building and urban boosterism of the 1920s, the new Jim Crow churches, schools, and hospitals endowed their clientele with "modern" values that upheld the virtues of racial separation. As these institutions bestowed education and molded separate group identities, they reflected the mores, laws, and the political economy of their region.[1] Every type of segregated institution evolved a distinct character. Educational segregation, for example, was able to incorporate an expanding number of public school students and held firm, even with the gradual ascendancy of the four-year college in American society.[2] In medicine, however, segregation struggled to adapt to the challenges posed by a burgeoning health care industry. As the business of health care grew, medical schools and hospitals saw massive changes — in technical infrastructure, in the rise of capital-intensive techniques, in the advent of increasingly specialized theories of health and illness, and in the growing interconnections among universities, hospitals, clinics, research facilities, and government agencies supporting medicine. These developments moved black hospital care and medical education farther and farther to the margins of American life, setting the stage for health crises, protests from disenchanted middle-class African Americans, and political upheaval after World War II.

As the health care system itself grew more complex, health care politics also became more complex and contentious. Health care touched on an expanding set of human concerns. As medicine came to be more closely associated with effective therapies, segregation in health insurance, medical care, and medical education carried many more apparent life-and-death implications. The battle against illness had continuing spiritual resonance, as well as easily discernible economic and political implications for the national well-being. But health was now also big business, for pharmaceuticals and health insurance were regarded as growing, market-based commodities in the private sector. At the same time, public sector government agencies exercised increasing power in the protection, regulation, and provision of health care, regarding health, in some measure, as a political right.[3] Amidst these sweeping changes, the segregation of blacks and whites in southern health care became a vexing political problem.

By the late 1930s, Americans had begun to invest heavily in institutional medicine. They looked upon hospital care and university research in urban centers as the places where they could find the best knowledge of disease and the greatest therapeutic power. They saw the rise of a health insurance industry in the 1930s and 1940s as a beneficial force, a system for increasing their access to treatments in time of need.[4] Only a tiny percent of Americans entered the 1940s with any kind of health insurance. But by the end of the decade, labor unions had begun to negotiate health care benefits for their members, and enrollment in private health insurance had begun to climb.[5] Reading these trends, Vice President Harry S. Truman would make national health insurance a presidential campaign theme in 1948, and his critics would label it "socialized medicine."[6] Good health, although still regarded largely as an individual matter, became increasingly a collective concern in the 1940s — and a crucial legislative matter for national, state, and city governments.

World War II had inspired many of these changes. The war had endowed American medicine as a significant healing agent and a protector of soldiers and citizens. For example, the invention of blood plasma transfusion and the wartime production of the new drug penicillin highlighted the intimate connection between medicine, the war against fascism, and the defense of democracy. The relationships of doctor and patient, institution and disease became politically charged and freighted with symbolic meanings: the future of free enterprise, the defense of democratic society, the fight for equality, and the march of totalitarianism seemed to be at stake in the structure of American health care. The war accelerated the pace of medical specialization and the stature of specialists, promoting a new public appreciation for the intricacies of medical knowledge and for the fact that specialists spoke a very different language than the layman. Health expertise entered a new phase.[7]

This chapter focuses on the ways in which black health was transformed in this eventful decade. The involvement of African Americans in the war effort produced a new discourse on race and health, a discourse that was tinged with disturbing questions about inequality, democracy, and citizenship. In localities across America, a new racial politics created worries for Jim Crow medicine. In Memphis the war had powerful local effects as the city became a national laboratory. Because the military was deeply interested in the treatment of malaria in tropical regions, the Mid-South region (which had never fully vanquished this malady) became a focus of malaria research. Municipal hospitals like Memphis's John Gaston also became training grounds for army physicians, providing valuable clinical material for their education. The war resulted in a dramatic expansion in federal spending on science and medicine at the local universities — a process that would expand in the 1950s and 1960s. By the mid-1940s, wartime mobility meant that the state's black population was now a majority urban population.[8] In the midst of these and other changes, Memphians were forced to reconsider whether their segregated institutions could survive — and, if so, under what circumstances. Moreover, in a booming postwar health care economy, black Americans could now effectively argue that their dwindling health care options had grave implications for democracy itself, and they lobbied at city hall and in their communities to participate equally in, and to share the benefits of, modern health consumerism.

War, Health, and Economic Expectations

While sweeping developments in science and medicine — antibiotics, blood plasma, and, of course, the atomic bomb — provided tools for a successful war effort and redefined Americans' sense of their power in the world, several smaller ventures, all seen as vital in the fight against fascist dictators and Nazis, redefined the relationship between local civic culture and national war goals. In early 1943, for example, the John Gaston Hospital became a training ground for army radiologists when the army's X-ray school relocated to the city and affiliated with the University of Tennessee. The army had moved its training school to Memphis for strategic reasons. It needed to anticipate medical and surgical emergencies abroad, and Memphis served as a fitting site for testing new technologies. As one local doctor noted, "We have an unusually large service of traumatic cases that will be important in their instruction program."[9] At the same time, the city's arrangement with the radiologists brought an influx of highly trained faculty and high-powered diagnostic tools into the declining municipal hospital. In anticipation of war in the tropics, the army also sought out Memphis as an ideal place to study new treatments for malaria. Indeed, it seemed that the region's very "backwardness" — its inability to fully eradicate malaria and its high incidence of trauma cases — became a virtue in the army's perspective.[10]

Even as outsiders streamed into Memphis to retool for the war in its hospitals, many of the city's own citizens ventured beyond its parochial confines, crafting new habits of mind. The experiences of Memphians traveling abroad for military service also altered their city. Annie Pope Van Dyke's sons, for example, wrote to her about race relations, military life, and their concerns for America in the postwar era. "We now have Negroes with us," wrote Robert Van Dyke in October 1943, "although the only contact we have with them is in the latrine. They are well educated naturally or they wouldn't be in this company. I just don't like the idea though. Naturally, there is nothing I can do about it."[11] Military service itself had imposed a new order, and Robert bemoaned the fact that he was compelled to adapt. William Van Dyke was more prescient about what events abroad and at home augured for race relations. "I was in a cold fury the other day — a boy in my tent got a new 'Life' . . . which was devoured by all," William wrote to his mother. Racial violence in Detroit had caught his eye. "When I read about the race riots in Detroit it really made me mad," he wrote. "I thought it was to prevent stuff like that that they've got 2½ million of us over here." William directed his anger at how the "white mobs acted," and he had an ominous message for his mother in Memphis: "I've talked to dozens of boys over here, and everyone seems to think that the race problem will burst in our faces after the war. There are thousands of negroes whose point of view is being decidedly changed by the army. They're getting equality like they never dreamed of, and I believe it'll have far reaching effects. The ignorant, bigoted, poor-white trash in the South will create the big problem if and when we start to arbitrate the race question."[12] As such impressions flowed back to the Mid-South, they described, better than observers at home could, the slow transformation of expectations and the dark clouds of racial conflicts on the horizon. Cities like Memphis faced daunting postwar challenges, chief among them "arbitrating the race question."

The soldiers' experience of health care also sent ripples through the homefront. Viewing with concern the rising cost of health care and seeking to support soldiers' families, the U.S. Congress appropriated funds in 1943 to pay for health care for soldiers' wives and children, thereby establishing new expectations about the government's role in providing health security. In Memphis alone, the wives of over 200 servicemen applied for maternity and infant medical care under a new national law making such care available, since the servicemen's "salaries [were] not adequate to cover the cost of medical care of their dependents."[13] Here was another instance of federal paternalism, of an expanding national government stepping in to protect vulnerable Memphis families. While some Americans envisioned these measures as merely "emergency" wartime provisions, others feared (and some hoped) that such legislation was only the beginning of federal intervention to ensure affordable medical care.

Lemuel Diggs, whose interests had never been parochial, left Memphis briefly during the war, taking a temporary wartime post with the Armed Forces Institute of Pathology. The Institute, a national repository of pathological material from around the world, introduced Diggs to several other specialists who shared his interest in the still-obscure disease, sickle cell anemia. According to Diggs, the Institute's director "had been to Panama and he had collected a whole bunch of cases of sickle cell anemia, was interested in it himself, but then he put it in a barrel and brought it back to Washington with him . . . didn't have time to look at it."[14] For Diggs, this collection of case reports was a treasure trove of valuable data, and he used it to build up a vast knowledge about the rare disorder.

At the same time, Diggs continued, sickle cell disease had became "very important to the Armed forces . . . [for reasons related to national security] so they appointed me as a paid consultant for many years."[15] The military's surprising interest in the malady stemmed from an obscure scientific debate about the fitness of people with sickle cell trait as soldiers. In one inflammatory medical article, a physician named Julius Bauer had stridently asserted that sickle cell trait—a little-known, largely benign condition—posed "a distinct danger particularly as our armed forces are concerned." He believed that "having sickle cell trait, [the soldier] may become the victim of his constitutional biologic inferiority and succumb under circumstances which are innocuous to average normal people."[16] Such views created the need for an independent assessment at the Institute, which had been established precisely to study such issues.[17]

The sickle cell trait controversy was overshadowed by another race and blood controversy that had arisen in 1942. The American Red Cross's policy of labeling "Negro blood" and "non-Negro blood"—and separating them for transfusions—had inspired national debates and protests. Anthropologists, the National Association for the Advancement of Colored People (NAACP), and liberal newspapers had all expressed dismay about the practice, charging that blood segregation reflected deep-seated racist prejudices about the intermingling of blood. Not only did such practices have no basis in accepted science, they seemed to undermine national solidarity and the goal of equal participation in the war effort.[18] With the war as a crucial backdrop, critics of these practices could effectively portray segregation as mindlessly uninformed, undemocratic, and insulting to African Americans who sought to contribute to the national welfare. The blood controversy gave reform-minded Americans a visible symbol of the weakness of the segregationist position in health care. Segregation was presented as superstition in a scientific era and as counterproductive in the nation's war against Nazis and their own racist ideology.[19]

Nationally and locally, the controversy over segregated blood seemed to symbolize the future of democracy and civic participation in America, and it revealed the illogic of Jim Crow medicine. One cartoon in a New York newspaper portrayed the cost of this policy as twofold: it could lead to the loss of white soldiers' lives as well as to the undermining of black patriotism (see illustrations). The first segment showed an injured, bleeding white soldier being refused a transfusion because the doctors "had nothin' but negro blood left." The scene suggested that white soldiers were dying because physicians—hamstrung by Red Cross blood labeling and military segregation policy—were reluctant to intermingle their blood supplies even if it could save lives. The second scene pictured a spectacled scientist scratching his head because the labels "Negro Blood" and "White Blood" had fallen from two bottles of blood. It highlighted that scientists themselves could not differentiate without the labels, for the blood samples were identical. The third scene presented one outcome of this practice: a portrait of "reverse discrimination" in which the "colored lads" got plenty of transfusions while whites were denied care. It suggested that white soldiers saw and understood that this segregated system was working against their own interests. The last picture offered the final moral. It portrayed an injured, bedridden African American soldier being held in the arms of a white doctor. In a gesture of selfless heroism he begged the doctor, "Give me anybody's blood . . . so long as I get back to the front."

In late 1943 the Red Cross would decide (amidst public pressure from the NAACP and other reform-oriented organizations) to abandon its blood labeling policy. But the blood transfusion debate had a lasting impact, putting the American system of health care and segregation on public trial. The notion that hidden dangers lay nascent in "Negro blood" or "Jewish blood," or that special virtues existed in "Aryan blood" or "white blood," came under an international microscope.[20] Wartime controversy revealed the extent to which national groups — including the American Red Cross, the U.S. Army, the NAACP, and academic groups like the American Association of Physical Anthropologists — were willing to criticize segregation in health care. As a result of such national debates, black Americans (particularly those who had served in the military) had higher expectations about the possibilities of ending such unsupportable segregation practices. Many now argued that segregation was akin to Nazi racial ideology, for it too was anchored by an irrational, unscientific, and unsupportable myth.

Stories of blood, racial prejudice, and health care segregation resonated with meaning in cities across America. Black Memphians, for example, indulged in a local version of the blood transfusion story, highlighting that Jim Crow medicine had life-and-death implications for whites and blacks in the Bluff City. Memphis disc jockey Gatemouth Moore personally witnessed a telling incident when Memphis's ambulance companies were segregated (Thompson's for white people, S. W. Quall's for black people). Moore was a prominent gospel voice on a local radio station, WDIA, the first station in the country broadcasting an "all black" theme.[21] As he recalled, "I was on my way to the station, and when I come around the curve there was the ambulance from S. W. Quall's with the door open, and there was a white lady laying in the ditch, bleeding. And they were waiting for Thompson's to come and pick her up. . . . I guess I waited thirty or forty minutes and still no ambulance. They tell me that the lady died."[22] Moore remembered "telling the tale" on the radio and using the station as a bulletin board for discussing the issue. " 'Look here,' I said. 'Black folks put their hands in your flour and make your bread, they cook the meat, they clean up your house and here's this fine aristocratic white lady lying in the ditch bleeding and they won't let black hands pick her up and rush her to the hospital.' "23

The radio personality's story of the unintended effects of Jim Crow ambulance service had a double irony, revealing that even as segregation came under attack, the tradition of racial paternalism was still very strong. Not only did Moore assert that Jim Crow ambulance service harmed well-to-do "aristocratic White ladies," he also drove home his point with a conservative appeal — evoking the image of black public and domestic subservience to whites. Segregation, in his account, stood in the way of blacks serving whites and saving their lives. The appeal apparently worked, according to Moore, for "the next week they changed the law. . . . I got that changed on WDIA."24

In between gospel music and blues recordings, there was a great deal more to protest on WDIA. Memphis's John Gaston Hospital buckled under the burden of migration from the countryside, and, as the largest hospital providing care for African Americans, it strained to meet the rising expectations of middle-class blacks. Postwar farm mechanization would greatly accelerate the flight from farms to the city, even as soldiers returned home. The tractor — a new technology for the farm to match new technologies in the hospital — transformed farming.25 It did away with the need for large numbers of field hands, and it provoked a massive redistribution of laborers, who now headed for the prosperous metropolis. Memphis's population skyrocketed in the 1940s, and institutions like John Gaston Hospital were not prepared for the growth.

A sad paradox of the postwar years was the fact that even as Gaston became more crowded with the poor and its facilities deteriorated, it increased in value as a site for medical research. Memphis physicians and visiting doctors continued to perceive the institution and its patients as valuable clinical material. In September 1947, for example, the *Memphis Medical Journal* reported that a University of California medical school professor, Hamilton Anderson, had launched a cooperative research study with Memphis's own John Gaston Hospital and the University of Tennessee. According to Anderson, "Memphis was selected because of the unlimited clinical material and general interest of the staff of the Medical College."26 His study focused not on patient care per se, but on the life course of a particular parasite causing amebic dysentery — a problem open to extensive study in the region because of its deplorable health conditions. The journal's editor commented that, in the Memphis area, "the numbers of patients harboring *endamoeba hystolytica* in whom the infection was not suspected is amazing. Dr. Anderson hopes to follow some of these patients who die of other causes to autopsy in an effort to gain information relative to the controversy as to whether or not *endamoeba hystolytica* can live in the intestinal tract of man without producing lesions."[27] The likelihood of death itself made the research possibilities even richer for Anderson. Such cooperative research arrangements, linking Memphis with the California-based researcher, suggested that the Memphis medical community was quite willing to advertise the city's health problems as research opportunities. Indeed, in an era in which biomedical research expanded without explicit regulations — a "gilded age of research" — institutions with such marginal patients were valuable repositories of clinical material.[28] John Gaston Hospital provided a mother lode of research opportunities for physicians like Anderson.

Gaston welcomed new research projects even as it struggled with the demographic influx and with the growing dissatisfaction of middle-class blacks about the hospital. Except for the CME's Collins Chapel Hospital, none of the black hospitals built in the 1910s had survived the Depression. Even Collins Chapel struggled to meet the new needs. By the early 1940s, John Gaston had become the only large institution providing health care for Memphis's black people, both the poor and those who could afford to pay. But in the eyes of those who could pay for health care, it was an institution unfit for their families and children. Once seen as a center of benevolent charity care, the hospital was now pervaded with the stigma of poverty and an aura of municipal dependence — and the stench of political and economic corruption.[29] For Memphis's black middle class, the hospital had come to symbolize their economic entrapment within the petrified system of Jim Crow medicine.

By the close of World War II, then, for all of these reasons — the broader symbolism of blood transfusion segregation, demographic and economic shifts in cities, and the emergence of new consumer ideals about health care — Jim Crow medicine was headed for troubled times. At the same time, however, the health care system was seeing massive growth, with infusions of dollars, specialists, and technical resources. The health of children — perceived as the future of democracy itself — stood prominent among new health concerns, especially for the parents who produced the post–World

War II "baby boom." Congress lost no time in addressing these concerns and adapting to the new political environment, considering a vast array of health legislation — including the Hospital Survey and Construction Act of 1946, as well as Truman's eventually defeated national health insurance proposal.

Federal activism such as the Hospital Construction Act (known as Hill-Burton for its sponsoring legislators) proved to be a boon for the South and for Memphis, but such activity was also unsettling.[30] The act provided $75 million in matching grants, over five years, for states to build new hospitals and expand urban health centers. C. E. Thompson, the president of Tennessee's Hospital Association, saw nothing wrong with this infusion. He estimated that "47.8 per cent of the funds will be divided among the fifteen less wealthy states, the majority of these being in the South. The South therefore will benefit materially from this hospital distribution."[31] Some $2.6 million would be distributed in Tennessee alone.[32] "It should be clearly understood," Thompson stressed to his conservative medical colleagues in Tennessee, that this measure was not "socialized medicine."[33] Moreover, many southerners like Thompson saw Hill-Burton as consistent with the preservation of segregation, for although it included a nondiscrimination clause, the legislation allowed states with separate facilities for separate populations to ignore the clause if they could prove that the facilities were "of like quality."[34] Despite the act's value for Tennessee, Thompson must have known that new hospital construction posed a threat to local medical culture. Cautious general practitioners regarded new hospitals and more specialists as unwelcome competition; they looked upon national health initiatives with hostility, and they braced themselves for the trouble such federal activism might stir up.[35]

The time was ripe for the remaking of health care institutions according to a new model. Whatever new institutions might emerge would have to be built against this paradoxical background of deterioration and growth, of black pressure for increased accommodations and white hostility toward any policies intended to benefit Memphis blacks. It was precisely as William Van Dyke had predicted. Memphians now promoted their city's good works on behalf of its black citizens. To meet the new needs, for example, the "beautiful halls of the old General Samuel T. Carnes home . . . where once Memphis' elite met [would] become halls of health and mercy for Memphis' negroes."[36] This kind of expansion recognized the need for new facilities in a rapidly growing city. But there was significant community opposition by those who felt that the city's African Americans, particularly the growing group of middle-income blacks, should build their own hospitals and not rely on municipal assistance.

The Plight of the Black Consumer

Health expectations among this post–World War II generation rose fast. Parents were now encouraged to consider the emotional and psychological health of their children as well as their physical well-being—from birth to adolescence—as a national health priority. Numerous experts like Dr. Benjamin Spock emerged to guide and calm anxious parents concerned about child rearing and the preservation of good health. Polio epidemics created havoc with parents' sense of security, however. Even those who distanced themselves from "socialized medicine" admitted that government had a large role in the preservation of health—and that "the health of American children, like their education, should be recognized as a definite public responsibility."[37] Large-scale national health programs, from niacin enrichment in bread to the pursuit of a polio vaccine, were widely popular, though not without controversy. In step with these national trends in public health, Memphis's Lloyd Graves would soon take up the fight for fluoridation of the city's water supply. But local physicians fought him, fearing this public health measure as a surreptitious attempt to usurp the role of doctors through a kind of "mass medication."[38] Such issues only increased the general visibility of child health and its dependence on medical goods and services.

The availability of Hill-Burton hospital construction funds, along with urban growth and the focus on the child, converged in Memphis in the late 1940s with the creation of a new hospital, LeBonheur Children's Hospital. An elite Memphis women's club, a group that previously had devoted its energies to tea parties and horse riding, shifted civic course after the war and spearheaded the hospital plan. Media coverage of their quest to improve child health was uniformly positive. In July 1949 one local paper praised the group's determination, noting that "regardless of how long it takes to obtain funds, LeBonheur expects to build a children's hospital in Memphis."[39] Indeed, these women placed themselves at the center of a new urban health politics. Their methods suggested a new postwar civic activism: a public campaigning for health that was focused on overcoming local political obstacles while exploiting new federal funds. The women of LeBonheur pushed to obtain Hill-Burton funds even though city hall initially refused to provide support for their mission.

Justifying the need for a children's hospital was not difficult in the midst of the boom in births and the rising faith in medical science. To fulfill their dreams of building a hospital, the women of LeBonheur allied themselves with local pediatricians like James G. Hughes. Writing to state officials in charge of administering the federal Hill-Burton program, Hughes evoked images of a city that had outgrown its institutions. He insisted that "Memphis and West Tennessee have outgrown their hospital facilities for sick children . . . beds for chronically ill children are almost totally lacking . . . private pediatric beds in the City of Memphis are equally insufficient for the needs of the population."[40] Hughes spoke positively about Memphis's responsibilities to the surrounding states, using the city's proximity to Mississippi and Arkansas as justification for new facilities. He also invoked the image of neglected children with chronic diseases — rheumatic fever, congenital heart disease, convulsive disorders, diabetes, cerebral palsy, and others. He noted that "lacking the drama of acute disease, their illnesses progress insidiously, but nonetheless importantly, to produce irreparable and avoidable damage."[41] This double neglect could be addressed, it seemed, by building LeBonheur. In order to win state support, Hughes also pointed to the teaching and research value of such patients: "Many problems concerning chronic diseases of childhood remain to be solved . . . [and the hospital] would enable profitable investigations to be carried out."[42] Eventually the LeBonheur appeal was a success. One-third of the construction costs were covered by the Hill-Burton program, and much of the remaining funds were raised in a speedy, well-organized public campaign supported by physicians, women's civic clubs, and Memphis businessmen. In the face of such success the city eventually agreed to rent the property on which the hospital would be built for the sum of $1 per year.[43]

The determined, well-connected, and resourceful LeBonheur members raised money from all parts of the city — including the black community, which was promised a role in the civic campaign as well as a place in the new facility. When they turned to middle-class black Memphians, the women asked for $15,000 for the hospital, in exchange for which some "12 or 14 beds" would be provided in the new 100-bed hospital.[44] The *Memphis World* — the city's leading black newspaper (soon to be joined and overtaken by *the Tri-State Defender* in 1951) — embraced the challenge. The black community's professionals and businessmen rallied to the call, seeing the new hospital as a sign of civic progress in race relations — and as an occasion for their own involvement in remaking health care in the city.

All over the city, there were signs of subtle change in booming times —

small gestures by civic leaders and elected officials aimed at opening parts of the city to black civic participation and at offering African Americans new roles in segregated society. In 1948 the city hired its first black policemen to patrol Beale Street. There was growing pressure to open city parks and art galleries to black citizens, if only for one evening a week.[45] Challenges to strict segregation were evident everywhere — in the redesign of hospitals, in the practice of ambulance services, in the police force, and in access to parks and public schools.[46] In this context, a new question emerged. Was it not time for a new black hospital that would provide a viable alternative to the Memphis General Hospital, especially for African Americans who could afford to pay?

Middle-class African Americans had gained greater visibility in Memphis. If whites could ignore the existence of blacks in earlier decades, they could not do so after the war.[47] While blacks organized to support LeBonheur, they also called upon the city to redesign the deteriorating municipal hospital and to build a new facility. Their very prominence, however, could also be used against African Americans. As one angry white physician noted in the local newspaper, "The negro group is making more money than ever in its history. Many are making more — and paying more in taxes — than thousands of white people who would be required to build and maintain the proposed new hospital. I see and hear of many driving their Cadillacs, Buicks, etc." This unsympathetic writer believed that even this well-off group was too quick to depend on handouts and deserved no help from the city. "The negro as a race in public matters has been riding 'piggy back' for some 200 years," he concluded.[48] Visibility and economic gains could thus inspire new levels of animosity and stereotyping, creating new postwar tensions over the question of who would take responsibility for black health.

If the city could support the LeBonheur effort, could it not also support the construction of a new black hospital? This issue became a key focus of civic debate in the late 1940s. All could see that the situation at the Memphis General Hospital had worsened. The CME's Collins Chapel Connectional Hospital had also deteriorated, and its future was unclear. Its leaders had raised $282,000 from regional Colored Methodist Episcopal congregations, with the intention of expanding the small facility. Church leaders also organized to apply for matching Hill-Burton funds — as had the LeBonheur women. At the same time, a variety of civic groups acknowledged that renovating Collins Chapel would not address the problem. Black physicians (separately organized in their own Bluff County Medical Society because they were not admitted to the Memphis Medical Society) pushed for a new hospital, believing it would attract young doctors to the city. The black medical society was supported by the white doctors of the Memphis and Shelby County Medical Society and by the Chamber of Commerce, who saw the facility as economically beneficial. But Mayor Watkins Overton resisted. Overton regarded any plans for an all-black hospital as "not sound business or policy."[49] He argued that the problems were overwhelming, particularly the questions of how to staff such an institution and how to obtain trained black nurses and physicians when the University of Tennessee did not admit blacks for professional training.[50] Overton believed that a black hospital not only would pose administrative problems for segregation but also would draw attention away from other public projects.

By July 1949, however, Overton was under heavy pressure to address the issue. Memphis's congressional representative, Democrat Cliff Davis, wrote: "I am just about as aggravated as I know you would be about this drive being made on you to build immediately the negro hospital." Davis saw the reform-oriented newspaper editors as instigators in the affair, noting that "experience has shown in the past that the *Commercial Appeal* will be knocking on this proposal once or twice a week from now on." He suggested that Overton use an "old-time technique" and meet in his office with the most interested parties (the editors, the head of the Chamber of Commerce, "the white doctors, the negro doctor, and a few others who have been so outspoken"). Such a meeting would lay out the figures and put the activists on the defensive.[51]

Overton tried to take the offensive against his critics, challenging them to document the problem — if one existed at all. "You speak of 'the crying need for more adequate hospital facilities' for negroes," he wrote. "This I cannot subscribe to if you refer to the public facilities." He insisted that John Gaston was a fine institution — and, indeed, that it was a costly de facto "negro" institution that drew considerably on the city's resources, on taxpayers' dollars, and on the city's charitable goodwill. "I do not think," he said, "any city in the South offers as good hospital facilities as does Memphis to its negro citizens who cannot pay for private hospital care."[52] The *Commercial Appeal* responded to the mayor's defense of the city's benevolence by admitting the strong record of "attention to the needs of its negro residents . . . [with] parks, playgrounds, swimming pools, schools and the like." But the editors turned the argument back on the mayor, insisting that "the good will and good intention of the community in respect to the hospital here in mind were proved by the overwhelming vote for the bond issue. The time has come to start on an institution."[53] By the middle of

August, backed into a corner, Overton did what other mayors had done in the past—he launched an outside study. Basil MacLean, one of the most widely known national experts in hospital consultation, was brought to Memphis to study the problem.

The MacLean Report on Memphis

The MacLean study, like the Oppenheimer study of infant mortality in the 1930s, was guided by the interests of the Chamber of Commerce, Memphis civic leaders, and politicians. But now, unlike earlier decades, the economic interests of the business community diverged from those of the elected officials. Such controversies were not unique to Memphis, for other cities also struggled with race-related hospital deficiencies. Harlem's Sydenham Hospital, for example, was embroiled in a similar crisis.[54] Built in the mid-1920s, Sydenham had become Harlem's only "interracially operated hospital," allowing both black and white physicians to walk its halls and care for its patients.[55] Through the 1930s debts mounted, and annual public campaigns addressed these shortfalls. "We managed to pull through," noted one hospital spokesman in 1948. "But you can only go to the public on a crisis level just so many times."[56] The postwar era brought new crises. Higher technical standards in hospital care highlighted the fact that Sydenham still carried its original equipment and lacked facilities to accommodate modern specialists. In March 1949 the city of New York took over the hospital. The takeover was orchestrated "to preserve the interracial practice of the hospital in connection with private patients."[57] To do otherwise would have put Harlem in the exact situation in which Memphis now found itself.

In 1949 black Memphians obtained the small concession from Mayor Overton to finance MacLean's study of black health care. In October the hospital consultant arrived in Memphis, treading the ground carefully and redefining the issue in subtle but important ways. He praised the city for taking seriously the main problem, which he saw not as health care per se, but as the need to train African American practitioners. The issue was not *patients* (which could put paternalistic Memphians on the defensive) but building a facility for the production of *doctors and nurses* (an economic problem of supply and demand). The burden, MacLean proclaimed calmly, was not Memphis's alone to bear. "There are no quick or magic remedies for national shortcomings in providing health facilities," he noted.[58] Local newspaper editors echoed the point, reassuring their readers that Memphis was not to blame for national disparities in the distribution of doctors. Nor, they warned, should Memphians feel besieged by the presence of this outside consultant. The *Commercial Appeal* explained to its readers that "there is no disposition to disparage what Memphis has done and is doing to provide hospital care for negroes. The fact is, for all that, that there is no place here where young doctors, nurses, and technicians can be trained." The challenge, as the editors saw it, was to promote upward professional mobility, so that trained African Americans could learn to take care of their own. The paper insisted that the hospital deficiency in Memphis "tends to discourage capable negroes who would otherwise find it profitable to settle here for practice."[59] And what Memphis seemed to need most was capable black leadership.

MacLean's study revealed much about the changing commodity status of health care in the late 1940s. His findings also highlighted specific consumption gaps in black health care, many of which were aggravated by local race politics and southern custom. Some northerners believed that southern governors and mayors were finally "waking up to the health needs of the Negro" and realizing the necessity of training black professionals for the new health care regime.[60] MacLean shared many of these assumptions. He believed that building up black health care consumption and the production of physicians was good for the economy and for a stable society, and he gently prodded Memphians to adopt his view.

During his visit, MacLean collected information showing that Memphis had done well—but could do better. Local death rates for diseases like pneumonia and tuberculosis had dropped precipitously from 1938 to 1948. The pneumonia death rate had fallen from 159 per 100,000 to 52. The tuberculosis death rate had dropped from 221 to 105. These declines were linked, in part, to the growing use of antibiotics, but cities like Memphis could certainly take pride in the numbers. However, MacLean found continuing large gaps between black health and white health; these were particularly severe in the availability of health facilities and in the use of health services. For him, black membership in Blue Cross plans—insurance against hospitalization—became a crucial indicator of the problem. Based on Blue Cross statistics, black Memphians appeared slow to join the growing ranks of health care consumers. MacLean alleged that the consumption gap could be explained, in part, by the "Negro's . . . preference for free care."

But MacLean's report concluded that medical segregation also limited black health care consumption. "As long as the only semi-private and private hospital accommodations available to Negroes in the Memphis region are in the present Collins Chapel Hospital," he suggested, "the Negro enrollment [in Blue Cross] will be small."[61] By contrast with Memphis's black membership in Blue Cross, MacLean pointed to cities like Richmond and New Orleans which had achieved 21 percent and 13 percent membership in hospital insurance plans. The consultant saw the problem in stark economic terms: here were frustrated or unaware consumers who needed encouragement to spend their health care dollars. They were quick to purchase new cars and new homes, but not health care and hospital insurance. How could Memphis best make use of this dormant market of consumers?

Nationally as well as in Memphis, the subject of hospital insurance for black people had become a contentious issue, and MacLean merely echoed some of the common themes of the debate. Even in 1937 T. O. Fuller had recognized that "the laborer is anxious for wages sufficient to meet the demands of living a normal life . . . with money for insurance against sickness, accidents, and lay offs, for church dues, taxes, and facilities for recreation, saying nothing about a decent funeral when the end comes."[62] A decade later, concerned that the war had heightened these expectations, Lloyd Graves acknowledged that "hospital insurance plans which have been entered into by so many people in recent years have brought more hospital service within the reach of a large group of the middle and lower income classes of our population." "Such plans as the Blue Cross plan," Graves continued, "will make a great contribution to the public health by providing hospitalization for large numbers of people who heretofore have found it difficult to secure these services."[63]

The reasons that African Americans could not secure these services were simple. National insurance companies like Metropolitan Life had long avoided providing policies to African Americans as a "high-risk" group. But companies were increasingly pressured to rethink this policy, for where did this practice leave middle-class blacks in the prosperous postwar years? Invoking the image of an "iron curtain," one official at the black-run Atlanta Life Insurance Company, one of the South's leading black insurance enterprises, insisted that insurance segregation was inconsistent with the ideals of a true democracy. "The life span [of black people]," he wrote, "is shortened by segregated housing, like that set up there in New York City." Black people were "divided by America's great iron curtain of segregation and racial superiority. This iron curtain . . . in the North and South, leads to ghettos in housing, education, hospitals, schools, travels, and liberty, and happiness of colored people."[64] Insurance practices themselves — another part of the complex web of Jim Crow health care — helped fortify this iron curtain.

If hospital insurance and health care consumption were problems according to MacLean, so too were the meager supply of black physicians in Memphis and their advanced age. In 1949, of the forty-six black doctors in Memphis, 40 percent were between forty and sixty years old, and an astonishing 60 percent were between sixty and eighty. One noted black physician was still practicing at the age of ninety-two. As one doctor commented to MacLean, "The young doctors are conspicuous by their absence. We are simply not getting any young negro doctors and this is a source of grave concern not only to the people of Memphis and Shelby County but to the people throughout the entire Southland. The younger men are simply not coming here to practice."[65] The reason for the lack of younger physicians under the age of forty was also simple — it was related to the changing structure of the medical education system. Medical education and specialization had grown to require residency training in hospitals after the first four years of medical schooling, but all of Memphis's residency programs were located in hospitals that did not allow black physicians to work in them. Without residency programs and professional access to well-equipped hospitals, young African American doctors would never locate in Memphis. Other cities like Chicago, Nashville, Washington, D.C., and New York had at least one hospital where this training could take place. Memphis had none.

In this new health care economy, the hospital was a lynchpin institution. It was the focal point for federal loan funds, for insurance plans, for residency programs, and for specialty practice. MacLean's final recommendations for Memphis were eleven in number, and at the top of his list was the hospital problem. He called for the construction of a new private hospital for blacks adjacent to John Gaston Hospital — a move that would solve the problems of health care consumption, access to care, and physician production in one sweep. As MacLean envisioned it, the new hospital would be run by the university medical school and city authorities, and it would "provide adequate hospital interneship and residency training for Negro medical school graduates."[66] African American consumers and practitioners would be well served by the arrangement, as would the local economy. MacLean also encouraged the construction of a parallel nursing facility, and in the long term he envisioned "training facilities for Negro dieticians, occupational therapists, and medical technicians."[67] The Chamber of Commerce and Memphis's black community could not have asked for a stronger endorsement of their plans.

In MacLean's thinking, the continued growth of this city-university health care complex was far preferable to another, more ill-conceived plan — the expansion of the "unsuitable" Collins Chapel Hospital, run by the CME congregation. The church hospital was then awaiting the results of its Hill-Burton application, but MacLean vigorously opposed the extension, recommending that "the City Administration discourage . . . Collins Chapel . . . from continuing further with plans to build a new Negro hospital."[68] Moreover (and somewhat bizarrely), MacLean suggested that the funds already raised by that hospital might be donated "to build the required nurses' residence" adjacent to the hospital envisioned in his plan. Not surprisingly, the head of Collins Chapel and the CME bishops objected to this aspect of MacLean's report.[69] In a letter to the bishops, Collins Chapel's W. S. Martin wrote that the bishops should continue to raise funds to complete the hospital's expansion, for this was part of a regionwide religious commitment. The hospital, he noted, "serves the Tri-State area, and is our church hospital ministering to the sick and afflicted of our race. Memphis . . . is its home." Rejecting the MacLean plan, Martin called upon the bishops in surrounding communities to try to raise the $45,000 balance to begin the planned construction. "The diverting of funds is morally and legally impossible. Any recommendation of this [MacLean] survey concerning Collins Chapel presumes upon the submission of the church to its recommendations."[70] Clearly, these two different visions of black health care clashed with one another — one proposing to draw black health care into the new health care economy, the other proposing to build upon the clergy's strong regional religious commitment to aid the suffering. Memphis newspapers sided with MacLean, criticizing the church for its "regrettable" and "shortsighted decision."[71]

Yet some officials, like Lloyd Graves, supported Collins Chapel, hoping that "conditions will permit the construction of a new Collins Chapel Hospital within the near future."[72] Any hospital expansion at all would certainly help to remedy the severe shortage, Graves reasoned. Black medical students in places like Meharry regarded Memphis as a professional graveyard. But the MacLean hospital plan, which framed the case in economic terms, had gradually won the support of Memphis newspapers and, begrudgingly, the city administration.[73] The controversy over Collins Chapel seemed to be resolved finally when the hospital's request for Hill-Burton funding was rejected. One concerned Memphis woman observed that "some persons allege the state rejected it and it is dead; others that the federal government did so; some that it just lying doggo and neither the city nor the state mean ever to act on it . . . some say the city applied in good faith. . . . I report this so you can see the kind of confusion in people's minds." In her thinking, the issue had become a political one, "the whole matter being made a political football, Collins Chapel figuring as the Anti-Administration independent plan and the City's plan as the Machine plan."[74]

The MacLean study unquestionably raised expectations among African Americans in Memphis, even as it pitted the Collins Chapel vision of black health care against MacLean's corporate plan. When the Bluff City Medical Society announced its support of the MacLean plan in the *Memphis World* and the white press, the physicians were quick to note that this endorsement "was in no way connected with proposals to rebuild the Collins Chapel Connectional Hospital."[75] Numerous other civic and business organizations followed suit, and expectations for a new hospital reached great heights as the decade came to a close.[76] Against the backdrop of a postwar boom in urban development and the health care economy, MacLean's report had done an exceptional job of chronicling important unseen disparities between health care options for the city's black citizens and physicians and its white citizens and practitioners. Memphis newspapers acknowledged the disparities and dramatized the human dimensions of the issue, framing the crisis in terms of citizenship, economic growth, and family stability. One newspaper editorial, for example, began by asking Memphis citizens to put themselves in the "negro citizen's" shoes, noting that "it is easy for us to imagine the anxiety that would come over a negro citizen if he thought of what he could do if he or his family became seriously ill."[77]

The MacLean report on Memphis offered many anxious Memphians — white and black — a promising plan for a new era. If carried out, the plan would preserve Jim Crow medicine, but it would incorporate large numbers of African American consumers and practitioners into the burgeoning health care system. In many respects, the MacLean study was an index of how a prosperous economy brought an end to nearly two decades of shortages and national poverty, and how prosperity provoked middle-class anxieties about the postwar economy, equality, and social order.

A New Landscape of Visible Diseases

In the early 1940s, Lloyd Graves, Memphis's well-established authority on public health, had offered a familiar, pessimistic, and stereotype-filled refrain on the city's health. "There is no city in the United States the size of Memphis with more health problems or a more trying public health history," he complained. "Besides all the general problems common to other communities we have malaria, a large rural non-resident element, and an almost forty percent Negro population, with its well-known high-rates in tuberculosis, syphilis, maternal and infant death, poor nutrition, poor housing, etc."[78] As in the 1910s and 1920s, geographical circumstances and the African American population continued to be portrayed as the principal reasons for Memphis's poor disease ratings.

But even Graves acknowledged that the disease landscape had changed greatly and that these changes had altered familiar associations between race and disease. "The breeding of Anopheles mosquito has been suppressed," he noted, "to the point where malaria transmission is practically nil."[79] Indeed, Graves was compelled to acknowledge that the face of death in Memphis — as throughout America — had begun to grow older and somewhat alter its complexion. Heart disease and cerebral hemorrhage topped the list of Memphis deaths in 1939, he noted, with tuberculosis now in third place, cancer in fourth, and pneumonia fifth. The new disease profile told the story of aging, prosperity, and changing times. As Graves pointed out, "It will be noted that three of these [cancer, heart disease, and stroke] belong to the group of so-called degenerative diseases which naturally increase as deaths from infectious diseases and other causes of death in younger age groups decrease."[80] Only a year earlier, physician Ernst Boas had characterized these diseases as an "unseen plague" that became fully visible only in the wake of the decline of childhood infectious diseases.[81] Although tuberculosis and pneumonia continued to rank high on the list of Memphis pathologies, Graves predicted that they would continue to decline with the use of the new sulfa drugs.[82] The new disorders appearing in the wake would occupy the attention of Americans for decades to come.

In the 1940s the disease landscape appeared to be in a slow, deliberate transition. Child health continued to be socially and politically important to Americans, but by the late 1940s other "new" childhood diseases captured public attention. The rise of childhood leukemia seemed sudden and dramatic in the 1940s. Some associated the doubling of case rates with new diagnostic technologies, others with modern consumer conveniences themselves — the use of X rays and radiation and exposure to waste material, gasoline fumes, cosmetics, and suspicious chemicals, for example.[83] The disease seemed all the more mysterious because it did not fit neatly into older racial and economic explanations about disease prevalence. Polio also confounded age-old stereotypes about class, race, and disease. Surveying Memphis's alarming polio outbreaks in 1946 and 1949, one public health official, S. L. Wadley, noted that "there were some cases reported with Memphis addresses that did not live in the city." But the number was tiny, he admitted. The case load was overwhelmingly white, for "of the 114 cases [in 1949], 98 were white and 16 negroes."[84] Polio thus posed a puzzling paradox to those comfortable with the "natural" association of African Americans with disease. Its profile suggested that new analytical tools were needed to explain disease prevalence, since "the negro attack rate has been consistently lower than for whites . . . but no one has offered a valid explanation of its significance."[85] Wadley concluded, with a sense of irony, that polio may have favored those in less sanitary neighborhoods. "The theory has been advanced that negroes living in less favorable sanitary surroundings and in more overcrowded houses acquire the disease at an earlier age [when it manifested itself as a] subclinical infection that is not recognized."[86] These kinds of anomalies in leukemia and polio signaled to some southerners that familiar explanatory models needed revision in order to make sense of this "new" disease landscape.

By wide public agreement, modern, technically up-to-date institutions were necessary to recognize and handle these new ailments. This basic assumption explained the public's enthusiasm for the LeBonheur Children's Hospital — an enthusiasm that would carry through to the building of the St. Jude Children's Research Hospital for leukemia within a decade. It was not racial or religious self-preservation that gave rise to these new hospitals in the 1940s. Rather, it was a powerful civic activism combined with the federal financial commitment and the expansion of health care insurance. This confluence of forces promised to bring the benefits of science to every patient in every region of the country. The re-creation of the health care system brought new diseases to public light — diseases of children, of the aged, of consumers of all kinds. As Graves observed near the end of the decade, "One reason for the increase in demand for hospital service is the fact that the majority of the population is making more money at the present time than ever before. They are, therefore, seeking hospital care for conditions for which they would not have thought of going to the hospital a few years ago."[87] This high profile was not available to African Americans, however. For the time, their "new" ailments remained invisible to the system. "In Memphis," Graves noted, "so far as the negro population is concerned, with the exception of two or three very small and poorly equipped institutions, the John Gaston Hospital is the only institution in which negro patients may be treated." This situation was particularly frustrating, he noted, for those among the 150,000 African Americans in Memphis who "could pay for their treatment if good hospital service was available for them."[88]

This apparent conflict between economics and racial politics was one of the key worries of Jim Crow medicine. Experts like Basil MacLean saw clearly that the black middle class had to be incorporated into the emerging health care system, but there was much disagreement about how that incorporation should be managed — and whether any change at all would undermine segregation. What new disease problems might emerge if African American patients were brought into this new system? And what might their incorporation mean for medical education, for the health insurance industry, or for patient care? There were no clear answers in the late 1940s.

A decade earlier, malaria, typhoid, and tuberculosis had dominated Memphis's civic concerns. In the intervening years, these old diseases had begun to disappear, and new ones began to emerge. In September 1948 the editor of the *Memphis Medical Journal* recalled that "many of us remember when, at this season of the year, the wards of the old Memphis General Hospital were literally filled with cases of malaria and typhoid fever. At the present time, we do not have enough cases of this disease to demonstrate adequately to students." The reduction in tuberculosis was deemed "phenomenal."[89]

Even as Memphis physicians bemoaned the lack of good clinical material for teaching, new pedagogical possibilities lay just on the horizon. In 1949 Linus Pauling and his colleagues published an article in *Science* entitled "Sickle Cell Disease — A Molecular Disease." Pauling's article offered a new molecular biological explanation for the disease, transforming it into a cutting-edge scientific puzzle. Here was a disease tailor-made for the new era, a disease that could also fit the label of childhood chronic disorder, and a malady that was rising in prominence with the decline of acute infectious disease. At the same time, new diagnostic technologies promised to enhance clinicians' ability to discern the malady. Sickle cell disease would be vaulted into importance in medical schools across the nation. For Memphis physicians and citizens, the disease would become a key symbol of African Americans' fight for recognition in the new health care system, providing a new focus for black civic activism.[90] Its rising visibility would be closely associated with the struggles of frustrated African American consumers — and with the continuing challenge to reform Jim Crow medicine.

4 The Commodification of Black Health

In February 1953 the *Memphis Commercial Appeal* reported that "automobile dealer, Herbert Herff presented Dr. [Lemuel] Diggs and the University of Tennessee [a grant of] $8,500 to expand research into sickle cell anemia, a serious and painful disease prevalent among Negroes."[1] A year later, Herff renewed the research grant, which was aimed at learning more about the "strange malady" that was apparently "widespread among Mid-South Negroes."[2] The donation exemplified the increasing public support for research, as well as emergent liberal sympathy for black health concerns.

In all of Memphis's earlier community activism around race and child health, seldom were any specific disorders like sickle cell disease invoked as centerpieces of reform. Herff's private bequest followed in the tradition of John Gaston's donation, decades earlier, to rebuild the general hospital. Four years before Herff's gift, the LeBonheur women's civic club had established another standard of health activism. The women organized local money for the construction of a general children's hospital through public campaigns, pressured the city to obtain an inexpensive land lease, and even raised funds from Memphis's black community in exchange for accommodating a handful of African American children in the new facility.[3] In the same year, organized popular pressure had pushed the city to study the black hospital crisis in Memphis. Against this backdrop, the Herff grant represented a new gesture—local dollars donated by a lone successful businessman going toward research on a specific racial malady.

What had happened since 1949 to launch this disorder into the local headlines in 1953? What did its notoriety signal about Memphis's new social relations? And how would this "strange," "serious," and "painful" malady be used in the 1950s to frame a broader awareness of race relations and health care? This chapter explores how the drive to accommodate African Americans into the burgeoning consumer health care and research systems helped to catapult the strange malady into local headlines. New health care institutions (from the E. H. Crump Hospital to Lemuel Diggs's sickle cell disease research center at the University of Tennessee) were formed to give black patients a place in this changing system — a place to purchase health care and a chance to develop emotional stakes in the research system. Liberal Memphians sympathetic to the cause of racial reconciliation seized upon black health as an important social cause, particularly if they shared a sense of common cause with blacks. The Herff grant — from a noted Jewish businessman who advertised his Ford automobiles in many places, including the African American *Tri-State Defender* newspaper, and who depended on African Americans consumers — was one window on a shift in attitudes and society. With this grant came the promise of new social alliances in the Bluff City.

The obscure disease's new visibility reflected several other liberal developments in a city that was struggling with changes in health care and race relations. Child health again became a focus of philanthropy and social activism, as it was in the 1920s, and Memphis would see a wave of new pediatric hospital construction in the 1950s.[4] But the individuals speaking on matters of disease in public forums had changed since the 1920s. More important, the social meaning of "disease" had changed. With the birth rate rising and municipal population growing rapidly, the health status of middle-class children became a pressing cultural concern.[5] Particular childhood disorders — from polio to leukemia and sickle cell anemia — were now rallying cries for the upwardly mobile, socially active, and anxious middle classes. Middle-class Americans bought up copies of Benjamin Spock's bestselling *Baby and Child Care*, and they awaited Jonas Salk's every pronouncement, hoping that his research would discover a vaccine for polio and end their fears of this recurrent summer plague.[6] If black children were still peripheral to these mainstream health concerns, the push for racial equality and school integration would make them increasingly visible in the 1950s.

The rising social awareness of sickle cell disease reflected a convergence of racial politics and a new disease economy. First and foremost, sickle cell disease would become visible in the academic health care complex, itself embracing novel disease challenges and expanding rapidly with an influx of federal research grants and Hill-Burton construction dollars. The fate of people with sickle cell disease in places like Memphis became inextricably bound to the university hospital. In a gesture that was driven by long-standing clinical and scientific curiosity about the malady, as well as by interest in the social plight of African Americans, Lemuel Diggs organized a sickle cell anemia center at the University of Tennessee. Diggs's clinic was perhaps the first of its kind in America, and it became the beneficiary of increasing local patronage and federal research support — a key part of boosting local awareness of the disorder.

In the 1950s, then, the automobile dealer Herbert Herff, the research scientist Lemuel Diggs, various African American supporters of the clinic, and sickle cell disease itself all became prominent symbols of new urban possibilities. Together they moved the pain and suffering of patients to the forefront of public discussions, making the malady into a recognized cultural motif — a metaphor for an African American social experience. What processes transformed the obscure malady into a notable cultural marker on the streets of Memphis? The disease documented the existence of suffering in the black community, and postwar biomedical discoveries corroborated this tragic condition. The existence of clinical pain grabbed the conscience of some Memphians, calling upon them to discuss and understand the black experience. For a time, this malady replaced older, similarly encoded diseases like syphilis, malaria, and tuberculosis in civic discourse.

Looking out onto the Delta in 1955, everyone could see that malaria had disappeared — it no longer surrounded and defined Memphis as it once had. New medicines and new disorders had created a new health care environment. As local columnist Paul Flowers noted, "Quinine has gone out of style in the Arkansas Delta thanks to mosquito control and the antibiotics which have made malaria mostly a memory. Chills and fevers, once so prevalent where standing water afforded breeding places for anopheles, are the exception rather than the rule today."[7] If patients in modern Memphis suffered from recurrent shakes and spells, few would leap to a diagnosis of malaria as they might have in earlier decades.[8] Newspapers no longer followed the trail of this declining disease. Instead, they followed the new scientific dramas, the mysteries of emergent disorders like sickle cell anemia, and turned hopefully to research in university clinics to expose and conquer these novel maladies.

The Culture of Medicine in the Fifties

Speaking before Memphis newspapermen, radio broadcasters, and television personnel in 1952, one journalist captured the scientific optimism of the era. "It seems obvious from readership surveys," Don Durham stated, "that medicine and health news can't be kept out of the papers."[9] Durham sought to convince physicians of the virtues of publicity. He urged them to embrace and encourage the public's interest in their work, for the public was prepared to be amazed by the wonders of American medicine. "Industry in this country has been amazing . . . but tremendous as is the job of industry, it has been outperformed by the march of the magic men of medicine and the service given by our hospitals," he wrote.[10] In Don Durham's mind, not only was medicine leading the fight for better health, it (like industry) was also vital in keeping communism well behind democracy in the great rivalry of the age.[11] The issues confronting medicine — the fate of "socialized medicine" and segregation in medicine — were powerfully symbolic and demanded public engagement between physicians and an interested lay audience.

Public consumption of medicine was nurtured through radio, popular magazines, newspapers, and (now) television. The intense hunger of the media gave the medical profession opportunities to promote its achievements and to rally the public around health campaigns. As the editor of the *Memphis Medical Journal* noted, "In 1952 and 1954, by popular request under the auspices of the *Commercial Appeal* and WMC, a Medical Forum was held at the Goodwyn Institute . . . questions on medical subjects, uppermost in the public's mind, such as arthritis, hypertension, etc. were answered." Television provided another, even more powerful venue. "In 1956 and 1957 television programs were telecast over WKNO to enlighten the layman. In 1956 [the] society co-operated with the polio foundation and the local health department in mass inoculating the schoolchildren of Memphis against poliomyelitis, gratis, and others at very low charge."[12] The new media were crucial to winning support for public initiatives, establishing new norms of health behavior, and shaping consumer demands.[13]

Even as they profited from the media exposure, doctors were skeptical about the media and the atmosphere of lay health activism that also fed press reports. One local Memphis newspaper reported in 1959, for example, that the local medical society was "disturbed by the increased number of fund-raising drives." In response, the society launched an investigation of local agencies.[14] Organizations promoting awareness of polio, muscular dystrophy, and other disorders were urged to curb their activism; some were accused of not rendering the services they promised. The medical society complained that the existence of two muscular dystrophy foundations constituted "an unjustified duplication." While the society praised the nation's premiere voluntary health organization, the National Foundation for Infantile Paralysis (NFIP), the physicians complained of being overpowered by the Madison Avenue, media-savvy techniques of such organizations and condemned the NFIP for its "air of indifference . . . toward the medical profession."[15] Voluntarism and civic activism around disease could be a mixed blessing in the view of the medical society. In Memphis, as elsewhere in America, physicians struggled to marshal these popular trends in ways that served their interests.[16]

One of the nagging problems for physicians, the media, and all Americans (especially those holding up their democracy as a model for the world) was racial segregation; indeed, the issue marked the South in particular as a backwater. The black hospital crisis of 1949 had brought the problem home to Memphis, forcing local politicians, physicians, and civic leaders to address the deficiencies in their own way — by endorsing the construction of a new, technically up-to-date, Jim Crow hospital. The city's leaders hoped that the new facility would relieve the frustration of middle-class black patients, allowing them to dissociate themselves from the charity cases at the municipal hospital. Municipal leaders spent much of their time worrying over issues like the new hospital, public housing construction, public health initiatives, and the fate of segregation.[17] Amidst mobility and economic growth, they struggled to maintain the status quo, supporting the idea that "the bulk of the Negro population be confined to definite districts."[18] Many white and black Memphians continued to hope that updated Jim Crow institutions would satisfy the rising desire for racial equality while preserving the basic structure of segregation. But African Americans in Memphis were not so easily channeled and controlled.[19]

When the E. H. Crump Hospital opened its doors in 1956, it responded to the rising socioeconomic ideals of African Americans in Memphis even as it sought to fortify racial segregation. The new teaching hospital promised a rebirth for Memphis. "Boss" Crump himself had died two years before the hospital's completion, and with his death had come the end of his political machine. But as one historian has explained, "Crump's death left a political vacuum among Negroes, for it broke their main tie with the white community."[20] After Crump's death in 1954, many black citizens found themselves estranged from urban machine politics at the very time that they were fighting to build new political coalitions. The building of Crump Hospital suggested that new processes were at work in Memphis and in cities throughout the South, a region cognizant that it was widely perceived as a stagnant backwater of the America democracy.

In Memphis, Mayor Edmund Orgill saw Crump Hospital as a social balm. It promised to heal the wounds and remove the scars of middle-class blacks who deeply resented the pain of exclusion from white hospitals and despised the stigma of being labeled as welfare cases at John Gaston Hospital. Many Memphians hoped that the hospital would represent a new phase of racial reconciliation. At the 1953 groundbreaking ceremony, former Mayor Frank Tobey predicted that the hospital would be "outstanding [even] 100 years from now." Lemuel Diggs was on hand, and he proclaimed that the hospital was a perfect opportunity for African Americans "to serve themselves and one another."[21] In short, the institution promised to reinforce an ethic of social service and to fortify civic order for years to come. But other Memphians were not so generous. Many perceived Crump Hospital not as a balm, but as a further opening of a wound — an extravagant concession to the belligerent blacks who refused to accept their place in society. Against the backdrop of liberal attacks on segregation through cases like *Brown v. Board of Education*, even small concessions to local black citizens seemed to threaten the very basis of white rule. Crump Hospital was a political quagmire for Orgill — and for those white citizens who supported his middle-of-the-road policies.

For black Memphians, however, the hospital problem was only one aspect of systemic social inequality, and their strategy for confronting such inequalities now employed stepped-up public pressure and legal attacks. These were the crucial years of economic boycotts, quiet protests against segregation, and increasing public visibility.[22] Black civic activists, like the physicians and the women of LeBonheur, saw that the mass media — television and radio — played an increasingly important role in shaping public awareness.[23] A new black newspaper in town, the *Tri-State Defender* (an offshoot of the popular *Chicago Defender*), soon gave voice to their frustrations, beginning publication in 1951, shortly after WDIA began its own "all-black" programming. Both new media counterbalanced the city's conservative black newspaper, the *Memphis World*, vying for the hearts and minds of a growing young audience. These sources of information dispatched provocative new ideas about city politics, about health care, and about social life. They made the black presence more visible, and they played a crucial role in organizing the African American assault on segregated institutions.[24]

In the 1950s Memphis faced the headache of expansion and equality. Describing the city's transformation, one journalist at the *Defender* noted that "after World War II, many defense workers who had found jobs in Memphis decided to stay here. The veterans returned home, residents of Arkansas, Mississippi, and other states moved here hoping for suitable conditions, and as a result, the population from 1940 to 1950 increased

50 percent."[25] New public facilities sprang up to answer the increased demand, and the shortfall in hospital beds became noticeably worse.[26] As historian Christopher Silver has noted, new racial tensions over the boundaries of segregated neighborhoods blossomed as "a direct result of an aggressive postwar development drive."[27] The question of where to place white and black federal housing projects provoked public anxieties — in Memphis as elsewhere in the South — not unlike those that bubbled up over the creation of Crump Hospital. Everywhere, the underlying concern was how much visibility black people should have, and where they should be seen.[28] Throughout his tenure, Orgill mediated these controversies, walking a difficult tightrope, attempting to accommodate frustrated African Americans while reassuring angry whites that segregation would stand. But Orgill's liberal position was increasingly untenable, for there were too many tensions in Memphis — between the consumer expectations and middle-class democratic ideals of African Americans on one hand, and the deeply rooted desire of many white Memphians to maintain supremacy in a Jim Crow system and "keep the Negro in his place" on the other.

In the same year that the U.S. Supreme Court took up the *Brown v. Board of Education* school desegregation case and one year before Rosa Parks challenged segregated public transportation in Montgomery, Alabama, many subdued conflicts over the legality of Jim Crow were already evident in cities like Memphis. One debate swirled around the Memphis and Shelby County Medical Society (MSCMS), as local newspapers focused on its membership policies. The society, it seems, had only one African American member. The situation would have been unremarkable except for the consequences of urban growth. The city's plans to construct E. H. Crump Hospital forced an awkward reconsideration of MSCMS membership policy, since membership indirectly determined who could and could not work in local hospitals. "The reason all this came up," suggested the public relations chairman of the society, "is because of the new Negro teaching hospital."[29] Black doctors could not be granted privileges in the hospital, it appeared, without being recognized by the national American Medical Association. But membership in the national medical organization depended upon prior membership in a recognized state and regional medical society. Thus racial exclusion from the MSCMS meant that black physicians would not be allowed to work in the new Crump Hospital. The dilemma exposed the organizational entanglements of Jim Crow medicine, for the local medical society was the gateway into respectable hospital work and national recognition.[30] For black Memphis, this was yet another public insult.

Faced with the problem caused by its membership policies, the medical society's president suggested an awkward change in policy: in order to forestall a staffing crisis at the soon-to-be-built Crump Hospital, black doctors would be admitted to the MSCMS "on a scientific level." The move conceded that black and white doctors would be permitted to engage in scholarly discussion and scientific interaction. But in a revealing bow to local prejudices, the president insisted that their involvement "would not include mixing at social functions."[31] By July 1955, as the construction of Crump Hospital progressed, the society formalized its new policy.[32] Scientific discussion was designated to be an acceptable basis for racial interaction, but "social functions" were not. White Memphis physicians — like other citizens — thus struggled to uphold the old social order, even as they were compelled to adjust to new developments in medicine and society.

Disease and the Booming Research Economy

In conjunction with institutional changes, new technical developments began to undermine and destabilize the old social order. As the new field of molecular biology made previously obscure diseases like sickle cell anemia and leukemia the focus of intensive investigation and community activism, public attention was drawn to them. In part because of newly discovered scientific and clinical features, sickle cell anemia was gradually transformed into a mysterious and challenging problem — in the clinic, in the research laboratory, and in the community.

To many clinicians, sickle cell anemia was gaining recognition as an "often misunderstood" disease. As early as 1950, Memphis physician Russell Patterson had identified 142 sickle cell patients at the John Gaston Hospital (17 of whom had been admitted to the surgical service because their pain suggested appendicitis or some other "surgical" disorder). Patterson had written a short clinical account of these cases to inform his colleagues about the disease's typical features and to avoid such diagnostic misunderstanding. New drugs and tests were incorporated into medical practice, altering the ability to clinically recognize these patients. "In general," Patterson wrote, "surgeons have failed to realize the surgical significance of sickle cell anemia." They tended to believe that "febrile episodes in which the patient has severe, incapacitating [abdominal] pains" was a surgical symptom; as a result, many "unnecessary operations have been performed."[33] Moreover, Patterson noted, "the bone and joint pain [have often incorrectly suggested] . . . rheumatic fever."[34] In keeping with a clinical reformer's role, Patterson drew his readers' attention to the need to properly understand this enigmatic disorder. Indeed, his article was one of the first Memphis-based accounts to identify the problem of "misunderstood pain" so directly as a crucial feature of the malady.[35] Patterson's article suggested a new clinical awareness and a sensitivity to the nature of the patient's experience in the John Gaston Hospital. Yet it also highlighted the ways in which sickle cell anemia had become a valuable topic for clinical researchers — useful in building disciplines like molecular biology and specialties like pediatrics, and helpful in reshaping diagnostic awareness within medical institutions and civic awareness throughout the city.

By the early 1950s, widening interest in sickle cell disease made the malady into a commodity. Illness and disease have always had a peculiar exchange value to university-based physicians because they are necessary for training students. Patients with diseases served both the faculty and the student body, bringing the young learners "into intimate contact with practically all the diseases that they will [later] be called upon to treat."[36] In the 1950s diseases took on increased value as university medicine became much more research-oriented. Since the 1920s Diggs had been fascinated by the intricacies of the disease process in sickle cell anemia, but he was more or less alone. Indeed, when Diggs first arrived in Memphis, "the [medical school's] Dean more or less said, 'we are mainly interested in you teaching . . . and running a good program for these patients. Research is not a major effort here.'"[37] But by the 1950s the significance of his research had grown. For this generation, Linus Pauling's discovery of the molecular mechanism of sickled red blood cells was nothing short of revolutionary. It revealed that disease processes, previously unseen, existed within the red blood cells at the molecular level. Pauling's discovery immediately made sickle cell disease into a researcher's cash crop, opening the way for clinicians like Patterson to work in the wards where Lemuel Diggs had labored for decades. In the aftermath, sickle cell disease became a researcher's commodity for doing science as well as a social commodity for building awareness of the African American condition. At the same time, it continued to be a commodity of increasing value in medical education, highlighting the links between molecular biology and clinical medicine.[38]

The malady's growing prominence was not merely a matter of its social significance or its new intellectual appeal, for new drugs had already altered its visibility by making its sufferers better known in the clinics. The sulphonamide drugs of the 1930s and penicillin in the 1940s had a dramatic impact on the way many diseases, including sickle cell anemia, were visualized. Penicillin (a rare drug in the early 1940s, but later widely available due to wartime scaling up of production) allowed physicians to treat a broad spectrum of well-known childhood infectious diseases.[39]

Pediatricians saw that many children who were dying of tuberculosis, pneumonia, and other infectious diseases could now be treated with the powerful antibacterial agents. But it also became clear to these practitioners that some of the children continued to be sick, for they had developed infectious diseases primarily because of underlying or preexisting disorders like diabetes, cystic fibrosis, and sickle cell anemia (to name only three).[40] Overwhelming infection tended to obscure the existence of these underlying disorders. Penicillin and a growing armamentarium of antibiotics thus exposed a new spectrum of diseases for study and treatment, constructing a new clinical population. Penicillin also helped physicians to recognize a long-standing dimension of the sickle cell disease experience — that infection was a primary cause of death for sickle cell patients. As one St. Louis doctor wrote in 1951, "Since it has been shown that intercurrent infections are the most frequent cause of death in sickle cell anemia, it is logical to assume that antibiotics and chemotherapy may be of benefit in prolonging life in those afflicted with sickle cell disease."[41] As the pall of infectious disease lifted, the new malady's complex profile became more distinct in clinics across America.

It was Linus Pauling's research in molecular biology, however, that quickly made sickle cell anemia into a "star" disease — a disorder at the cutting edge of new science. As one researcher stated about this optimistic era, "There was a flurry of activity in the cellular and molecular biology. The war . . . had given a boon . . . to biomedical research. Sputnik [later] had enhanced this profusion of research. The scientific climate was exuberant. . . . Much of what was going on related . . . to hematology: the structure of hemoglobin, the story of sickle cell disease."[42] Indeed, sickle cell disease was the quintessential stock example of how molecular-level mechanisms could lead to clinical disease. The malady's unique molecular characteristics drew sickle cell patients into a new economy — one in which the drive to publish new findings, get grants, and build research programs increased the value of the patients themselves.[43] Sickle cell patients were no longer merely bodies writhing in recurrent pain, nor were they simply educational opportunities for demonstrating clinical and postmortem facts. They were now at the locus classicus of scientific literature and therefore were useful in extending areas of scientific investigation — and in shaping the careers of the researchers in those fields. Molecular biology was only one field that thrived upon the high profile of sickle cell disease. Specialists in pediatrics, radiology, cardiology, and ophthalmology also saw people with the malady as important research opportunities. These sufferers became valued, at least in part, because of the way they legitimated research agendas. Sickle cell patients could be studied by geneticists, pediatricians, hematologists, and pathologists as they struggled to develop the insights of molecular biology in their own fields. In the context of America's race with the Soviets for scientific and technological advantage, federal support for such research expanded dramatically, as did dollars for studying disease mechanisms precisely like those in sickle cell anemia.

The appeal of child health and molecular biology merged in the case of sickle cell patients—and in local pediatric institutions the significance of children with the disease expanded. In the 1950s the cache of patients at the John Gaston Hospital became an ever more valuable resource for the University of Tennessee. In 1954 two university pediatricians, James Hughes and James Etteldorf, oversaw a two-floor addition to the children's wing of the municipal hospital.[44] The pediatricians also staffed the new section, and because of their affiliation they came into intimate, day-to-day interaction with sickle cell patients. Over the next three years, these doctor/researchers (who had previously taken little interest in sickle cell anemia) would publish nine articles on the disease, all based on patients they had studied at John Gaston.[45] The expansion of medical research at the municipal hospital meant that readers of the *Tennessee State Medical Journal* as well as far-flung readers of journals like *Pediatrics* and the *Journal of the American Medical Association* would follow accounts of sickle cell patients at John Gaston. This outpouring of new knowledge also contributed to the higher professional visibility of the disorder.[46]

These trends should not be seen as narrowly scientific, for they were part of the economic and ideological transformation of the region in the 1950s. Federal dollars and the university's promotion of research had opened the South to new influences. "The most apparent change in the South's political economy," historian Randall Miller noted, "has been the movement away from their preoccupation with maintaining white supremacy and social stability toward the promotion of business and industrial development."[47] Like the promotion of business, the promotion of research in Memphis boosted the city as a whole, for research medicine meant new construction, new jobs, and local revitalization of urban infrastructure.[48] Research also captured the public's attention, drawing resources from civic groups and federal agencies; research spurred urban boosters and fed municipal activism.[49] Thus, for the University of Tennessee, Lemuel Diggs's work quickly came to represent the institution's commitment to knowledge and to community — and this dual appeal explains why men like Herbert Herff could see the sickle cell disease clinic as a worthy focus for financial support.

In Memphis as elsewhere, the medical research enterprise expanded dramatically in the 1950s. The University of Tennessee built eight new buildings, demolishing adjacent neighborhoods in the name of urban renewal.[50] Researchers encountered few of the bureaucratic constraints associated with research on patients today. There were no institutional review boards overseeing research, no formalized informed consent procedures to be sure that patients knew the difference between research and therapy, and no federal agencies regulating research ethics.[51] This "gilded age of research," as historian David Rothman has labeled it, was an era of free-wheeling, laissez-faire research expansion fed by the massive growth of funding and leading to the physical enlargement of urban medical complexes.[52]

This powerful convergence of social, economic, and technical forces — new antibacterial agents, expanding government funding for research in fields like molecular biology, the growing population of cities, and middle-class civic activism — thus created a new culture of research, and it was this culture that transformed obscure diseases into cutting-edge concerns. As research findings poured out of urban academic centers across the country, Memphis could now claim to be among the cities contributing in a major way to new knowledge about pain and suffering in African American children.

Birth of a Clinic

All across America — in the writings of pediatricians and social scientists, in the arguments of litigants in the 1954 *Brown v. Board of Education* case, and in the case of the children involved in the Little Rock school crisis of 1957 — it seemed that the fate of democracy itself depended on the treatment, image, and social life of the black child. These years gave rise to a wide range of ideas on the crisis of black childhood, all with significant implications for the social order. "The Negro child *is* different from other children," wrote Margaret Anderson in 1958, "because he has problems that are products of a social order not of his making. . . . The Negro child comes to us an overburdened child, taxed in a hundred ways that make him old beyond his years."[53] Such theorizing suggested a pervasive interest in how the black child was formed, what experiences molded his or her spirit, and whether changes in society could have long-term consequences for the child and the nation.[54] Not surprisingly, it was the now famous "doll studies" — studies of black and white children's attitudes toward black and white dolls — that provided the data on how segregation destroyed the self-esteem of black youth that was crucial in *Brown v. Board of Education*.[55]

Sickle cell anemia emerged in this social context, offering its unique insight into the hardships of black youth. It stood beside diseases like leukemia and polio as a family nightmare, exposing, in this family-centered era, profound anxieties about the untimely death of children.[56] Polio, for example, intensified the fear of public swimming pools, theaters, and common community places. Like leukemia, polio also exposed fears of the sudden destruction of the nuclear family by unseen forces. With the development of the Salk vaccine, the fears of polio began to subside by the late 1950s, but leukemia continued to sow the seeds of fear. And in 1959 the case of a young woman with sickle cell disease would be featured in *Time* magazine as a portrait of "the sickle threat." The story of Marclan Walker, set "on the campus of integrated Marshall College in Huntington, W. Va.," told how she grew from childhood through high school "living from crisis to crisis, and being pulled through each time by blood transfusion." The short article reflected the anxieties of the era, but it was also a portrait of how life-saving transfusions were making a "normal life" beyond childhood and a college education possible for this stricken black girl living "on borrowed blood" (see illustrations).[57] These diseases — now associated with ideals of economic security and upward mobility — became the basis for voluntary health organizing, fund-raising, institution building, research, and civic education. Such diseases provided the rationale for building new child-oriented hospitals and clinics in Memphis and elsewhere in America.

In July 1952 the LeBonheur Hospital had opened with fanfare and a strong sense of civic accomplishment, imbued with the power to preserve and protect the family.[58] Well-known professors of pediatrics from New York, Nashville, and Durham, North Carolina, converged on Memphis for the opening ceremonies. The women of LeBonheur received high public praise for their initiative. But there was also praise for others who made the hospital a reality. Of the $2.3 million raised, "nearly one-half was given by the Federal government under the Hill-Burton Act; about one-fourth was provided by the state of Tennessee and the remainder was raised by LeBonheur . . . philanthropic organization."[59] The hospital's planners had complained that "there [was] no children's hospital in the offing for any of the neighboring states."[60] To the planners, preserving the mother-child relationship was also a central justification for LeBonheur. "The idea behind the one-hundred percent children's hospital," noted one writer, was that it was "designed for the mother to hover close by." The child's emotional development had assumed crucial significance in health care, so "the child's psychology was considered along with his treatment." Memphians had "decreed . . . that LeBonheur would be different — that here parents could be present and would be provided for."[61] With the birth of this clinic, Memphis celebrated and upheld these family bonds.

A few years later at the University of Tennessee, another children's clinic was being born. Between 1953 and 1959, the small sickle cell disease center became a beneficiary of much more modest financial patronage. Not only had Herbert Herff donated a significant amount of money, but by 1958 he had renewed the grant and several other citizens had joined the effort. The women's auxiliary of the black medical society supported the research.[62] The active Alpha Kappa Alpha black women's sorority at LeMoyne-Owens College gave $200 to establish an "anemia research fund," a small sum targeted for the purchase of an electrophoresis machine. By the mid-1950s, electrophoresis had migrated out of the obscure confines of the molecular biology laboratory, becoming essential to hemoglobin analysis — and thus to diagnosing cases of the "molecular disease" that might go unrecognized.[63] Like penicillin in the 1940s, electrophoresis aided the visualization of the new disease. Even the *Memphis Medical Journal* agreed that such funds and instruments were needed "to maintain the clinic . . . to keep accurate records over the period of years, to maintain a library of knowledge, to perform essential tests and follow leads in diagnosis and in treatment."[64] In this clinic, a compelling detective drama was unfolding around the suffering black child.

In the years since the war, one newcomer to Memphis had joined Diggs in the hunt to unravel the mysteries of sickle cell disease. Physician Alfred Kraus became Diggs's research colleague and, ultimately, one of the city's most prolific authors on the malady, matching and then surpassing even Diggs. Born in Vienna in 1916, Kraus had emigrated to the United States in 1938. After completing an M.D. at the University of Chicago, he had arrived in Memphis in 1950 for work in the Veterans Hospital. Two years later, he accepted a post as an assistant professor at the University of Tennessee medical school.[65] Like Diggs, Kraus was attracted to the excitement surrounding sickle cell disease. He was fascinated with the molecular basis of the sickling process, and his early research focused on using electrophoresis to authenticate the existence of the abnormal hemoglobin (HbS) in patients suspected of having the disease and in carriers of sickle cell trait.

What slowly emerged from such electrophoretic scrutiny was a new image of the disease — based on the realization that abnormal hemoglobin molecules came in many varieties. Moreover, not all abnormal hemoglobins actually caused clinical disease. Thus the migration of the instrument into the hospital had created a new mystery: Why did some abnormal hemoglobins result in severe disease while others did not? How many "abnormal" hemoglobins were there? And why did some patients with HbS experience only mild pain and symptoms, while others with the same HbS experienced a severe and lethal disorder?[66] These were only a few of the compelling scientific problems Kraus and Diggs tried to unravel in the 1950s and 1960s.

As the disease gained a greater social profile, however, Kraus turned to a problem at the intersection of these scientific mysteries and matters more vital to patients: the relationship between the sickling process and the "crisis and episodic pains" experienced by patients. Thus, over decades, a research program that began by simply looking for new molecular manifestations of the disease gradually evolved, converging with questions that were increasingly crucial to patients and the local black community. Kraus (like other biomedical scientists of his generation) built much of his career around this disease. He wrote only four articles on sickle cell hemoglobin in the late 1950s, but during the decade he became codirector of the sickle cell anemia clinic. In the 1960s Kraus went on to produce some sixteen articles on the disorder, followed by thirty-three articles of new findings in the 1970s.[67] Pain and suffering, for Kraus, were certainly experiences to be treated, but this particular pain and suffering were also the basis for building new knowledge in biology and medicine.

In the 1950s a third children's clinic — the St. Jude Children's Research Hospital — was in its early stages of conception. Long before its completion in the early 1960s, however, St. Jude had become a force in the growing visibility of childhood disorders like leukemia and sickle cell disease. The research hospital represented something dramatically new in the city, especially because its construction was driven by outside forces, and because its mission called for the welcoming of the sick and indigent from beyond the boundaries of Memphis. This was a notable shift away from the city's historical ambivalence toward sick and indigent outsiders.[68] Here was a new hospital, the brainchild of actor / comedian Danny Thomas, promising free care for catastrophically ill children wherever they might live. The apparent generosity was made possible by the new research economy—and by the prospect of financing the hospital operations through public donations and federal research grants.

Yet, at its core, the new research hospital—named for the Catholic patron saint of hopeless causes—represented the arrival of national forces that would alter health care arrangements in Memphis. The inspiration for such a hospital was Thomas's, but it was financed by a confederation of American Lebanese and Syrian charity groups from across the country who, like the Lebanese American Thomas, were seeking to return America's support and investment in them. By the late 1950s, the St. Jude project became a mission for Thomas and for the American Lebanese and Syrian Associated Charities (ALSAC); although the name of the hospital reflected Thomas's Catholicism, the hospital was to be a nondenominational institution.

As historian Robert Orsi has noted, devotion to St. Jude had taken on a particular significance for this generation of American Catholics—a group that would soon take pride in Americans' acceptance of John Fitzgerald Kennedy as the first Catholic president. The once-obscure figure of St. Jude appealed to these second-generation immigrants trying to mark their place in American society. Now in their adulthood, Orsi notes, they found themselves somewhat estranged and distant from their parents' religious icons and traditions, yet they sought ways of affirming their faith. As Orsi explains, "They had to find new ways of honoring family ties they had been raised to respect because the old ways had become impossible or irrelevant to them."[69] The image of St. Jude provided a powerful outlet. The Memphis research hospital represented one aspect of this devotion; a new cause—leukemia—gave medical credibility to the ALSAC mission, and the hospital channeled the patronage into the heart of the American South.

Appropriately enough, well before the hospital was completed ALSAC channeled funds to the sickle cell clinic—a gesture that demonstrated the ever-widening appeal of the Diggs-Kraus clinic. "Before they actually started building the hospital," recalled Kraus, "they supported some of the sickle cell work" with a grant of some $25,000 to the clinic.[70] In 1959 local pharmaceutical entrepreneur Abe Plough added yet another $10,000 to the research funds. Plough's grant placed "particular emphasis on [studying and alleviating] the recurrent crises which characterize this condition." The Herff and Plough grants came from two of Memphis's better-known Jewish businessmen, and, together with the ALSAC grant, these tens of thousands of dollars represented a formidable, symbolic identification across racial and ethnic lines with the pain and suffering of black children in Memphis.[71]

If the sickle cell clinic appealed to African American civic groups, it also appealed to a widening orbit of Americans who were sensitive to the pain of discrimination and to the slights of ethnic intolerance in the 1950s. Their "economy of gift exchange"—from business gains into the research economy and thereby to patients, research subjects, and the alleviation of suffering—proved to be a potent builder of new coalitions.[72]

Racial Animus, Liberal Sympathy, and Disease as Social Cause

One cannot ignore the social symbolism of sickle cell anemia—for Diggs, for Herff, for the organizers of ALSAC, for Abe Plough, for the Alpha Kappa Alpha sorority, and for numerous others—as it earned a place among Memphis's notable diseases. This generous patronage flowed in an era of increasing racial tension and animosity, at a time when public segregation was under attack and when the existing racial order was beginning to crumble at the edges. Yet institutions like the University of Tennessee School of Medicine still defended their right to refuse admission to African American students, and municipal officials across the South fought to preserve segregation while also promoting racial harmony.

Charitable sympathy for pain and suffering contrasted sharply with racial animus in Memphis. Where moderate and liberal white citizens saw charity as a social balm, conservatives perceived these same acts as evidence of the imminent breakdown of social order. In the turbulent wake of the *Brown* decision mandating school integration, for example, reform-oriented Mayor Edmund Orgill was overwhelmed by a seemingly small controversy that framed the high stakes of racial politics in the city. Orgill was cut from similar political cloth as Tennessee's newest U.S. senator, Estes Kefauver, a Democrat who had won election in 1948 despite the opposition of Crump's chosen candidate. Kefauver's victory opened the door for anti-Crump forces in Memphis, and Orgill had reaped the benefits of the change.[73] The mayor became known as a liberal on racial matters, a middle-of-the-road negotiator who visited black groups and spoke often on racial reconciliation throughout his tenure. But in 1956 one of his seemingly minor gestures—a hospital appointment—highlighted both the tenuous position of white liberals who negotiated with blacks and the political danger posed by "massive white resistance" to integration in cities like Memphis.

Orgill had suggested appointing J. E. Walker, the noted black physician and founder of Universal Life Insurance in 1923, to one of the five positions on the Board of Directors of the John Gaston Hospital. The mayor hoped that this gesture would "secure stronger support on the part of right-thinking Negroes . . . [about] our City Government, and this would have a tendency to preserve the harmony . . . and defer the day when lawsuits will be filed to permit Negroes to attend *our* public schools and use *our* public parks."[74] Walker, who had considerable standing among Memphis's African American community, would be the only black member of the board. In the early 1950s Walker had run unsuccessfully for a seat on the Memphis Board of Education as part of a push by Memphis blacks to win municipal representation. Orgill hoped that the small reform would help, in the long run, to preserve the existing social order. The mayor's modest gesture won praise from many black ministers and civic leaders; it was an encouraging sign that he was concerned about black representation in civic government. One accommodating black minister agreed that the move "would help to strengthen the morale of the Negroes." He also concurred that "the question of integration could be delayed for a longer time if there was some way to place a Negro on the Board."[75]

By contrast, however, unbridled hostility poured from many sectors of white Memphis, ultimately forcing the pragmatic mayor to back away from his appointment. In the heart of the Delta, white resistance was building against all such plans to accommodate and integrate. The virulently racist Citizens' Council had been launched and was publishing the *White Sentinel* newsletter. In Memphis, numerous conservative civic organizations like the Citizens for Progress dedicated themselves to fighting all manner of integration. Memphis's powerful Council of Civic Clubs also called for a continued strategy to maintain "segregation at all levels."[76] "Give them [blacks] one inch," one council member concluded, "and they'll take a mile. So don't give them anything."[77] To such groups, Orgill's conciliatory gestures were nothing but concessions to integration, "race-mixing," and "mongrelization." One outraged Memphis physician responded to Orgill's proposal as if it were an act of civic treachery. "Edmund Orgill," he wrote, "in order for you to give a Negro a feeling of belonging to John Gaston Hospital you will take away the feeling of belonging from the white patients . . . a great idea mayor you will be making a lot of white people sick."[78] For this physician, the choice was stark — either the promotion of black health or the promotion of white health, but not both. Another Memphian objected by making bold appeals to white supremacy and racial purity: "Let's keep America white instead of submitting to integration which will surely lead to mongrelization please think of your descendants."[79] Yet another irate respondent objected that "Orgill is stirring up racial hatred by going around to negro civic clubs promising them" access to all sorts of civic services, including "the zoos seven days a week." In the eyes of segregationist forces, the mayor's willingness to make concessions to blacks made him "guilty of racial hatred and rabble rousing within our county."[80]

White citizens heaped additional scorn upon the mayor when the municipal-financed Crump Hospital finally opened its doors to the black public in 1956. In contrast to the lavish opening ceremonies for LeBonheur a few years before and for St. Jude a few years later, the opening of Crump Hospital was a modest but upbeat affair. The mayor was pictured in the local newspapers holding open the front door for well-dressed African American men and women. The image only inspired further hostility toward Orgill, whose efforts to preserve "harmony" and whose very public gestures — such as holding doors open for blacks — violated customary lines of racial deference and paternalism. One citizen clipped the photograph from the local paper and sent it to Orgill, with this mocking warning written across the top: "Did you shake hands with all the 'gentlemen' and give each one of the 'ladies' a sweet kiss? I'm one who voted for you, but would never vote for you again" (see illustrations).[81] Even if Orgill's act was aimed toward the long-term preservation of Jim Crow, many white Memphians saw the image through the eyes of white supremacists. To them the gesture was a sign of how the racial order was being overturned — and proof that blacks wanted nothing better than to subordinate whites, forcing white Memphians to hold doors for them and serve them as Orgill did.

In sharp contrast to this animus toward integration, racial reconciliation, and liberalism, the modest civic donations to the University of Tennessee's sickle cell center represented a gesture of goodwill, a safe step toward better health. Charity and gift-giving for "the alleviation of pain and suffering in black children" suggested one route out of the racial troubles of the 1950s. Newspapers sympathetic to the cause of sickle cell research dramatized the gift-giving and highlighted the fact that some of the funds would be used to "obtain the services of a well-trained [black] chemist and technician" — a worthy example of "Negroes helping themselves." The mysterious malady was now on the map of local childhood diseases (second only to leukemia), and it owed its prominence in part to the new political currents that had begun to transform Memphis.[82]

Sickle cell disease was now part of several different kinds of social relationships and cultural exchanges. A driving force behind black middle-class activism was the desire for recognition and visibility, and in this context the new malady could serve larger goals.[83] White liberals sympathized, to some extent, with these middle-class aspirations and with black people's aspirations for their children and could, by extension, rally to the cause of sickle cell disease. In the prosperous 1950s, moreover, various other civic groups, physicians, researchers, and public health officials turned to organized fund-raising activities, using the disorder to gain strategic advantages in the new economic climate. New and tragic maladies, far from being civic blemishes or social burdens, were now positive centerpieces of social, political, and economic relations. The research university was also at the center of this new exchange system, for in the process of shining a light on the pain and suffering of African American children, researchers like Diggs elevated themselves in the world of professional medicine. In promising to unravel the mystery of disease, these physicians also suggested that the painful experiences of sicklers in their communities would be understood with compassion in the clinic — and that research would ultimately bring relief.

The integration of people with the malady into research medicine was essential to the success of the enterprise — and this fact provides additional insight into the commodity status of disease in the university economy. The Diggs-Kraus clinic became a crucial nexus of scholarly activity. The clinic did not claim, however, exclusive rights to study its patients. Diggs opened the clinic to many other researchers, making a gift of his patients to the university research community at large. "We not only tried to study this disease ourselves," he later noted, "but we tried to get everybody else at the University interested in it."[84] He welcomed orthopedic doctors, eye doctors, pediatricians, neurosurgeons, radiologists, gastroenterologists, pulmonologists, and the "kidney people" into the well-financed clinic, offering a place for them to do their own studies and to learn more about the strange disease. As Diggs noted, "The Sickle Cell Center became a focal point in which we spotted and diagnosed and did the laboratory work on these patients, and then passed these patients on to other specialists for the study of their own field of interest."[85] The diverse symptoms and the complexity of sickle cell disease sustained work in all of these fields, making the disorder well suited to the emerging economy and culture of university-based research medicine. In turn, the open-door policy "made the Sickle Cell Center much more productive" and far better known. Sharing patients only enhanced the disorder's profile. "I didn't try to monopolize," noted Diggs.[86]

To most Memphians, these kinds of developments inside the clinic — amounting to a commodification of black health — were obscure, and far less interesting than the public story of pain and suffering. Stories about this strange new malady in the local papers were much less controversial than the appointment of Walker to the John Gaston board or the creation of E. H. Crump Hospital. Accordingly, many Memphians came to know and praise Lemuel Diggs for his work as a researcher on sickle cell disease and for his help in bringing St. Jude to the Bluff City. By contrast, many saw Mayor Edmund Orgill — the man who helped make E. H. Crump Hospital a reality — as a racial problem himself. Away from the public spotlight, however, a new economy was taking shape in Memphis institutions by the late 1950s, and in the creation of new hospitals, the city was slowly refashioning its self-image.

While these developments in urban medicine — and the new, specialized ways of thinking about disease — seemed powerful to some, they appeared esoteric and strange to others, including many medical practitioners. One Memphis physician argued that "a patient is not an eye, or an ear, or a heart, or a broken bone; he is a human being in toto and hence has many areas from which danger signals can flash the presence of disease."[87] Specialization, it seemed to him, had brought a loss of the appreciation of human identity. Certainly, as sicklers became a multifaceted clinical novelty in the 1950s, one could see these trends at work. The Diggs-Kraus clinic represented a balancing act — at once studying molecular mechanisms, unraveling the many clinical features of the disease, and promising to address the pain of patients. In the emergence of specialized perspectives on the malady in the clinic, one could see the academic center seeking — in the coded language of research medicine — to highlight and address problems of human suffering.

The sickle cell center at the University of Tennessee symbolized a new civic economy and a new approach to patient, disease, and race relations. In the 1950s all such activism around black health in Memphis was part of the broader politics of racial accommodation. In admitting "colored patients above a certain income," the E. H. Crump Hospital had sought to reconcile frustrated blacks to a modified Jim Crow society. The hospital created a tenuous compromise between the new economy, with its middle-class consumer ideals, and the old tradition of racial segregation.[88] The LeBonheur Hospital, the St. Jude Research Hospital, and the Diggs-Kraus sickle cell center also represented strategies of accommodation. In particular, the sickle cell disease clinic wedded the fate of sufferers to the promise of relief within university-based research medicine. But in venturing into the Diggs-Kraus clinic, patients also unknowingly entered a new economic system. Their pain, their infections, their complaints, and the other characteristics of their disorder were becoming increasingly useful — in raising community consciousness, in mobilizing resources, in building institutions, and in creating research programs. Inside and outside the clinic, the meaning of disease had shifted markedly, especially since those years in the 1930s when Ella Oppenheimer studied infant mortality in Memphis and saw a community deeply offended by the presence of indigent outsiders laboring under the strain of disease. In sickle cell anemia, Memphis discovered a promising new proxy for black health. The disorder's rise to visibility owed much to the newly emerging civic culture in which activists in search of reform could affiliate with university research scientists to pursue compassionate, economically prudent, and utilitarian goals.[89]

Amidst battles over the future of segregation in health care and in public accommodations, university researchers of this era could be viewed as both objective and also deeply engaged with the subjective experiences of their patients. They perceived the "real," yet hidden, condition of suffering African Americans, and their studious attention to the sickle cell patients promised an antidote to racial tensions. The growing visibility of sickle cell disease reflected a liberal impulse in Memphis; a new civic culture was struggling to take shape, one whose desire for compassion was buttressed by its zeal for science and by the economic generosity of people like Herbert Herff.[90]

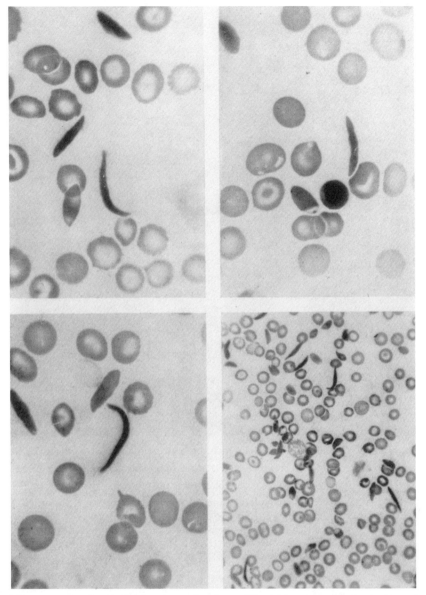

These images of sickled cells appeared in James Herrick's 1910 article in *Archives of Internal Medicine* and in countless articles since then. In America and the West, the new disease would take its name from the shape of these cells. In African cultures, as one critic later noted, the names given the disease (such as "Chwechweechwe") reflected the patient's experience of recurrent pain rather than the pathologist's fascination with cellular morphology. (Reproduced from Herrick, "Peculiar Elongated and Sickle-shaped Red Blood Corpuscles in a Case of Severe Anemia," *Archives of Internal Medicine* 6 [1910]: 517)

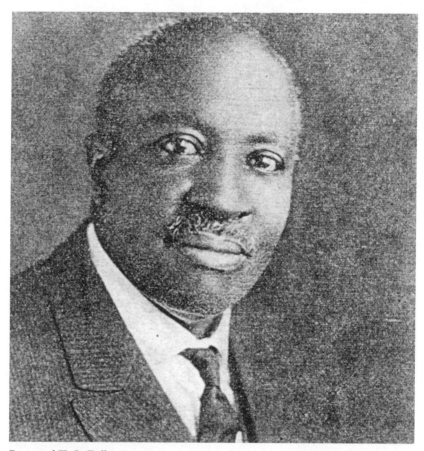

Reverend T. O. Fuller (1867–1942), pictured here ca. 1930, reflected the moderation and accommodation and the ideals of racial uplift charateristic of many Memphis black pastors in the Jim Crow era. Such ideas often brought them into conflict with other black Memphians and, occasionally, with their own congregations. (Reproduced from T. O. Fuller, *The Story of Church Life among Negroes* [Memphis: T. O. Fuller, 1938])

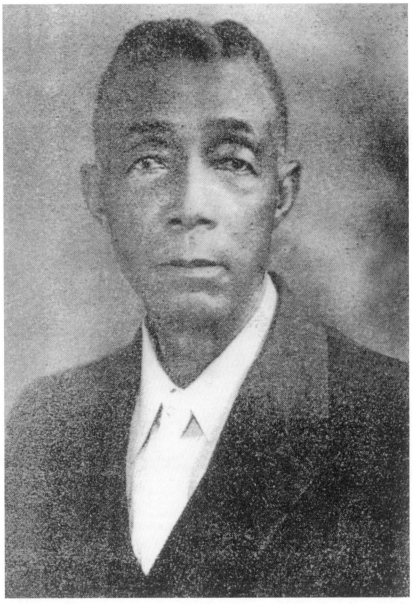

Dr. Miles Vandahurst Lynk moved his African American medical college to Memphis from a small town in Tennessee in 1912, shortly after the school was heavily criticized (along with four other black medical colleges) in the 1910 Flexner Report for its lack of training facilities. (Reproduced from Miles V. Lynk, *Sixty Years of Medicine* [Memphis: Twentieth Century Press, 1951])

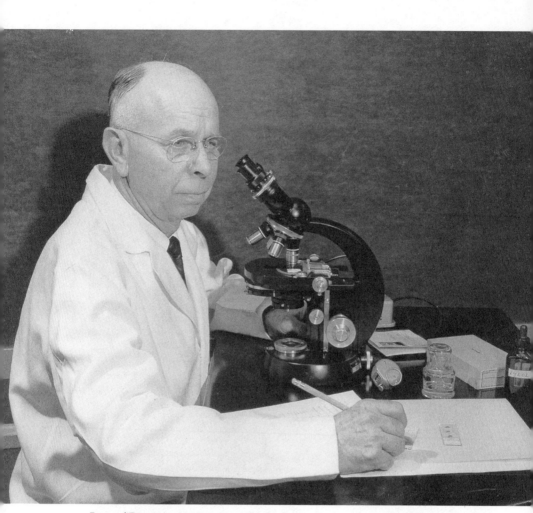

Lemuel Diggs (1900–1995) was Memphis's premier expert on the clinical aspects of sickle cell disease. From before his arrival in Memphis in 1929 and well into his nineties, Diggs continued to be an active researcher and writer — following his curiosity about the disease wherever it took him. Often that meant that Diggs was drawn into controversies around race relations in Memphis or regarding the health implications of having sickle cell trait. (Reproduced with permission from the Diggs family)

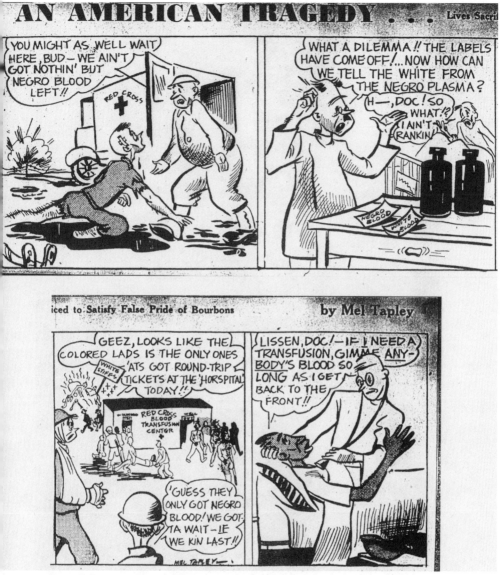

"An American Tragedy." As the controversy over the segregation of "white" and "Negro" blood plasma raged during World War II, commentators such as cartoonist Mel Tapley sought to dramatize the issue for New York newspaper readers. This image appeared in an unspecified paper, possibly the *New Amsterdam News*, and argued that blood segregation killed white soldiers and hampered the war effort. It also spotlighted the heroism of the black soldier and his willingness to see past "race" and to sacrifice for his country. (Reproduced with permission from Alexander Gumby Collection, Rare Book and Manuscript Library, Columbia University)

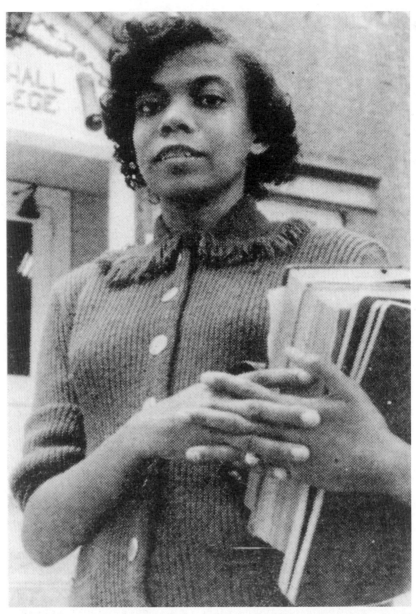

"Marclan Walker — On Borrowed Blood." This image and the caption beneath told the story of a young African American woman with sickle cell disease aspiring to a college education. In her quest, she was assisted by "borrowed blood" — a reference to her need for frequent blood transfusions. Such images of upward mobility conveyed the ways in which medical therapy and sickle cell disease became part of a larger cultural narrative about integration and African American aspirations in 1950s America. (Reproduced from *Time* magazine; photograph by Mike Shea)

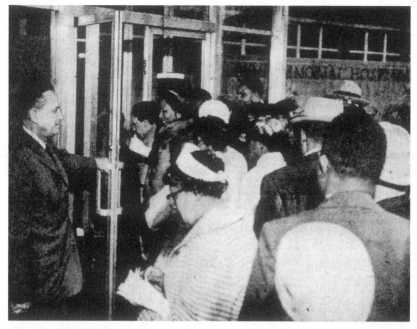

"Step Right In." Mayor Edmund Orgill was pictured on the front page of the *Memphis Commercial Appeal* in March 1956, holding open the door of the newly completed E. H. Crump Hospital for African American men and women. It was to be a segregated hospital for the paying "private patients." An irate Memphian clipped the photo and sent it to Orgill with a handwritten note scrawled across the top reading: "Did you shake hands with all the 'gentlemen' and give each one of the 'ladies' a sweet kiss? [I am] one who voted for you — but would never vote for you again." (Reproduced from Edmund Orgill Papers with permission from Special Collections, McWherter Library, University of Memphis)

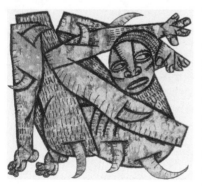

The caption beneath this image (from a 1993 article on sickle cell anemia) stated: "Before you can get past the agony, you have to get a doctor to believe it's real." Entitled "The Pain Game," the article explored the dilemma of sickle cell patients seeking pain relief in urban medical centers. Increasingly throughout the 1990s, stories appeared of how such patients were dismissed as illegitimate fakers or (because of their need for frequent pain medication) stereotyped as another kind of "inner-city" drug addict. (Reproduced with permission from *Discover* magazine)

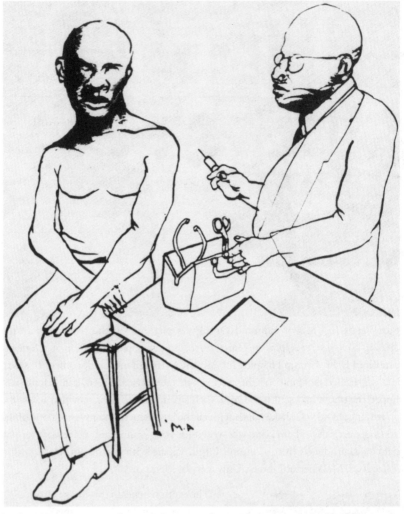

In the 1980 *Nation* article accompanying this image, reporter Richard Severo asserted that DuPont engaged in the practice of testing its black employees for sickle cell trait and using the results to screen for employment. His article exemplified how carriers of the trait became the focus of public policy debates in the 1970s and 1980s and how questions of social discrimination swirled around these individuals. (Drawing by Marshall Arisman; reproduced by permission)

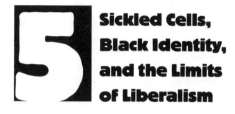

Sickled Cells, Black Identity, and the Limits of Liberalism

By the early and mid-1960s, race relations and health care had become deeply unsettling and fractious issues for Americans. Both would explode into contentious national debates over the Civil Rights Act, the Voting Rights Act, and Medicare legislation. They shone the political spotlight on social inequality, highlighting the fact that economic progress had actually increased the gap between elderly and young, rich and poor, black and white. More important, the concerns of both the elderly and African Americans revealed that more and more Americans expected that federal intervention could restore equality in a prosperous but unjust society. In these two seemingly disparate issues of health insurance for the elderly and civil rights, Americans confronted a similar problem — what to do about those people locked out of "the system," denied the benefits of citizenship, and prevented from being consumers in a time of economic growth and prosperity. Faced with these national crises, increasing numbers of Americans in the 1960s embraced reform and activist government.

The poor health of southern African Americans was a particularly vexing political concern, attracting the attention of social critics, reformers, and revolutionaries. Black southerners seemed to be more infirm and at greater risk for death than either whites or their northern counterparts. The plight of poor southern blacks revealed an especially vicious pattern, whereby racial segregation and poverty aggravated the racial disparities in sickness and mortality for which the region had become well known. Reformers from outside the region flocked to the South to rally for black voting rights, to march against segregation's injustice, and to participate in the creation of a truly biracial democracy.[1] Federal investigations pushed this process along — interrogating regional values, calling southerners to task for their continuing race policies, and seeking explanations for the enduring disparities in health care and mortality.[2] Such outside investigations as the 1962 U.S. Civil Rights Commission hearings in Memphis were far more confrontational than had been the U.S. Children's Bureau studies or the U.S. Public Health Service surveys in earlier decades. Unlike surveys and studies, hearings would provide a stage for local testimonials and dramatic accounts of the plight of disenfranchised southerners; these accounts would uncover the complex ways in which sickness and health were intertwined with economic and racial inequality.

Where the 1950s saw the rise of peaceable and polite accommodation politics, the 1960s brought its tumultuous end. The question of black health care would be transformed by confrontational protests, by lawsuits and court decisions tearing down segregation in health care, by the government's use of the Medicare entitlement to help promote a race-blind system, and by other efforts to legislate equality and enforce inclusion.[3] Challenges to racial segregation brought the South to an economic and cultural crossroads. In Memphis, as public pressure spurred businesses to embrace integration, powerful anti-integration forces like the Memphis Citizens' Council insisted that black participation in a consumer society threatened the city's economic future. Richard Ely, the Citizens' Council president, argued that the white backlash against such businesses was also a stultifying force. "Thousands of accounts have been closed with the establishments that have integrated," he claimed. Ely warned that racial integration would bring economic disaster, and he threatened that "the merchants who have given in to the pressures from NAACP, the two newspapers [the *Commercial Appeal* and the *Press-Scimitar*] and certain other liberal elements may yet regret their decision to flaunt the wishes of the majority of the people who want racial integrity preserved."[4] He reminded Memphians that the city's "growth and prosperity were created under . . . segregated conditions" and that its economic future was threatened by racial accommodation.

Against this backdrop a new face of sickle cell disease, and of sicklers themselves, began to appear. As scholars fleshed out their understanding of racial differences in mortality and health in the region, they began to use the experience of specific sickle cell patients and sufferers to dramatize the life-or-death implications of racial exclusion, to highlight the new economics of health care, and to construct new images of the "African American patient." Recognition of the disease experience itself—of recurrent pains often misdiagnosed—tapped into the anxieties of the era, and into the psyche of many African Americans. The disease was a powerful case in point for all those whose pain was unrecognized, and for all who continued to be misunderstood and shut out from access to medical care.[5] At the same time, scholars also fleshed out a portrait of the mysterious sickle cell disorder that emphasized its historical origins in Africa, thereby connecting the malady with other aspects of African American self-understanding. Because of its evolutionary origins in Africa, the disorder was increasingly understood as an African inheritance, a trace of authentic African identity among American blacks.

It is not surprising that both the misunderstood pain of the disease and the theory of its African origins became more widely discussed in the 1960s. The disease became, in microcosm, an index of African American history and experience. The case of the sickler now meant far more for social policy and social reform than it had meant in previous decades. Stories about the difficult lives of patients injected an experiential and clinical particularity into abstract debates about race and health policy. Having achieved local and clinical significance in the 1950s, the malady in the 1960s was elevated to the status of a national symbol of pain and suffering in the black community. Those who invoked the symbol discovered that it had power not only in politics but also in medicine. Soon, for example, the question of appropriate pain management appeared on medicine's radar, revealing the ways in which the politics of disease and pain heightened clinical sensitivity to the patient's experience and spurred new approaches to therapy.[6]

This chapter examines how sickle cell disease, by the late 1960s, had become a disorder with extensive social entailments, a popular pathology that was used to highlight a wide range of issues — from black history and black identity to the problem of chronic pain and the need for therapeutic reform. For some, the malady could justify sympathy for the African American social condition and could be used to explain the need for liberal, compassionate remedies for racial inequality. But its trajectory through the 1960s also illuminates Americans' changing understanding of race and the limits of liberalism in medicine, in Memphis, and in American society.

Testimony on Race, Health, and the Economy

In the 1950s and 1960s white Memphians increasingly were forced into the uncomfortable position of explaining disparities in health care between blacks and whites in socioeconomic terms. Confronted by stinging charges that restrictions against black patients in white-only hospitals were responsible for the poor health of local African Americans, white citizens felt besieged. Many pointed defensively to poverty as the real culprit. Indeed, the assault on southern racism prompted even conservatives to stress the poverty issue. They believed that economic disparities—more than racial discrimination—explained the inequalities in mortality and health care. This economic link between class and health would become more widely employed in Memphis and, in turn, would come under increasing scrutiny.

This style of reasoning was quite familiar in the region, and Memphis civic leaders had always employed a mixture of moral condemnation and economic analysis to explain health disparities. In the decade after World War II, for example, as farm modernization and migration of poor rural blacks to the city produced obvious new class tensions, Memphis experienced an "unexpected rise in the infant death rate," after a steady decline in previous decades.[7] Among conservative Memphians, one popular theory held that rural immigration, increased illegitimacy, and teenage pregnancy were to blame. Lloyd Graves, now a senior public health official, issued a reprise of these views, and he also laid blame for the increase at the doorstep of the black population, noting that "the death rate among negro newborn was almost double that of white births in 1958." But Graves could not ignore the fact that the problem also seemed intimately related to economic disparities. "There are many factors influencing infant death rates. . . . Nutrition, medical care, housing, education levels, all these things play a part," Graves pointed out. He acknowledged that "Memphis does have a fairly large negro population," but he concluded, "You always find a higher rate among lower economic and social groups. On the whole, they don't receive quite as good medical care."[8]

Thus, when the U.S. Civil Rights Commission was dispatched to Memphis in June 1962, the topics of economics, race, and health shared center stage alongside criminal justice, education, employment, and housing. The hearings were chaired by prominent Catholic theologian Theodore Hesburgh, which only heightened Memphians' sense of being under intense moral scrutiny. Many civic leaders, both defenders and critics of the city's health care system, stepped forward to testify, all of them highlighting the close relationship of health to the poverty and inferior purchasing power of African Americans. These factors, they argued, were the key causes of health inequality.

Throughout the hearings, aggressive questioning put white civic and health care leaders on the defensive, while giving a few black professionals a sympathetic hearing. The city's leading health care professionals explained how Memphis had worked to accommodate African Americans in the growing health care economy as workers, as patients and consumers, and as administrators. But the dean of the University of Tennessee School of Medicine was taken to task for the racially restrictive admissions policies of the hospital and the school. The chief of the public health department was grilled about gaps between health services for blacks and whites, and about the demand for such services. Amidst the barrage of questions, the commission sought to determine whether Memphis had lived up to its promise to promote integration and equality—and if not, why access to city services had not expanded for blacks.

Questioned about disparities in immunizations, Nobel Guthrie, assistant director of the Department of Health, suggested that the problem was not the city's commitment; rather, it was "primarily a socioeconomic situation. It's a matter of money, and partially, of course, there's always the lack of information, motivation, and such as that enters into it, but this all goes with being in a lower socioeconomic group."[9] For such officials, African Americans' inability to pay, as well as their ignorance that the service existed and a lack of interest in immunizing their children, accounted for inequalities in health care. Guthrie suggested that the economic status and purchasing power of black Memphians were gradually changing, but "initially there were no private facilities for Negroes because I think there was no demand for them. They could not afford them."[10] Guthrie pointed with optimism to the recent rise of a "statistically recognizable group of middle class or well-to-do Negroes in Memphis"—who were both able and willing to pay. Looking to the future, he suggested that their growing numbers and influence would be a crucial factor in reducing health disparities. Put on the defensive by accusations of racial discrimination, Guthrie, like many white Memphians, clung to the argument that poor health was an unfortunate by-product of this failure of consumer demand.

Civic leaders attributed Memphis's other failures to the poor supply of black professionals. While some implied that Memphis's health system purposefully deprived African Americans of access to jobs as nurses and doctors, Guthrie and others pointed to the inadequate supply of qualified workers. He admitted to commission members, for example, that the six registered black nurses on his own staff were the "smallest number we've had for some time." But the problem here was that such nurses were in increasing demand in other agencies: "A good many years ago we were . . . one of the few that employed professional Negro nurses, and since that time other institutions have been employing them." At the same time, he noted, "We have simply not had qualified applicants."[11]

These civic leaders resorted to similar explanations—the failure of the marketplace rather than willful discrimination—when discussions turned to the lack of hospital privileges for black physicians and to hospital admissions policies. Asked whether there had ever been a white patient at the city's Crump Memorial Hospital, city hospital administrator Oscar Marvin replied, "To my knowledge, there never has been." Nor did blacks receive care in Memphis's historically white-only hospitals—but these policies were portrayed as matters of consumer choice. Asked if it would be possible for a black doctor to become a member of the staff at the city's John Gaston Hospital, Marvin replied, "No sir. Under the contract with the university only members of the active staff [of the university] are engaged in caring for patients at John Gaston."[12] Marvin's comments passed the responsibility to the University of Tennessee medical school dean, M. K. Calleson, who in turn pointed back to the problem of physician supply. The university, Calleson noted, simply did not have any black faculty members, but there was a small black courtesy staff. These failures were not specific to the Bluff City, Dean Calleson noted, for there "is a shortage of Negro physicians everywhere, not just in Memphis."[13] Where the commissioners might see the specter of racial exclusion in these institutions, Memphis health care officials argued that the problems stemmed from economic matters beyond their control.

The hearings unearthed these lingering frustrations with racial exclusion and put a spotlight on issues of poverty, supply, demand, and the changing health care system. While critics saw segregation and stonewalling behind the disparities in health care, defenders of Memphis saw impersonal economic factors. In an era of activist government, what was the proper role for federal intervention in breaking through these barriers? Called to testify, one well-established member of Memphis's black community, physician Stanley Ish, insisted that the federal government could use the power of the purse to alter these local practices. Ish testified that local economic pressure from black consumers had brought quick, smooth changes in some parts of Memphis: "To mention a few, the buses have been desegregated; the downtown lunch counters have been desegregated; department store facilities, airport, train and bus terminals have been desegregated."[14] But in his opinion the university medical school had fallen behind—taking only the smallest steps by admitting "one Negro student who will be able, if qualified, to do an internship at John Gaston Hospital." Ish called upon the federal government to use the carrot of education funds more aggressively to reshape hospital and university admissions practices. "I would recommend," he noted politely, "because of the court's change in viewpoint toward the separate-but-equal policy, that the Hill-Burton Act be revised so that hospitals built with Federal funds can be constructed for people and not for races and, in fact, that all hospital facilities in Memphis for the training and the care of patients be opened to Negro patients and to Negro physicians."[15]

Ish's concerns were those of a frustrated but respectful black professional — and though the strategy he outlined would be employed by government agencies throughout the rest of the decade, his polite manner of appealing for help would become less reflective of his own increasingly angry community. Indeed, by the mid-1960s many black activists would be as frustrated with their own leaders' polite appeals as they were with white intransigence. But in the early 1960s it was individuals like Ish who spoke for their fellow professionals — and, by extension, for patients and for all of black Memphis.

Inside the hearings infant mortality attracted attention, but there was no mention of sickle cell anemia, which had begun to capture the interest of many black Memphians outside the hearings and in local newspapers. In these public venues, Memphians were busily reframing their discussions about the disease in terms of the economic rhetoric of the day. Charles Dinkins, president of African American Owen College, called upon others in the community to be "aware to the importance of sickle cell anemia as a health and economic problem." In his mind, the disorder was an opportunity for the black community to mobilize itself economically — to create, perhaps, a community fund to support medical research on the disease.[16] For other observers, sickle cell anemia was an index of smoldering resentment in the face of racial barriers and economic hurdles. Local journalist Moses Newsom, for example, bemoaned the fact that "while much of the nation fiddles in unawareness, a mysterious and crippling blood disease of considerable prevalence burns unchecked, causing much pain and suffering." Newsom also insisted that researchers were "hampered by a stumbling block" of insufficient funds.[17] Thus, even as the Civil Rights Commission heard polite testimony about the supply of health care services, consumer demand, and racial exclusion in health care, a more searing rhetoric was rising up around this metaphorically and literally "crippling" disease.[18]

Disease and African American Identity
Indeed, sickle cell disease proved to be especially malleable in the late 1950s and early 1960s. As each of its dimensions was explored and analyzed, the malady found its way into national popular consciousness. In the pages of *Time* magazine or the new black lifestyle magazine, *Ebony*, it could be used to reflect several dimensions of the African American experience — to

convey the strivings of African Americans for upward mobility against great odds, to relate stories of black vulnerability, or to speak about the preservation of African identity in black Americans.[19]

Building upon the status of sickle cell anemia in the biological sciences, scholars in the human and social sciences constructed new theories of black identity around the disorder. In the fields of evolutionary biology and physical anthropology, theories of the disease emerged that gave the malady a far wider currency—and a greater popular resonance. The extensive use of modern electrophoretic methods of testing hemoglobin structure confirmed that some 10 percent of African Americans carried the abnormal hemoglobin associated with the usually benign sickle cell "trait," and that close to 1 percent of the American black population had the disease (caused only if children inherited the trait from both carrier parents).[20] With the rise of medical genetics and population genetics as fields of study, new theories arose to explain these numbers, and to relate them to the prevalence of the disease and the trait on parts of the African continent. The disease thus became a crucial intellectual problem for human evolution and a case in point for the construction of population genetics theories. In short, by the early 1960s, as scholars studied the disorder, it was rapidly becoming a focal point for discussions of race, evolution, heredity, and racial differences in health, just as tuberculosis and venereal disease had been in an earlier generation.

Sickle cell anemia became an archetypal disease—with different lessons for different observers. From the standpoint of molecular biology, for example, sickle cells were an important example of the molecular origins of a disease—a case study of how a single change in the huge hemoglobin molecule could result in disease. From such a scientific standpoint, sickle cells were less important for the pain and suffering they caused than for the window they provided into human biology and into the role of hemoglobin anomalies in causing disease. Based on this new understanding, some scientists wondered whether molecular cures were not just a step away.[21] Other biological scientists and anthropologists extended these findings in the early 1960s, when they began to echo British researcher A. C. Allison's theories about the prevalence of sickle cell trait and disease in Africa. Allison had suggested that the abnormal hemoglobin variation causing sickle cell trait (the carrier status) persisted because these carriers "might have some advantage in survival over those who lacked the trait."[22] Using the widely discussed principles of population genetics, Allison argued that the gene must have provided its carriers some adaptive advantage. He suggested that perhaps "it protected its carriers against some other fatal disease — say malaria." Allison believed that this survival advantage would continue to be handed down from one generation to the next because of its value for surviving the particularly severe *falciparum* form of malaria. Unfortunately, this also increased the likelihood that two carriers might meet, have children together, and produce a child with the deadly disorder. For scientists in the 1960s, this theory quickly became dogma: the disease, the trait, and malaria had evolved together, an exquisite example of what was called a "balance polymorphism" — a situation where the gene distribution could be explained by ecological circumstances.[23]

For such theorists, sickle cell anemia embodied an entirely different way of talking about race. Rather than speaking of "racial groups," it was far more accurate to speak of "gene pools" and "gene frequencies" in a multitude of discrete populations. Moreover, as similar hemoglobin disorders were found among many other groups across the globe, modern molecular biologists and population geneticists began to argue that the study of hemoglobin variations could yield new understandings about the evolution of gene pools — groupings of people who shared similar biological characteristics.[24] Indeed, in order to fully understand the prevalence of particular genes in specific populations, it was necessary to delve into history, evolution, geography, mating relations, and local ecology. Academic science in the 1950s and 1960s looked upon sickle cell disease in particular as a result of many thousands of years of interaction among malaria, genes, and patterns of marriage and reproduction. As early as 1953, Lemuel Diggs had sought to remind Memphians of this very point, noting that while sickle cell anemia was "extremely prevalent among Negroes [it was] not entirely unknown to whites."[25]

As it unfolded in the 1950s and 1960s, the story of the sickle cell gene and its evolution generated important new understandings about the situation of black Americans. Allison's research suggested that sickle cell anemia was, in the context of *falciparum* malaria, a helpful genetic adaptation. But he speculated that "when Negro slaves were first brought to North America from West Africa some 250 to 300 years ago, the frequency of the sickle cell trait among them was probably not less than 22 per cent."[26] This movement of enslaved black peoples to America in the seventeenth, eighteenth, and early nineteenth centuries brought Africans into contact with new populations and new environments and altered the gene's frequency. Allison further suggested that "with mixed mating with Indian and white people, . . . this figure was probably reduced to about 15 per cent. In the absence of appreciable mortality from malaria, the loss of sickle cell genes through death" further reduced the frequency to 9 percent. Allison reasoned that the absence of *falciparum* malaria, the deaths during migration, and the prevalence of racial intermarriage had already played a key role in the lower frequency of the gene among American blacks.[27] Based on such highly speculative models of disease evolution, sickle cell trait and disease became crucial pieces of evidence for thinking about the African American past— and, by extension, the African American present and future. If the interplay between genes, environment, and marriage patterns over the centuries could reduce the trait's prevalence from 22 percent to 9 percent, then could not this interplay eventually lead to its eradication?

While such theories were crafted, other observers spun out the social implications. Some questioned whether the trait that was supposedly evolutionarily beneficial was actually as clinically benign as it appeared to be— wondering whether high altitudes, for example, might provoke people with the trait to develop the disease or symptoms of disease. One physician, writing in 1958, suggested that "since a large segment of the population is involved, awareness of the problem should be encouraged among members of the medical profession, the air transportation industry, the medical services of the Armed Forces and among Negroes themselves."[28] The trait's importance for society widened at the same time that its significance for scientists expanded. For the general public and for scientists alike, its value lay in the way in which it opened such rich speculation and furthered the understanding of evolution, population biology, molecular genetics, and social policy.[29]

Through such discussions, the disease's historical roots and its hereditary characteristics configured a new narrative of black health in America. These theories refashioned familiar old concerns about the consequences of population migration, the racial peculiarities of disease, and the conditions of American blacks as "strangers" in their own country.[30] In modern theories of sickle cell disease, blacks appeared out of place in America—benefiting from a measure of assimilation and accommodation into the "melting-pot" American culture, yet still existing apart and carrying a vestige of their biological past that only weighed them down. In Africa they had evolved symbiotically along with *falciparum* malaria and the environment. But in America a new kind of evolution was taking place, and for academic scientists in the 1950s and 1960s, sickle cell disease seemed to provide a window on this new process.

Indeed, American anthropologists took the argument a few steps further, enfolding these theories of sickle cell genes into their own picture of African culture and history. Reasoning that it was the presence of malaria that created a welcoming, even nurturing, environment for sickle cell trait, they turned their attention to that disease. Malaria, insisted one noted anthropologist, was itself the product of African cultural evolution.[31] Anthropologists writing in the 1960s spun a new narrative of disease in which the rise of African agriculture was a crucial turning point in the story of the gene. The ancient shift from roaming hunter-gatherer communities to stable agricultural societies involved clearing land and, as a consequence, the creation of stagnant pools of water where the mosquito bred. Mosquitoes, of course, were necessary in the transmission of malaria to people, so only in the wake of the turn to agriculture could malaria and the sickle cell trait flourish. Sickle cell disease was thus intertwined with the changing African ecosystem and cultural history. By the mid-1960s, academics had given the once-obscure malady a rich history that intersected with many features of African identity. Sickle cell anemia became the basis for sweeping academic discussions of ecology, human biology, cultural evolution, and the changing African and African American identity.[32]

So compelling were these new theories that historians and social scientists would take them up in the 1960s and 1970s, using the peculiar and now widely known case of sickle cell disease to weave elaborate and far-fetched explanations of African American death, survival, history, and life. Some invoked the single disease to explain higher black mortality on American slave plantations.[33] Others used the supposed survival advantage of the sickle cell trait in malaria-prone areas to explain the rise of a rice and slave labor economy in colonial South Carolina — a specious theory to be sure, especially because the transition to rice cultivation occurred over mere decades and because of the absence of the specific form of *falciparum* malaria from the South Carolina rice fields. Nonetheless, such applications demonstrate the widening popularity of the story of this ecological African disease in American academic circles in these years.

Accounts of sickle cell anemia appeared in popular black magazines such as *Ebony* and *Jet* in the 1960s, but the topic of African evolution — standard fare in academic writings — was not highlighted in the popular media. Rather, the disease provided an appealing case study of black vulnerability, as well as an opportunity for raising consciousness about the struggles of contemporary African Americans to improve their social condition. One story focused on the plight of the Johnson family from upstate New York. The family had struggled "through ten years of hardships and deprivation" and "looked on helplessly while two of their six children have wasted away from the debilitating effects of sickle cell anemia, an incurable, hereditary blood disease predominant in Negro youths."[34] Their search for medical and social understanding sent the family from one hospital to the next, "scouring the nation by mail in attempts to find cures." Finally, they turned to the federal government and, in particular, to the National Institutes of Health in Bethesda, Maryland. It was there that Mrs. Johnson volunteered one child "as a 'guinea pig' in order to obtain tests free" and to ensure a measure of therapy and clinical study.

The article contrasted the profound social ignorance about the disorder against the sympathetic understanding of the research community. It portrayed the Johnson parents as stigmatized by friends who wondered where their children picked up the "germ." In the course of their own struggle to understand, the Johnsons worried constantly that their other children (all carriers like their parents) would develop the disease. Misunderstanding, ignorance, and fear stood in the family's path everywhere they turned. But a handful of new research institutes, from Washington, D.C., to Memphis, dedicated to people like the Johnsons were portrayed as "rays of hope" — beacons for sufferers around the nation. "Bleak as the future seems to be," noted the article's author, medicine's antibiotics had been able to successfully "combat the infections that once claimed so many of these vulnerable people." Research promised further breakthroughs. Singled out for special note were "the pediatrics clinics at Howard University College of Medicine and Freeman's Hospital in Washington, D.C.," and Lemuel Diggs's own sickle cell center at the University of Tennessee — "another focal point of research on this disease."[35]

In the 1960s, attention was turning to these beacons of intelligence and understanding — research centers that promised to wipe away society's ignorance and to uplift people like the Johnsons. Memphis seemed to have a natural interest in the disease. Founded in 1958, its center had been sustained by grants from the NIH and by the "Negro citizens of Memphis [who] organized a 'Sickle Cell Anemia Fund.'" The *Ebony* article also indicated that "interest in the disease runs high in that part of the country, for it is estimated that in Memphis and Shelby County alone, 40,000 persons have inherited the sickle cell trait."[36] The center's method of studying the disease as a family and community dilemma clearly appealed to *Ebony*, which reported that "one of the most important projects currently underway there is taking investigators into the homes of patients where they will try to determine the environmental factors that trigger crises." But most important, the financial implications of this disease seemed far-reaching, and the Memphis center was also addressing its economic impact. "They are also probing the impact of sickle cell disease on social and economic conditions in the community for many of the people and their destitute family have been reduced to welfare status due to chronic illness." *Ebony* readers would come away from this article understanding that it was not laziness or ignorance, but disease itself that drove some sufferers into poverty and welfare. In this national forum, the disease thus provided a new window on the impact of chronic illness on the downward economic drift of patients. In contrast to the stereotype of the unmotivated and uninformed black consumer, the Johnson family represented a persistent striving for relief against great obstacles.

As the disease came to symbolize these complexities of African American life and identity, the Memphis center took on great national and local importance. It was a research center asking all the right questions about race, economics, and disease in the heartland of the black South. Patients and patrons from across the country recognized its value. In 1961 ALSAC — the Lebanese and Syrian group that founded St. Jude Children's Research Hospital in Memphis — had poured thousands of dollars into Diggs's sickle cell anemia research.[37] In the same year, the U.S. Public Health Service awarded a grant to Dr. Marion Dugdale at the University of Tennessee for a three-year study to develop "new laboratory procedures for the study of the coagulation mechanisms in sickle cell conditions."[38] Another grant from a local African American sorority was used "for the development of visual aids, including lantern slides, dealing with sickle cell anemia and related diseases."[39] The following year, Diggs received a $57,000 NIH award, in large part "because of the availability of patients."[40] In 1963 a local community fund was launched when "leaders in the negro community, aware of the importance of sickle cell disease as a health and economic problem, . . . formed an organization to support certain facets of research at the Sickle Cell center." The chairman of the fund drive, Owen College president Charles Dinkins, stressed that the money would be aimed at Memphis's ray of hope — the sickle cell center. Particular emphasis was placed on retaining a new African American member for the research team at the center.[41] For local Memphians, then, sickle cell disease could also highlight the need for African American inclusion into the university — not only as patients, but also as physicians, researchers, and laboratory technicians. Lemuel Diggs had already turned his attention to a particularly symbolic concern — "the treatment of the crisis," the painful, recurrent episodes in sickle cell anemia.[42] He would soon be praised by the *Tri-State Defender* also because he "not only created job opportunities for Negroes, [but] he has set a good example for good community relations."[43]

Public discussions of sickle cell anemia, "Negro disease," and African genes had begun to transform the discourse on black health.[44] As sickle cell anemia was being reconceptualized by biologists and anthropologists as one aspect of the complex, global African diaspora, it was also being reconceptualized by community leaders and the black media as a crucial aspect of the African American experience. On one level, its identity as a disease (with links to the African subcontinent and to thousands of years of evolution) became more and more widely discussed in college classrooms and medical lecture halls. On another level, the painfulness of the sickle cell experience continued to reflect an important truth about black experience. On yet a third level, discussions about the ways in which the disease led to disability, aggravated poverty, and weighed down on families also came to highlight a need for understanding and compassion. With Arkansas and Louisiana continuing to segregate "Negro blood" from "white blood" in the 1960s, and with all of the southern states awash in racial animosity, the Memphis sickle cell center was a beacon of academic enlightenment.[45]

The Coming of St. Jude

How would researchers in Memphis respond to these trends and begin to address the range of issues associated with black health and sickle cell disease? The coming of St. Jude Children's Research Hospital represented one kind of response, pointing the city economically and metaphorically toward a new era in health care. The new research hospital highlighted not only the symbolic importance of health care, but the power of the new health care economy to reshape race relations. The coming of St. Jude also highlighted how the continued expansion of research medicine — driven by forces from inside and outside Memphis — led to a new understanding of the meaning of sickle cell disease.[46]

Even as the U.S. Civil Rights Commission, *Ebony* magazine, and others focused on health and disease in the city, the St. Jude Research Hospital was breaking new ground. According to the official St. Jude history, television celebrity Danny Thomas "had come to [Lebanese Americans], his people, because never in the history of this country had people of their ethnic background joined together as a group to honor their forefathers who had come to America seeking a new world for their children. Nor had they done anything as a group to say 'thank you' to America."[47] By 1958, Lebanese and Syrian Americans in ALSAC had raised "over $159,000 from 142 chapters in 35 states."[48] Thomas himself led a spirited campaign, raising thousands of dollars for underprivileged children around the country and for "the less fortunate children at the St. Jude Research Hospital who were afflicted with the dreaded Leukemia."[49] The figure of St. Jude was a powerful factor in the fund-raising, for the saint had become a popular devotional figure for many American Catholics in the 1950s; the opening of the children's research hospital in the early 1960s thus brought Catholics, Thomas, Lebanese Americans, and Memphians together at a new crossroads.[50]

For local researchers the coming of St. Jude symbolized the maturity of Memphis as a medical center — a center now worthy of positive national attention on matters of health. Lemuel Diggs himself was one of the hospital's key proponents, and in his own fund-raising and promotional efforts, he insisted that "Memphis as a medical center and St. Jude Research Hospital have unlimited potentialities of development." For Diggs the presence of a major research hospital reflected well on the intellectual caliber of the city's physicians and scientists, and on the city's people: "There is no reason to think that all of the superior mental chromosomes of the country are localized in Boston, New York, or Baltimore or medical centers elsewhere and that no scientific good can come from Memphis. St. Jude will give to Memphis the opportunity of joining other cities as a center for scholarship and scientific investigation."[51] The coming of St. Jude was thus redemptive for Memphians as well as for Lebanese Americans. But in the process of coming to Memphis, St. Jude would alter both research and race relations in the city.

Diggs recalled that the decision to locate St. Jude in Memphis was not without controversy since Thomas's first intention had been to build a general pediatrics hospital, and "Memphis physicians . . . did not welcome the establishment of another pediatric hospital for LeBonheur was, at the time, struggling to survive and all the other hospitals . . . had strong pediatric units."[52] Diggs and a group of research-oriented doctors recommended that Memphians might be swayed by a plan for a research hospital, especially if it was dedicated to the study of catastrophic childhood disease. As the official history noted, "They preached the gospel of research and Danny Thomas listened." The venture proved appealing to the medical community wary of competition, to the staff of the medical school interested in research, and to practical businessmen as a boost for the health care economy. Its proponents believed that "a national hospital would draw patients and staff from across the country and would be a definite asset to the city."[53]

St. Jude was to be a nondenominational hospital despite the image of a Catholic saint looking over sick children, and this represented a new trend in Memphis. Diggs emphasized that ALSAC members were "of various religious faiths, Roman and Greek Catholic, Protestant, Moslem, Jewish, as well as atheist." Indeed, he portrayed the cause as a unifying force, for the research hospital had already "helped to unite these various Arabic religious groups and have them pull together in a common cause."[54] Diggs hoped that, by extension, it would do the same for Memphis.

As Diggs described the research hospital, it was an "outgrowth of a pledge made to St. Jude by Danny Thomas," but it was also to be a factory for producing new knowledge and testing promising therapies. The architecture thus reflected a mix of religious imagery and research efficiency: "Radiating outward from the hub [a central, circular set of offices] will be wings in the form of a five-pointed star." One arm of the star housed the research subjects, and the others contained food services, surgical wards, and research laboratories. None of St. Jude's therapeutic services were unique to this institution, and all could be found in other hospitals. Its uniqueness was its dedication to research — understanding the mechanisms of disease and testing unproven therapies. "One of the difficulties which is anticipated," Diggs noted, "is the education of the public to the fact that . . . the difference . . . is that basic and clinical research will be conducted at St. Jude in the *hope* of the development of superior methods of treatment."[55] Hope, expectation, and faith in the future pervaded such new institutions, and it was this intense faith, in part, that brought desperate patients from across the nation to St. Jude and that drove the scaling up of the research enterprise.

In many ways, the creation of St. Jude offered a sharp break with Memphis's past — a break with its civic disdain for "indigent outsiders" and with its previous low national profile as a research center. St. Jude welcomed indigent cancer patients to Memphis; it was able to do so because federal research funds were plentiful, more than paying the cost of patient care and research. Thus it was not a new altruism that defined this welcoming attitude to indigent outsiders. Rather, St. Jude was the product of the expanding academic research economy, which looked to foundations like ALSAC, to civic supporters, and to federal grants for financing — and to local and national universities for intellectual capital. As Diggs noted, "The individual patient admitted to the hospital will not be charged for his care," because the high cost of research could not possibly be carried by patients and their families. The research economy required the generous support of outsiders. He also pointed out that "patients admitted for study will not be considered charity cases but will maintain their dignity as individuals."[56] In this economy, the indigent outsider was thus subtly transformed in value and significantly elevated in stature.

Sick patients — now thought of as research subjects — were part of an expanding research economy that also added value to local universities. "Men trained in medical research techniques and the medical care of children are most often employed by universities and have university faculty appointments," noted Diggs. "In order to obtain such men it will be necessary to offer faculty appointments at the University of Tennessee, for the most desirable and most dedicated men are interested in maintaining their academic status."[57] By attracting academic researchers, St. Jude would raise the level of medical education in Memphis and enhance the city's reputation as an academic research center.

The research hospital also challenged racial segregation in subtle as well as direct ways. The planning of St. Jude began as Memphians were debating the desegregation of public facilities. For Memphians like Diggs, who sought to subsume issues of race to broader communal goals of children's health, "the petty matters of race pale[d] in unimportance in the face of catastrophes of . . . [leukemia]."[58] This meant that racial segregation could not be practiced at the new hospital. Since the hospital was being spearheaded by like-minded Memphians and liberal-minded outsiders, the original hospital plan did not call for segregated wards, bathrooms, or dining services.

Such decisions by a major new hospital sent ripples through the city. For example, local motels were looking forward to an upsurge of business from the expected influx of sick children and their parents. The original St. Jude plan involved building a motel "with efficiency kitchens on the hospital grounds to house the families of medically indigent patients so that [some] children can remain with their relatives for the majority of the time."[59] But the owners of the nearby Claridge Hotel hoped to capture the out-of-town business, and they strenuously objected to the St. Jude plan. With pressure from the Claridge and the local business community, St. Jude planners relented, deciding not to construct their own motel.

The apparent concession to local business, however, soon created an unexpected dilemma for the Claridge, which was now compelled to reconsider its own segregation policies. African American economic pressure against public and private establishments had already forced the public buses, public libraries, and public spaces like Overton Park to desegregate in 1960. In 1961 a black boycott of stores had prompted further desegregation. Schools too had been desegregated. And even as St. Jude was planning to open, the movie theaters were being pressured to integrate.[60] The business generated by the children's research hospital proved to be a useful tool in further eroding formal segregation at the nearby motel. When Don Pinkel, St. Jude's first director and a newcomer to Memphis from Buffalo, New York, insisted that any motel facility used by the families of its patients must be nonsegregated, the Claridge Hotel balked. As author Hazel Fath describes the situation, "The first attempt to register black children and their parents at the Claridge caused a furor," but Pinkel insisted that "if the black children and their parents were not allowed to stay in the hotel, the hotel would not be used for any patients."[61] The hotel management first conceded that blacks could stay, but it sought to make their presence invisible by stipulating that they would not be permitted to dine in the common dining room — African Americans would be restricted to eating in their rooms. But the hospital stood firm, and, concerned about the loss of business, Claridge's finally conceded. Within a year, the hotel was fully integrated — a clear demonstration of the power of the new medical research economy in reshaping local race relations.

The ALSAC support for leukemia research also sent ripples into local research on sickle cell disease. Because of its working relationship with Diggs, ALSAC made a commitment to supporting research in sickle cell anemia as well. In publicizing its support for Diggs's center, ALSAC drew clear connections between the two disorders — noting that sickle cell anemia was "comparable to leukemia . . . in the economic and family problems that it creates," and that it was "more common in the mid-South area than all primary blood diseases, including leukemia."[62] In the early 1960s, the two research enterprises moved forward together. Diggs acknowledged that "the aid given by ALSAC in starting hematological research in [the sickle cell clinic] was instrumental in enabling this department to obtain additional research grants from the U.S. Public Health Service."[63] He explained that "St. Jude had placed in the 'scientific dough' the leaven which is actively working" to leverage more research funds and to promote the rising profile of sickle cell disease.[64]

The coming of St. Jude thus pointed to the ascendancy of research medicine with its new economy, an economy with the ability to change the local conception of the infirm as well as to influence local values. St. Jude also exemplified a commitment to medicine "without regard to race, religion, or place of residence." And it represented a consolidation of public attention and cultural authority around new and feared childhood diseases, and around the specialists who studied them. These trends all reflected the influence of the outsiders who were coming to the South and shining a light on the ugly, concealed corners where economics, segregation, and health intersected.[65] In Memphis, as the debate over segregated accommodations moved from the local department stores and downtown shops to St. Jude, these problems gained increasing visibility. Indeed, throughout the region, the civil rights movement was uncovering appalling racial injustices and thrusting them into the light of American national politics.[66]

The new emphasis on research was not without its critics, for there continued to be a real gap between studying disease processes in research subjects and caring for patients. To some, St. Jude and other institutions like the University of Tennessee School of Medicine represented a disturbing trend. Noted one Tennessee physician, Addison Scoville, in 1963, "There can be no doubt that the emphasis in the medical profession has shifted away from treating everyday illnesses of ordinary people to the glamorous field of specialization and, particularly, of medical research."[67] Not all physicians appreciated the rise of the novel and the "glamorous." Scoville believed that by embracing research, universities were gradually relinquishing "their time-honored functions as clinical centers for ministering to the sick and training medical students." "Instead," he argued, "they have become medical scientific research institutes, consequently deemphasizing the ordinary problems of medical care."[68] Scoville's concerns reflected a common anxiety among some physicians as the research economy heated up and as diseases like leukemia and sickle cell anemia ascended in scientific importance. "As interest in scientific medicine grows," he warned, "devotion to people, sick with ordinary and unexciting diseases, wanes."[69] As Scoville rightly observed, the rise of a new research economy had direct implications for the relative visibility of diseases.

With the coming of St. Jude, "exciting" new diseases gained both scientific acclaim and wide cultural legitimacy. But what was the relationship between the researcher's curiosity about such diseases and the goal of improving the health of "ordinary" sick people? This question would continue to hound researchers through the 1960s. In the case of sickle cell anemia, however, the researchers had a quick response. Theirs was not merely an interest in a new, exciting disease. They could point out that sickle cell disease was truly a reflection of the complex history of African Americans, an indicator of the recurrent pain of the people, and a window on the experience of African Americans in general. For those who believed in the promise of research, this argument sufficed. But through the decade, researchers would be compelled by a skeptical public continually to explain and justify how their curiosity about hemoglobin molecules, genes, and African history would actually address the concerns of the ordinary patient.

Racial Pain and Hemoglobin Memphis in the Sickle Cell Center

In the early 1960s, there was in Memphis a significant faith that black and white civic leaders could work out the major problems of race and health in the city. Many Memphians, however, wondered how to stabilize local relations when race relations were transforming all around them. With mounting public protest and brutal police reprisals in other southern cities like Selma, Birmingham, and Little Rock, Memphians braced for marches, sit-ins, and mass demonstrations, and many of their leaders struggled with the problem of how to communicate in an era of mass protest and massive response by conservative whites. In this tense environment, academic medical pronouncements on health and disease would be measured for social relevance. Increasingly, even the research in the University of Tennessee sickle cell clinic would be compelled to speak to stepped-up demands for justice, immediate reform, and radical social change.

In May 1964, as the landmark civil rights bill wound its way through the U.S. Congress, the nation's eyes fell for a moment on Memphis, a city that seemed to stand apart from its southern counterparts as a model of "biracial leadership" and a calm spot amidst a growing storm. Reporters for the *New York Times* and ABC News documented tense but workable race relationships in the city. But the threats of violence, public demonstrations, and unruly protests were palpable, surrounding the city and underlying the apparent calm. According to the *New York Times* writer, the city "has all the ingredients to make it a racial trouble spot: Old South traditions, a large and restless Negro population and thousands of grumpy segregationists who have migrated from the Mississippi delta and the Arkansas lowlands."[70] Yet a small working coalition of black leaders and white liberals had formed and, for the time, had maintained the peace in the Bluff City. As segregation protests and anti-integration riots swept other cities, Memphians celebrated their city for keeping the peace through compromise — even as conservative whites, restless blacks, and other groups grew agitated.

Black and white moderates in Memphis hoped not only to preserve racial harmony, but also to distinguish their city from the rest of the South in the eyes of America. The face of moderation and reconciliation was the Community Relations Committee, a biracial group that included the editors of the two major white newspapers — Frank Ahlgren of the *Commercial Appeal* and Edward Meeman of the *Press-Scimitar* — as well as Hollis Price (African American president of LeMoyne-Owens College), Vasco Smith (a well-respected black dentist), and former reform mayor Edmund Orgill. Meeman said that "the committee had served as an arena of compromise, with everyone speaking 'honestly and candidly.' Once a decision is made, the group works quietly to put it into effect."[71] This quiet coalition of liberal Memphians saw themselves as a solid and respectful center, in opposition not only to the inflammatory, pro-segregationist Citizens' Council but also to the more "militant" black groups. Through their well-mannered, quiet work and their model of good conduct, the committee claimed to have created more employment opportunities for blacks and to have achieved the gradual integration of "most downtown hotels, restaurants, lunch counters and department stores."[72]

The peace, prosperity, and safety of the Cotton City contrasted with the turmoil in the Deep South. The president of Memphis State University (which had been exclusively white but had recently admitted 300 black students) proclaimed his pride "in the way we have conducted ourselves." Integration of the University of Mississippi in 1962 had precipitated rioting, but "during all the trouble at Ole Miss there was not one incident here."[73] The news reporters presented a portrait of a city still working out its relation to its Deep South neighbors, conscious of its image in the nation, and moving gradually in the direction of racial accommodation. Yet Vasco Smith noted that Memphians were also waiting nervously for national civil rights and voting rights legislation to take shape, for local alliances to strengthen, and for a potential backlash.[74] Asked what would happen if the legislation failed, Smith portrayed the dangers ahead for the politics of moderation: "Negro leadership will loose its effectiveness . . . it will have been repudiated and . . . the masses will take to the streets in a fearsome fashion."[75]

But many Memphians were already growing tired of this style of accommodation and leadership by committee, and their disenchantment sowed the seeds of greater racial discord. William Ingram had won the recent election for mayor without support from any of these leaders. Opposed by newspapers and most businessmen, Ingram had been backed by African Americans as well as white Citizens' Council members. One Memphian described this coalition as "an uprising of the unwashed" — groups that had grown weary, for different reasons, of accommodation, reconciliation, and moderation on the question of desegregation. Conservative whites and integrationist blacks were impressed with Ingram for very different reasons, and both rejected the advice of their "leaders."[76] Ingram's election was a harbinger of a populist uprising among the "unwashed" of Memphis — black and white — that pointed to increasing racial discord.

Inevitably, in this context the work of the sickle cell center in Memphis took on new meanings, and researchers were compelled more and more to address the concerns of ordinary patients and their communities. Lemuel Diggs would begin a set of studies of home remedies and of the day-to-day challenges of living with sickle cell disease, and he would hire an African American assistant named James Childs to work with him. It was also around this time that Diggs began to compile what would become over sixty volumes of writings on sickle cell disease, in an effort to make this knowledge available to anyone who was interested.[77] His colleague, Alfred Kraus, would turn to elucidating the mechanisms of sickle cell pain.[78] Diggs himself continued to promote the clinic's "particular emphasis on the recurrent crises which characterize this condition."[79] As a pathologist, he would focus most of his own research on rigorously documenting the various bodily lesions, pains, and ills that accompanied the disorder.[80] In so doing, he taught physicians and patients to visualize and recognize the telltale features of this still frequently misdiagnosed malady.[81] For Diggs, the disease's proper identification became even more of a cause than it had been in previous decades, for with proper clinical diagnosis came recognition and consciousness-raising within medicine, and this would have obvious implications for the advancement of patients — and of pathology as a science.

It was this goal of building clinical and community awareness that brought Diggs's laboratory technician, James Childs, into the offices of Memphis's Democratic congressman George Grider in November 1964 — an intersection of medicine and politics that revealed that, despite sickle cell disease's increasing cultural importance, it still fell well below the national radar of important political concerns. "He is an extremely intelligent Negro," wrote Grider, who "told me of the work that Dr. Diggs is doing on sicle [sic] cell problem among the Negroes . . . [with funds] from the Department of Health, Education and Welfare . . . and private contributions from Negroes."[82] James Childs's purpose in meeting with Grider was modest: "His main interest is making me aware of the problem . . . [and] at some future date . . . he may be able to come to Washington . . . to talk to me and Senator Bass."[83] But the matter went no further. Grider's major concerns in health politics would soon revolve around his defense of his support for Medicare legislation before conservative Memphians and his struggles with the Department of Health, Education, and Welfare (HEW) over the enforcement of the Civil Rights Act in hospital desegregation. Indeed, Grider was constantly on the defensive against Memphians hostile to integration. One citizen, for example, insisted that even Medicare was "not inspired by a desire to help the aged but simply another design on the part of the President and Congress to try to force white people into a close compoinship [*sic*] with negroes and get a little more of a strangle hold on the rights of the people."[84] Grider's moderate stance on such issues would draw intense criticism from his fellow white citizens and would lead eventually to his defeat by the conservative Republican Dan Kuykendall in the 1966 elections.[85] Thus, after meeting with Diggs's technician, Grider merely noted that "this [sickle cell research] seems like a very attractive and necessary activity and one that we ought to keep in our minds."[86] In the mid-1960s few national politicians like Grider kept their attention on sickle cell anemia, for its political significance was minor in comparison with civil rights, Medicare, and hospital desegregation.

After the summer of 1965, when rioting swept through Watts in Los Angeles, the politics of conciliation appeared to have reached its end.[87] One African American minister in Memphis suggested that all leaders were now challenged to speak a different language to black protesters. As Larry Haygood saw it, the "insurrection" in Los Angeles stemmed from the same forces that fed on poverty, ignorance, bigotry, and disease. The "Negro Revolution in L.A.," as Haygood called it, only highlighted the growing split among blacks themselves: "The masses of Negroes have been shortchanged in the entire Civil Rights struggle. . . . They are promised better housing, better jobs, better standards of living and better protection by law enforcement officers; nevertheless, they continue to go backward while the Negro Middle Class goes upward."[88] The disparity had left poor blacks like those in Watts "thoroughly disillusioned," wrote Haygood. "Not only do they no longer trust whites, but they no longer trust their own Negro leaders."[89] Moreover, rioters and looters had "manifested incivility, [in contrast with] the urbane, good manners that characterized the early demonstrations of the Negro movement."[90] As Richard King has recently argued, the militant "rhetoric of power" would soon supplant civil "freedom-talk."[91] From this point onward, black health discourse would reflect the shift in black political activism.

The scholarly output of Lemuel Diggs, Alfred Kraus, and Lorraine Kraus reveals much about the increasingly complex relationship between scientific knowledge of disease, clinical understanding of the sickle cell "crisis," and the social and political crises that raged in the 1960s outside the walls of the clinic. Through the early 1960s, the Krauses' research concerned the role of hemoglobin in disease and focused on making new hemoglobin-based discoveries that appeared to have little to do with patients' experiences. Writing on sickle cell disease in the 1966 edition of *Current Therapy*, for example, Alfred Kraus began his discussion of the disease by describing it as "a group of disorders having in common the presence of hemoglobin S [one variant of abnormal hemoglobin] in the red cells."[92] By contrast, one year earlier another author in the same textbook began by stating that "an understanding . . . of the types of crises in sickle cell anemia and some of its variations is essential for an approach to the treatment of these conditions."[93] For the Krauses (and Diggs), the two issues were closely connected, for they believed that the starting point for understanding any patient's experience with the disease was not the study of crises per se, but the study of abnormal hemoglobin itself.[94] Thus the discovery of a new hemoglobin variant in a patient in the Memphis clinic in the early 1960s was, in Alfred Kraus's view, a seminal event. The discovery of *Hemoglobin Memphis* added to the international cataloging of hemoglobin variations responsible for disease and put Memphis on the map of hemoglobin research at the same time that other laboratories were uncovering their own hemoglobin abnormalities. The new molecule became the focus of intensive investigation by Alfred Kraus in the mid-1960s.[95]

This study of hemoglobin was not without significance for patients, for Alfred and Lorraine Kraus both insisted that understanding the molecule would have far-reaching implications for the control of pain and the disease. They believed that knowledge of the basic mechanisms of disease, down to the level of molecular behavior, was essential for pursuing rational cures. They also assumed that the molecule somehow mediated pain. Between 1960 and 1969 Alfred Kraus published some sixteen articles on such hemoglobin variants, on the intricacies of various chemical interactions *within* the hemoglobin, and on how different hemoglobin molecules were manifested clinically as disease. Lorraine Kraus, a biochemist at the University of Tennessee, published similar studies. Her work too was built upon close scrutiny of *Hemoglobin Memphis* in the "propositus" — a scientific term for "patient zero," or the original person presenting the disorder whose case served as the basis for research. In one article, the Krauses suggested that manipulation of the red cells and the hemoglobin would naturally lead to alleviation of symptoms—pain, lethargy, infections, and so on. What was notable about *Hemoglobin Memphis*, they suggested, was that it did not follow the same "molecular behavior" as classic sickle cell disease when it was deprived of oxygen.[96] Looking closely at the interaction of alpha and beta components of these hemoglobin molecules, the Krauses' studies indicated that it was *intra-molecular* interaction that was "an essential part of the sickling phenomenon."[97] The Krauses' research thus pushed more deeply into the red blood cell, suggesting that this level of analysis might explain crucial differences among patients' experiences. As they reported, "The propositus and his niece, who have Hb Memphis/S [*Hemoglobin Memphis*], have little history of suffering from the typical painful crisis of the usual sickle cell anemia." Here was a milder disease associated with the new hemoglobin, suggesting that differences between the experience of patients were rooted in the hemoglobin.[98] As one 1967 overview of the research in the *Journal of the American Medical Association* noted, this work reflected the *possibility* of future therapies: "At the present stage of the work, Hemoglobin Memphis is characterized as an indication of a possible approach to gaining therapeutic control of sickle cell anemia."[99] But the discovery had no immediate implications for patients.[100]

Not surprisingly, given the tenor of 1960s politics, pressure was building for more immediate remedies. Pain management was quickly becoming one of the most important issues not only in science but in clinical medicine, as pain became the most central symptom in popular and professional representations of the malady. Sympathy for the pain of sicklers rose steadily, but Diggs and Alfred Kraus believed that there were clear limits (politically and clinically) on how far their clinic could go to alleviate pain.[101] From 1964 through 1967 all the articles on sickle cell disease in *Current Therapy* warned that "narcotics should be avoided if at all possible because of respiratory depression . . . and because of the danger of addiction."[102] Writing for the 1968 *Current Therapy*, Lemuel Diggs himself echoed this conservative warning, noting that "narcotics should be used sparingly in order to avoid addiction." Yet, unlike his predecessors, Diggs encouraged patients to use other home-based pain relief methods. "Home treatment of the minor painful episodes," he noted, "consists of hot baths, massage of involved areas if this gives comfort, forcing of fluids . . . every hour and alkalies by mouth."[103] But the 1969 edition of *Current Therapy* reflected a different perspective on pain in the profile of sickle cell anemia. Yale University pediatric hematologist Howard Pearson would document with great intricacy the nature of the crises, and he (unlike Diggs) voiced no objections at all to the use of possibly addictive medications.[104] In some contexts, then, liberal pain management might be endorsed—but in Memphis such therapy would remain controversial.

Such writing on pain and pain management continued to highlight the fact that the disease was an important "community relations" issue, but pain management would also test the limits of liberalism in medicine. The disease embodied other challenges in university-community relations as well. Articles in local papers suggested that a joint effort between the "University of Tennessee and Negro volunteers" against the malady was "helping to remove the stigma once attached to the disease and encouraging Negroes to work together to solve their problems."[105] One University of Pittsburgh hematologist recalled that in 1969 he "made a venture into the 'social' aspects of medicine" by starting "the Sickle Cell Society of Western Pennsylvania." "My principal motive," wrote Dane Boggs, "was based on what are now outmoded liberal type political beliefs; I thought I might prove more useful in that endeavor than in marching in support of 'open housing.'"[106] For his part, Lemuel Diggs argued that good relations between the university and the Memphis African American community had already helped to dispel the false notion that "our delving into it was a plot to make the race look bad."[107] Because the malady seemed to have broad implications for understanding the African American condition, many scholars felt compelled to extend their particular analyses of the disease (no matter how narrow) to touch upon questions of sweeping social significance—racial identity, black inheritance, and the problem of pain.

When asked in 1989 to recall the most important events in his research, Kraus noted that "one was the discovery of a new variety of hemoglobin which we named *hemoglobin Memphis*. We even made the *Commercial Appeal* at that time, had a picture in there."[108] But by the late 1960s, such discoveries and the promise of future pain relief were being challenged by calls for more immediate, tangible, therapeutic results. Scientific understanding, it seems, was not enough. By the end of the decade, the discourse of sickle cell anemia exemplified the rising importance of the patient's perspective on disease.[109] The pathology came to highlight not only the existence of pain, but also the problems inherent in pursuing a scientific understanding without also having immediate strategies for pain relief. In microcosm, the story of sickle cell disease exemplified a growing impatience with the pace of reform and a rising uneasiness among many African Americans about where liberal understandings of pain in black America would lead.

After 1968: Pain, Sympathy, and Black Power

In April 1968 civil rights leader Martin Luther King Jr. arrived in Memphis to support a strike of the city's garbage workers, and it was there that King was assassinated as he stood on the balcony of the Lorraine Motel. With one gunshot, the dream of peaceful racial accommodation seemed to end. In the wake of the assassination, the nation's eyes fell upon Memphis as a city that now symbolized racial hatred and intolerance, an archetype of the failure of southern race relations. White Memphians and their civic leaders struck a familiar, defensive pose. They believed they were being unfairly blamed for the murder of the civil rights leader; after all, King himself as well as his assassin, James Earl Ray, a man from Mississippi, were only visitors to Memphis. The tragedy, they believed, unfairly tarnished the city's good image.

The shocking murder motivated another wave of activism in race relations and black health care. As B. G. Mitchell, the president of the Memphis and Shelby County Medical Society saw it, "The tranquility of our community had been greatly disturbed by the horrendous murder of a national civil rights leader in our city." In the wake of the King assassination, "health care to the needy of this city remains a serious problem and one which deserves our attention."[110] One progressive commentator, J. Edwin Stanfield, wrote, "A former mayor is fond of saying that Memphis is 'always doing the right thing for the wrong reason,'" for "the city takes right action only when necessary to prevent a loss of its good image or economy."[111] King's assassination made the city and local institutions suddenly more vulnerable to criticism and thus more attentive to local suffering. St. Jude Children's Research Hospital began a malnutrition initiative and also jumpstarted a long-dormant sickle cell anemia research program, recruiting Dr. Rudolph Jackson to lead this effort and to do public relations work for the hospital.

For every era, there are characteristic diseases that attract public attention, and in every disease there are particular features that gain cultural currency and achieve high levels of popular visibility because they embody social concerns, cultural anxieties, and political realities.[112] As Lemuel Diggs later noted, "The main trouble with sickle cell anemia so far as the patients' discomfort is concerned . . . are what we call the sickle cell crises." These came "out of the clear sky oftentimes, very severe pains . . . in multiple parts of the body, but usually they are in the back or the bones . . . it makes them scream and cry . . . and it's the type of thing that occurs over again and really is the curse of the people who have sickle cell anemia."[113] It was not until the late 1960s, however, that sickle cell anemia developed this intricate social and clinical profile, driven by physicians' increasing attempts to identify with the anguish of African Americans who found themselves besieged by insidious, frequent attacks. One 1970 Memphis news story framed the disease as part of a people's struggle: "A Melrose High School student collapses with excruciating pain after playing basketball for three hours on a hot day, [another] boy wakes up screaming with pain in his back. A child continually sleeps in class, misses school because of illness, can't keep up with his school work, drops out. All are victims of an often misunderstood affliction — a biological quirk called 'sickle cell disease.'"[114] The sickle cell anemia experience thus took on political meanings, highlighting the need for understanding, sympathy in health care, and social relevance in research.

In subsequent years, the disease would acquire celebrity status, exemplifying even more dimensions of the African American experience — including black self-sufficiency, the dilemma of pain management and drug addiction, the role of the federal government in remedying racial and health inequalities, and the control of African American reproduction. Into the 1970s, the case of sickle cell anemia would inform these and an ever-widening variety of other social policy debates, from busing and special education to inner city drug abuse and black power. Sickle cell anemia would become a Black Panther Party concern and a rallying cry for black celebrities and sports stars. The disease would be thrust even further into the center of American popular culture, becoming a feature item on television and in motion pictures, as well as a campaign issue in national politics. In this context, pressure would build on the Memphis sickle cell clinic and others like it to deliver soon on the promise of therapy.[115]

6 Promising Therapy: Government Medicine on Beale Street

The year 1972 saw a new intensity of popular representations of sickle cell anemia in American society. The disease itself became a major political and media event. The vehicles of its popularity included a major motion picture starring Sidney Poitier, a made-for-television movie with Bill Cosby, several congressional hearings, and dedicated episodes of *Marcus Welby, M.D.* and *M.A.S.H.*[1] Along with this exposure and celebrity status came emphasis on different dimensions of the disease. As the malady became a national cultural symbol, many more groups with their own agendas entered the discussion about what it signified, reshaping the meaning of the disease both nationally and in cities like Memphis. In the Memphis tri-state metropolitan area (now an established center for biomedical research and health care), the meaning of sickle cell anemia moved outside of local control. It no longer had a predominantly local meaning as it had had in the 1950s. As the disease emerged as a national symbol through the late 1960s (reaching its peak in 1971–72), its public image reflected the political realities confronting African Americans. To understand the new face of sickle cell disease, it is crucial to understand the rise of black political clout in the wake of the Voting Rights Act of 1965, to examine how the disease experience became a cultural symbol for liberal Americans, and to explore the response of conservatives to the disease's celebrity and political significance.

In February 1971 Republican president Richard Nixon surprised many Americans by making sickle cell anemia part of his health message to Congress, thus putting it into the bright spotlight of presidential politics. In Nixon's portrayal, sickle cell anemia stood alongside cancer in defining the next major research challenges in biomedicine. "There are moments in biomedical research," he stated, "when problems begin to break open and results begin to pour in. . . . We believe that cancer research has reached such a point. . . . A second targeted disease for concentrated research should be sickle cell anemia." Using the image of a long-neglected disease, Nixon noted, "It is a sad and shameful fact that the causes of this disease have been largely neglected throughout our history. We cannot rewrite this record of neglect, but we can reverse it."[2] To remedy this neglect, he advocated that NIH set aside $5 million for sickle cell anemia research. The speech reflected the Republican president's pragmatism and his often-used strategy of pre-empting liberal domestic initiatives by co-opting aspects of the left's agenda into his own, while also appeasing conservatives and speaking for the concerns of a "silent majority."[3] One historian has labeled Nixon a "conservative in an age of change."[4] His embrace of sickle cell anemia along with the "War on Cancer" reflected this political maneuvering, and it also ushered in a new era in the national politics of disease research.

The years 1971–72 were eventful ones in the political economy of black health. They saw not only the enactment of national sickle cell anemia legislation by a liberal Democratic Congress and the Republican president, but also the discovery of the now notorious Tuskegee Study of untreated syphilis in black Alabama men. At the same time, a debate raged over Senator Edward Kennedy's proposal for national health insurance to cover large numbers of uninsured Americans. Political pressure on the medical research establishment was also rising, pushing health policy away from basic scientific research funding and toward medical care and research promising direct benefits to patients. Accordingly, these years saw an increased role for disease and health in American politics. Not coincidentally, these were the years in which sickle cell disease reached the pinnacle of its national visibility. Through the late 1950s and the 1960s, the symbolism of this disease — a malady defined by "pain and suffering long neglected" — had become well established in black communities. But the early 1970s brought new heights of cultural recognition in white communities as well as shameless politicization and celebrity for the once obscure disease. In the eyes of national politicians, many physicians, and other commentators, the malady seemed to illuminate "the race problem" itself in 1970s America.[5]

In this context, "victims" of disease emerged in greater numbers. Reform agendas formed around them, and advocates appeared to speak on their behalf when they could not speak for themselves. The 1970s saw the rise of distinctive patients' advocacy groups bent on shifting attention to patients' concerns rather than the promotion of research per se. Physicians and patients' groups both recognized the importance of lobbying politicians about the significance of particular disorders, and politicians in turn recognized the political appeal of particular disease stories.[6] Moreover, programs like Medicare had introduced a new type of consumer influence over local medical economies. As Tennessee's commissioner of public health, Eugene Fowinkle, noted in 1969, these programs provided "buying power for practically every person 65 years or older and enables them to go to a private market to purchase health care."[7] And by 1971 a new consumer health activism was maturing around women's health, abortion rights, and a wide range of health care issues.

The sickle cell patient was a particular kind of victim — an American consumer bearing a disturbing and disruptive cultural message. When the Ghanaian-born, British-educated sickle cell anemia researcher Felix Konotey-Ahulu gave talks in America in the early 1970s about the malady, he emphasized the "African-ness" of the disease, and later he came to stress the gap between Western medical understanding and traditional African knowledge of the disorder.[8] It was ironic to him that the West had only learned of this disease in the 1910s and had only recently begun to appreciate its links to Africa or the distinctiveness of the patients' experiences. In Ghana, he observed, the disorder had long been known and was named specifically for the intense and recurring bouts of pain that characterized the disorder. He wrote that "a peculiar syndrome of cold season rheumatism . . . [was] known to the inhabitants of the various West African tribes who gave specific names to the syndrome." All of these names, one of which was the Ga tribe's term *Chwech-weechwe*, "reflect the onomatopoeia of the repetitive gnawing pains characteristic of sickle cell crises."[9] Other names included the "Fante *Nwiiwii*, the Ewe *Nuiduidui*, and the Akan *Ahotutuo*."

This pattern of experiential naming became a clear example of the differences between Western medicine's fascination with blood cells and molecules and African medicine's historical concern for pain and the patient's experience. Konotey-Ahulu also emphasized the historical roots of knowledge in family lore, much of which anticipated modern medical understanding. "My forefathers knew that the disease tended to run in families," Konotey-Ahulu claimed, "and there was almost always an aunt who could be referred to as having the disease. . . . The conviction always was that the healthy parents [of the child with sickle cell disease] 'had it in the blood but did not themselves show it.'"[10] At the same time, Konotey-Ahulu suggested that African cultures had always been primarily concerned with the pain of sufferers. "Long before Linus Pauling found . . . that the hemoglobin of sickle cell anemia patients was molecularly different from normal hemoglobin A . . . our forefathers knew there were two common types of the *Chwechwechwe* syndrome which the Krobos called the *Gbagblaa* type (the severe one) and the *Pi-Gbagblaa* type (not so severe type)."[11] This tension between Western knowledge and African culture became a significant motif—for was the patient not best understood as a person with experiences rather than as merely a collection of cells and molecules? Such critiques of medical knowledge and its scientific discourses of disease became more prevalent in the 1970s and into the 1980s.[12]

Memphis sickle cell researcher Alfred Kraus recalled one other aspect of the disease politics of the time, noting that "this was the [era] of Martin Luther King and all the attention to blacks, and politically a situation where it was a good idea to look after blacks and maybe do something, so the politicians got into the game."[13] Indeed, few cities had felt the impact of civil rights and of King's assassination more immediately than Memphis. But federal agencies, recognizing the disease's political significance, had gotten "into the game" of sickle cell anemia funding well before King's assassination.[14] Yet, as Kraus noted, after 1968 national legislative attention to the disease would only continue to rise. Medicine was now central to Memphis's new economy, with the continuing decline in cotton and agriculture as the economic base of the Mid-South. In 1969 the city's hospitals provided over 2 million days of patient care per year. That year, the more than $250 million expended on health care made it the city's leading industry.[15] The hospitals employed 27,000 workers, a figure that grew with each year. At the same time, agricultural and manufacturing jobs steadily declined, throwing into even sharper relief the place of health care and medical research in the city's economic future.[16] Health and disease were therefore powerful issues in the local political economy, and any debate about health in the early 1970s attracted intense attention. Sickle cell disease became the focus of campaigns and public fund-raising efforts because of its immense value. In Memphis as in Washington, D.C., it was translated into a kind of cultural icon.[17] The malady's legislative history in 1971 and 1972 reflected wide recognition of this value, as well as the rise of black political power in the Democratic Party and the Republican Party's response to that power.

By 1972, sickle cell anemia had become entangled not only with political campaigning, but also with television, cinema, sports, and celebrity cultures. Like other high-profile diseases in the twentieth century (such as polio and AIDS, which both earned similar kinds of celebrity status), its significance was conveyed not by statistics or mortality rates alone, but by its image—by motion picture dramatizations, by made-for-television portrayals, and by fund-raising poster child appeals that played upon specific cultural anxieties of the time. Public attention to sickle cell anemia culminated in passage of national legislation in 1972, but to fully understand this legislation, it is important first to understand the ways in which the sickler was taken up and portrayed in American politics.

Black Celebrity and the Political War on Disease

By the 1950s and 1960s, celebrities had long been involved with disease causes. Danny Thomas's participation had been crucial, for example, in the founding and financing of St. Jude Children's Research Hospital, dedicated to research on childhood leukemia. His compassionate advocacy of these "innocent victims" followed in the tradition of stars like Eddie Cantor, who had taken a leading role in public campaigning against polio.[18] In the case of sickle cell anemia in the early 1970s, a number of African American personalities became associated with the disease, and through it they would represent the concerns of black communities. Celebrity status, however, was a double-edged sword, for it meant both wider visibility for the disorder and also the danger of hype and distortion that often accompanied fame.

Among those who took up the disease cause were sports stars, including champion boxers Muhammad Ali and Joe Frazier and acclaimed baseball players like Willie Stargell and "Doc" Ellis. Ellis was a particularly dramatic spokesman — he was not only an accomplished athlete but also a carrier of the sickle cell trait. Interviewed on a Washington, D.C., television station in August 1971 (in the midst of congressional hearings on sickle cell funding), Ellis gave personal testimony that he was one of the small number of people with the trait who actually experienced slight symptoms — occasional aching and "spells," as he put it. Even standing on the pitching mound in the midst of a game, he noted, "I have . . . [moments when] all the bones are aching in my joints. Plus I have fainting spells. I don't faint but I get faint. And like today during the first inning I felt that — faint, and the best thing that I did was to just stand still and try to shake it off."[19] As the interviewer concluded for her audience, Ellis had overcome these burdens and had done so dramatically, for "in spite of this, the trait has not affected his performance. Ellis is one of the National League's top pitchers with a record of 17 wins and 7 losses."[20] It was this image of success despite aches, pains, and adversity that drew the television cameras to Ellis and that drew Ellis's teammate Willie Stargell (along with thirty other athletes) to create the Black Athletes' Foundation for Sickle Cell Anemia.[21] At the same time, major movie actors like Bill Cosby and Sidney Poitier seized upon the drama of sickle cell anemia, crafting screen roles for themselves as the father of a sickle cell child (Cosby), or as the adoring lover of a beautiful, but ill-fated sickle cell victim (Poitier). Such staging impressed new meanings on sickle cell anemia as a disease of victims, as well as of heroes and survivors. As a new cultural icon, the malady was imported into popular entertainment, infiltrating a mass culture that sought ever-newer motifs to dramatize the black experience in America.

The targeting of sickle cell anemia for special legislation was in part a result of growing Democratic Party pressure for health reform, but it also reflected Nixon's political shrewdness and his overall fiscal conservatism.[22] As part of his "New Federalism"—a plan to limit the expansion of government—the president proposed to scale back spending, but he needed to do so in a politically feasible manner. In the case of medical funding, Nixon embraced research on a few important, high profile diseases like cancer even as he instructed the National Institutes of Health to reduce overall research expenditures. To pay for these initiatives, the president advocated no new expenditures, only a massive shifting of funds within a reduced NIH budget. By championing both the war on cancer and (surprising both his supporters and opponents) new research on sickle cell anemia in his February 1971 health message, he gained positive political attention for these bold initiatives while remaining true to his conservative ideals.

One researcher, writing to Memphis congressman Dan Kuykendall one month after Nixon's message, noted that the new, politically appealing focus on specific disease research was part of the president's compromise with "the Left." Researcher Marvin Sipperstein believed that "the philosophical change which is rapidly influencing the distribution of the NIH dollar [was] born of a . . . surprising ideological alliance between the 'new left's' demand for relevance in intellectual pursuits and the administration's press for the conquest of specific diseases."[23] The targeting of specific diseases had never before been imposed on the NIH so clearly from above. Rather, the Institutes had been given broad mandates and granted the freedom to determine research priorities. But a new agenda for research was taking shape in the political climate of the early 1970s—one that would have continuing implications for research politics in the 1980s and 1990s. The new agenda was born as Nixon responded to populist calls for "relevance" in research and acted to focus public attention on cancer and sickle cell disease rather than on cutbacks in research.

Nixon—and Memphis's Republican representative Dan Kuykendall, one of the president's staunchest congressional allies in the South—pushed vigorously for a fivefold increase in sickle cell anemia funding, thereby attempting to co-opt the celebrity cause. From the Democratic Party, Senators Edward Kennedy of Massachusetts and John Tunney of California supported even higher levels of funding, and they led the Senate hearings that would result in the passage of the Sickle Cell Anemia Control Act of 1972. The legislation proposed to increase funding for research, patient care, and reproductive counseling for parents at risk of having children with the disease. But it would stir deep resentment and controversy at both ends of the political spectrum. For many black Americans, the very term "control act" was an ominous indicator that the real goals of genetic counseling were eugenic in nature — a not-so-subtle effort to control black reproduction.[24] For some conservatives, on the other hand, this special legislation for a black disease represented a caving in to "special interests." Despite attacks from the Left and the Right, however, the act's passage served the political interests of Republican politicians like Nixon and Kuykendall, for they both had fostered a particular representation of the disease during 1971 and into the 1972 election year.

Their image of the malady was shaped by the new realities of electoral politics in the South and by the ways in which this new politics constrained the Republicans and forced them to co-opt liberal, Democratic issues, often in creative ways. In 1971–72, as the civil rights movement began to fragment, the voices of the Southern Christian Leadership Conference (SCLC) and the NAACP were overshadowed by those of Malcolm X's Black Muslim followers and by the Black Panther Party. This was true particularly in the North and West, but also to some degree in the South. The latter groups portrayed civil rights as a losing proposition, a benefit to the black middle class that held fewer tangible results for poor and working-class blacks. As Black Panther Kathleen Cleaver insisted, "It is the nature of a colonialist nation to create elite classes among its oppressed populations to exercise a form of indirect rule over the masses. The black bourgeoisie performs this function . . . in regard to the black masses."[25] It was in this context of fragmenting black social movements, when the power of revolutionary rhetoric was waning but still heated, that Nixon had called for sickle cell anemia legislation, thus allying his administration with the mainstream.[26]

The wheels of legislation moved quickly, for liberals, moderates, and conservatives all recognized the disease's potent symbolism. Even conservatives believed that legislation would show that government could address the concerns of pain and suffering in black communities, and many feared that without such legislation the poor and disenchanted would lend their support to "radical" and "revolutionary" causes. By October 8, 1971, bills calling for as much as $600 million for sickle cell anemia research had been introduced in both the House and Senate.[27] The Senate bill, introduced by John Tunney, had attracted a majority of senators from all regions and political positions as coauthors by the end of November. Some kind of legislation seemed assured. During the November hearings, a wide range of groups and individuals testified in support of the legislation, while the administration continued to oppose any bill that mandated additional spending. The Nixon administration (through Secretary of Health, Education, and Welfare Elliot Richardson) consistently argued that no new funds were needed and that it was well within the ability of NIH to reallocate dollars from its existing budget. This position was consistent with Nixon's 1968 campaign promise, and the president took pains to hold the line on spending as he looked to his upcoming reelection campaign. As historian Hugh Graham has noted, Nixon had been elected as a centrist in the 1968 three-way presidential elections "featuring Hubert Humphrey as the candidate of the liberal coalition and George Wallace as the protest candidate for disgruntled populists and Southern conservatives."[28] Throughout his first term, the president had practiced the politics of preemption, seeking to moderate and scale back rather than to repudiate entirely the liberal ideals set forth in Lyndon Johnson's Great Society programs.[29] Nixon's approach to health politics therefore reflected this position.[30]

Kuykendall, on the other hand, was a product of the increasingly disgruntled — and increasingly Republican — white southern voters, in a state that had swung dramatically toward the Republican Party. Until the mid-1950s, Memphis had been a solidly Democratic city, controlled by Boss Crump and his Democratic machinery. (While West Tennessee had always been Democratic, East Tennessee was staunchly Republican.) The battle over segregation and integration, however, had gradually transformed the party allegiances of white southerners. Whereas Memphis's Republican Party establishment in the 1920s and 1930s had been maintained by the city's leading black businessman, Robert Church, control of the local party was wrested from Church's supporters in the 1950s by angry segregationists with a wide and growing appeal. Kuykendall inherited this new Republican Party in the mid-1960s, with a firm backing of now-suburban white conservatives, who hoped he would hold the line against liberals and advocates of racial accommodation.[31] Yet many citizens thought the Republican Party was not conservative enough. Third-party presidential candidate George Wallace had done well in the Mid-

South in 1968. In 1970 Tennessee elected a Republican governor and placed a new Republican senator, William Brock, in office over the defeated liberal Democrat Albert Gore Sr.[32] Tennessee stood out even from other southern states at the time as solidly Republican in its leanings, but both Nixon and Kuykendall looked to the next elections in 1972 with some concern, for Wallace and his followers still represented a threat. Memphis, however, was a reliable Republican stronghold, in the midst of hostile Mid-South conservatism.

Kuykendall had built a close relationship with Nixon and with HEW Secretary Elliot Richardson and was a key coordinator of Nixon's Republican "captains," who would "fan out across the country, as time allows, to boost the 'Big Five'" issues, one of which was Nixon's health policy.[33] He was one of the most loyal of Nixon's followers, even in the darkest hours before the president's resignation in the face of the Watergate scandals.[34] Well before Watergate was a household word, Kuykendall openly promoted his allegiance to Nixon and made much of his involvement in national health politics — and of its benefits for the Memphis economy and citizens through 1971 and 1972. It was for local economic and electoral reasons as well as for national political reasons, then, that Kuykendall took up the flag of sickle cell anemia in 1971. In small part, Kuykendall merely climbed aboard a legislative juggernaut, hoping somehow to translate his support into some benefits for his Memphis constituency. But as we shall see, there were other pressing local reasons for his support of sickle cell legislation.

Speaking in the Senate on October 8, 1971, Tunney echoed Nixon's sentiments that "a deadly tragedy to thousands of black families in this country" had not been addressed. Sickle cell anemia, he said, "kills over half its victims before the age of 20." The poor record of support for this disease was made clear by contrasting research expenditures for sickle cell anemia with expenditures for other diseases. Senator Tunney noted that "sickle cell anemia occurs in roughly one in every 500 births of black children. Cystic fibrosis, a disease that affects primarily white persons, occurs with a frequency of one in 2,940. For muscular dystrophy [a disease with an apparently nonracial profile] the frequency is one in 5,000 and for phenylketonuria — commonly known as PKU — one in 10,000 births." Funding patterns in the private sector did not, apparently, coincide with this demographic profile. "In 1967, there were an estimated 1,155 new cases of sickle cell anemia," Tunney noted on the floor of the Senate, "1,206 of cystic fibrosis, 813 of muscular dystrophy, and 350 of PKU. Yet, in 1968, volunteer organizations raised $1.9 million for cystic fibrosis, $7.9 million for muscular dystrophy, but only $50,000 for sickle cell research."[35] Research knowledge and the spread of new diagnostic tests had highlighted the prevalence of these diseases, but because of massive disparities in private research funding, advances in treatment had not matched this diagnostic advance. It became the role of federal government to provide funding for care and research in order to redress such imbalances.

Just as many other commentators anthropomorphized sickle cell anemia, Tunney portrayed the disease as having *itself* suffered the neglect that black Americans experienced. "Sickle cell anemia for many years has been the victim of neglect," he noted. "That time must come to an end. No longer should black Americans be forced to wonder over the cause of that neglect."[36] Tunney insisted that the new legislation involved many voluntary initiatives for parents and sicklers — including disease screening, counseling, and family planning. By emphasizing voluntary participation, he hoped to avoid the impression of a heavy-handed, coercive federal effort to control the reproductive choices of black families. There was, then, some tension over what combination of methods — education, counseling, screening, research, therapy, and so on — would best accomplish the goal and control the disease.[37] But there was no doubt about *where* the war against the disease would be waged. As Tunney suggested, the malady was particularly an urban problem: "In cities with large black populations . . . sickle cell disease is not just another significant health problem, it is one of the more prevalent."[38] This meant that particular universities in urban centers stood to gain research dollars — and that there would be fierce political fighting for the funds.

The rapid movement of the legislation in 1971 and 1972 reveals the significance of the merging of disease funding politics with the politics of racial neglect — an issue that had cause some political embarrassment for the administration. It was in these very years that a memorandum by Nixon aide Daniel Patrick Moynihan (the liberal voice in the administration and later New York Democratic senator) suggested that civil rights issues would benefit from a period of "benign neglect."[39] Controversy soon followed Moynihan's remark. The statement prompted anger and protest among liberals and cemented their view of Nixon as cynical about civil rights issues, even those he embraced. The case of sickle cell anemia revealed, however, another side of the politics of neglect. For here was Nixon himself acknowledging a history of biomedical neglect and committing his government to reversing past wrongs, albeit in one small and symbolic area within the huge spectrum of racial and health care issues.

Municipal Medicine at the Pork Barrel

To fully understand Dan Kuykendall's support for sickle cell anemia in 1971, one must look to the local Memphis scene and to the local significance of the disease. Kuykendall's embrace of the malady signaled how much health politics had changed in America during the 1960s — and how much racial politics had changed in Memphis.[40] Racial animosity was still at high tide, and Memphians were still polarized — full of anger, resentment, and cynicism about government. Given the electorate's polarization, consensus was difficult to reach on any candidate, and Kuykendall's grasp on his own congressional district seemed tenuous. Certainly his embrace of black causes would not win supporters among Memphis's conservatives. White Memphians frequently complained to Kuykendall that they were fed up with even Nixon's racial accommodation. In April 1969, for example, one of Kuykendall's supporters wrote: "Even though I feel that President Nixon has done a much better job than the past two presidents. . . . I feel that he has, in his attempt to please the Liberals, lost sight of the 100,000 votes that Wallace received . . . and I am dismayed at the effort the Republican party is making to pamper the Negro and Ultra Liberal." The author also stressed that Kuykendall was in a tough electoral position. "Dan," he stated frankly, "I know your thinking well enough to know that you think the way I do, and I know you are in a ticklish spot and cannot say too much, but you are also in a spot where you can do a lot."[41] Clearly these supporters, wary of "pamper[ing] the Negro and Ultra Liberal," did not inspire the congressman's interest in sickle cell anemia.

Yet health and health care had become potent issues in local politics and local economics, and a congressman ignored them at his peril. Kuykendall's predecessor, Democrat George Grider, had lost public confidence over this very type of issue. In his time, the heated debates in health politics had been over Medicare legislation and the issue of Memphis hospitals' compliance with the Civil Rights Act.[42] Both had been his downfall. The dilemma at that time, as one newspaper put it, had been "how to increase the number of Negro patients in predominantly white hospitals — and vice versa — when the patients and the doctors who send them to hospitals don't cooperate." Memphians were slow to adapt to integration, while the federal government pushed for rapid change. This had placed Grider in an untenable spot. There would be a high cost in dollars for noncompliance; indeed, it was reported that "unless the hospitals come up with an answer within 30 days, they could lose millions of dollars in federal aid."[43] Grider was in the position of asking for time, understanding, and fairness from the Johnson administration while he struggled to explain the government's position and the economic consequences of inaction to local citizens.[44]

Kuykendall, by contrast, had built his conservative reputation by challenging liberal trends and government activism, beginning with an almost successful run for the Senate against Albert Gore Sr. in 1964. Kuykendall had earned a statewide reputation in that race, accusing Gore of deserting Tennessee with his moderate support for civil rights and attacking the Johnson administration for "galloping federalism"; he had also written off the black vote.[45] Having lost this bid, the Shelby County Republican turned his sights on the vulnerable congressional seat held by Grider. The district was growing increasingly conservative and was ripe for picking — not only because of the white backlash against civil rights, but also, ironically, because of the very redistricting that came in the wake of the Voting Rights Act.[46] Though more conservative and suburban than in the early 1960s, Grider's district was nearly 30 percent African American. So in 1966 Kuykendall was less dismissive of black voters than he had been in his statewide run, noting, "I certainly hope that we get more Negro votes than we have in the past and I have every reason to believe that we will, more this year than we did in 1964."[47] But in fact Kuykendall needed very little black support in sweeping Grider from office in 1966.

After entering Congress, Kuykendall (like all politicians in the 1960s) remained attuned to an explosive range of health care issues, among them the enactment — and the rising cost — of federal entitlements like Medicare and Medicaid in the late 1960s. Tennessee's decision to join the Medicaid program (a federal health insurance program for the poor that required state matching contributions) created a flow of dollars that put Memphis once again in a difficult regional position. The adjacent states did not act as quickly as Tennessee to provide matching state funds for Medicaid, and their slowness to accept the federal entitlement exposed old tensions between Memphis and people from Mississippi and Arkansas over indigent care. "I am in no mood to support a bunch of out-of-state freeloaders," wrote Memphian A. C. Halliday to the *Commercial Appeal* in 1969. Having just left one of the city hospitals, he stated: "My hospital bill was high because, in my estimation, I am paying the medical expense of a bunch of dead beats who are coming to Memphis for a free ride."[48] Such sentiments put the mayor of Memphis in the position of lobbying the state legislatures in Little Rock and Jackson to compensate his city for the care of their citizens when they crossed into Memphis seeking health care. Mayor Loeb estimated that the care of Arkansas indigents alone cost the city some $250,000 each year, and he threatened to "cutoff . . . treatment for nonpaying patients at Memphis city hospitals from Arkansas." Later Loeb "suspended the action [only] when Arkansas Senators agreed to sponsor a bill seeking more funds for Memphis."[49] By May 1969, bills to reimburse Memphis were moving through legislatures of both neighboring states.[50] Memphians also watched closely as the Mississippi legislature discussed whether to accept the Medicaid program. Some Memphians believed that "the Medicaid activity [in neighboring states] offers the best hope for financial relief for the city of Memphis hospitals."[51] In the years after Kuykendall took office, Medicaid was only the first among many controversies in health care politics.

The consequences of federal activism in health care were sweeping, altering the flow of patients and massive sums of money and reshaping regional politics. By 1971, when Kuykendall was entering his third term in office, elected officials were attuned to how decisions in Mississippi, Arkansas, and Washington, D.C., affected the flow of dollars and patients into their cities. Thus many of Kuykendall's positions on regional health care were designed to protect Memphis and to boost its booming health care economy. As long as health care was a subject in national politics, the congressman worked to ensure that Memphis institutions profited. In September 1971, for example, he fought vigorously at the statewide level against the creation of a new medical school in East Tennessee's Johnson City, "fearing any new facility would drain funds away from the state's only public medical school at the University of Tennessee Memphis."[52] At the same time, he lobbied fiercely for programs that brought federal grants to Memphis hospitals.

When new diseases like sickle cell anemia became the focus of political debate, Kuykendall examined the research and federal funding implications.[53] In his fourth term in Congress, now as an influential member of the House Commerce Committee and a vigorous supporter of the president, Kuykendall was in a position to craft legislation that brought more research dollars back to Memphis. The congressman boasted publicly about his ability to deliver for Memphis's health care institutions, for the Memphis economy, and for its citizens.[54] In early 1971, when St. Jude (which depended upon federal grants for 45 percent of its revenue) discovered that Washington fiscal belt-tightening would mean a large shortfall in its operating funds, Kuykendall had lobbied at HEW and resecured the funds for St. Jude.[55] The next May (a few months before the 1972 elections), he would attend a fund-raiser for the hospital with Danny Thomas and make "a surprise announcement of [an additional] five million dollars in federal aid for St. Jude." Asked how these "pennies from heaven materialized," Kuykendall bragged, "Let's face it. The White House is pretty deep in debt to me and I just cashed in a chip — a pretty big one."[56]

But perhaps the single most important factor explaining Kuykendall's embrace of sickle cell anemia was the changing electoral map in his congressional district after 1970. A nagging issue for the congressman throughout 1971 and 1972 was the problem, as one editorial put it, of "the changing complexion" of his district.[57] After the 1970 U.S. Census count revealed that Tennessee had experienced a loss of population relative to other states, it became clear that the state would suffer the loss of one congressional seat. Instead of nine representatives, as in the 1960s, Tennessee would have eight beginning with the 1972 elections — and the district lines would be redrawn before the elections. Kuykendall's Ninth District would be replaced by an Eighth District with a very different population profile.[58] As the Democratic-controlled state legislature took up the task of redistricting, one local columnist noted, "This puts Representative Dan K. in a peculiar situation." "Whatever the outcome of the district redrawings, [Kuykendall's district] won't be the 70 to 75 percent white nest of the past two elections. . . . That means that Kuykendall . . . must crack the black Democratic bloc . . . maybe by 15 or 20 percent, to hold the congressional seat." In Memphis, of course, it would be difficult for any Republican candidates "to win friends among Negro voters without . . . alienating their staunch white conservative supporters."[59] In his own words, Kuykendall was compelled to "build bridges to those in the Black community who share our sentiments about how the federal government should be run."[60] For Kuykendall and for Memphians in general, the rising issue of sickle cell anemia intersected with this new electoral map.

One of the ways Kuykendall intended to build those bridges was by appealing to a tiny core of conservative African Americans who had always supported the Republican Party. Another was the creation of a community liaison position, an emissary to the larger black community. The congressman (in conjunction with Republican U.S. senators Brock and Baker) hired a former police officer and GOP supporter named Edward Redditt to be their joint representative to several black community organizations. Redditt became the congressman's eyes and ears among Memphis's African Americans — defending Nixon as sensitive to black concerns whenever he was attacked, explaining Kuykendall's records, and also serving on the Memphis Sickle Cell Anemia Council.[61] Indeed, sickle cell anemia provided a final symbolic link between Kuykendall and the community — a convenient bit of masonry holding together this fragile bridge.

By now the malady resonated with meaning in Memphis's black community, but since that community was a diverse one, the meaning varied from group to group. A small community of black Republicans (businessmen, insurance executives, ministers, and the staff at the almost defunct *Memphis World* newspaper) shared Kuykendall's politics, gravitated toward Richard Nixon's message of black capitalism, and needed no additional coaxing or political symbolism.[62] But their influence both within the Republican Party and in Memphis was small. The more popular black newspaper, the *Tri-State Defender*, reflected the larger working-class black perspective — giving voice at the time to ideals of "black power," "self-sufficiency," and "social equality."[63] Where the *Defender* devoted much attention to sickle cell anemia in 1971 and 1972, a reader of the *Memphis World*, by contrast, might have missed the mere two mentions of the disease during the same period.[64] The *Defender* voiced deep skepticism about Nixon's and Kuykendall's motives. Its stories about sickle cell anemia emphasized black pride in the disease, the importance of self-sufficiency, and the value of building an accurate social awareness of the disease. As the debate over national legislation emerged, for example, one Tennessee state senator asked in its pages, "How can a President back a plan to spend $2.6 billion to conquer cancer, yet claim $5 million is enough to devote to a disease which attacks one in every 500 black children?"[65] At the same time, however, the *World* praised the president for his other initiatives. On one day in April 1972 when the *Defender* called attention to a local fund-raiser for sickle cell anemia, the *Memphis World* ignored the event, telling its readers instead about a *Wall Street Journal* article on the rising toll of heart disease — a disorder that killed many more Americans, black and white, than did sickle cell disease.[66] In general, then, readers of the *Tri-State Defender* would understand Nixon's "war on disease" as yet another cynical "power ploy," a gesture meant to "divide blacks with handouts to a few black elites."[67] The contrast between Kuykendall's representations of the disease and the *Defender*'s portrayals provides additional insight into these ideologies and into establishment Republicans' responses to these developments.

Widening public knowledge of the disease had already created unintended controversies. As early as January 1971, one researcher had noted that testing people for sickle cell trait could be misused and might pose psychological and social risks. Yet some scientists like Lemuel Diggs supported testing for the trait, not only because it was essential for the success of reproductive counseling, but also because (Diggs believed) the trait was not entirely benign for the carrier. Since the 1940s, when he did research for the Armed Forces Institute of Pathology, Diggs had believed that high altitudes posed special dangers for carriers. Other scientists disagreed. But in early 1971, the risks of high altitude to carriers became the focus of intense debate. Scientists, policymakers, and the public grew concerned about the possibility that sickle cell carrier tests could foster discrimination, since "these people will probably be excluded from such jobs as . . . airline pilot, and stewardess just when many opportunities are finally beginning to open up to blacks."[68] The plight of *all* black people applying for jobs and fearful of discrimination seemed to be symbolized by the question of testing for sickle cell trait. As one author noted, testing for trait and disease even had implications for the fight against poverty, for "not being able to enter the Armed Forces might be disastrous to a young man who wants to escape the ghetto if the sickle cell trait becomes a cause for draft exemption."[69] While thousands protested the draft and the Vietnam War, here was an imaginary scenario of a case where testing might actually prevent a young black man from serving his country and escaping poverty at the same time. In early 1971, then, representations of sickle cell anemia were intricately intertwined with African American aspirations, with debates about employment opportunities, and with the politics of discrimination. These very associations led, by mid-1971, to local television talk shows in Memphis — featuring Lemuel Diggs, Alfred Kraus, and Rudolph Jackson, the newly hired sickle cell researcher at St. Jude, as well as a medical representative of the NAACP — designed to address such concerns and "create community awareness of sickle cell anemia."[70]

Meanwhile, in hearings before House and Senate committees in Washington, D.C., Kuykendall and other Memphians showed that they too were aware of the malady — particularly as an economic issue. Memphis's geographical location and its large black population made it an ideal recipient for federal dollars for disease research. "[The disease incidence] varies in the United States," noted researcher Alfred Kraus. "There are pockets where the incidence is unusually high. One in North Carolina, for instance . . . Washington, D.C. has relatively lower incidence that Memphis . . . only about 7.5%. Washington is right between the northern cities like Chicago and New York." Memphis, however, stood out. "It is high here in the mid-south region . . . about 8.5% here, which is a little higher than the rest of the country."[71] Relative disease incidence and demography took on new significance in the competition for federal research dollars, especially with the envisioned cutbacks. In this competition, Memphis's disease burden, its proximity to poor states, and its status as a regional health care center was a great value, and in hearings on Capitol Hill, Memphians played up their regional role. "Actually," noted Kraus, "we are talking about an area encompassing part of Mississippi, Arkansas, Missouri, [and] a little of Kentucky. . . . Memphis has traditionally been the center of health care for that area."[72]

In his testimony in November 1971, Kuykendall echoed this line, but he also put his own conservative moral spin on the issue. Memphis, he pointed out to fellow congressmen, "has one of the largest concentrations of black people in the nation," as well as considerable research experience with the disease. But it was by connecting the malady with the drug problem that Kuykendall spoke a language that his conservative peers and followers could truly understand. He noted that "one of the byproducts of sickle cell anemia is a tendency to turn to narcotics because of the pain." In his view, this was a previously unseen face of the drug abuse problem, but he stressed that "sickle cell anemia victims turn to drugs not for the reasons that other young persons do, but simply to get relief from the excruciating pain."[73] In such statements, he wove the disease profile together with crime and drugs, themselves potent Republican issues. Nixon had made drug abuse a campaign issue, noting that some drug addicts were "victims" and warranted some small level of sympathy, while the drug dealers deserved only harsher prison sentences.[74] Kuykendall's implicit (if odd) commentary on sickle cell disease followed the Republican script, running parallel to Nixon's drug message. Both stressed that some preemptive therapy for victims was necessary unless these vulnerable people were to become casualties of the worsening drug problem.

Such concerns about drug addiction resonated throughout Memphis, shaping the character of television portrayals, church sermons, and even local clinical decision-making about pain relief. Indeed, addiction politics had found its way into church. One December 1971 Memphis television program, *Black Journal*, portrayed a Pentecostal church in Harlem so that local viewers could gain "insight into the life of an addict, the deterioration of his soul and body, the illegal methods of supporting his habit, and the struggle for mental and physical well being."[75] In addition, Alfred Kraus would recall that the use of potentially addictive pain management medications in the Memphis sickle cell clinic was something of a local taboo. The use of such drugs, Kraus observed, differed from one city to the next. "Chicago people [i.e., clinicians and researchers] may have done it differently than here," he noted. "I know the Oakland people disagree violently with what we do. They are very strong on management of the crises with pain killers, opiates and what-not. They feel that we under treat. We don't give it; we are too scared."[76] The political debate over drug abuse and addiction would only heighten the clinicians' fear. The power of Memphis conservatism reached directly into the clinic, revealing the sharp distinction between health care in the Bluff City and liberal Oakland, for example.

By early 1972, the mass media (television, radio, and motion pictures) as well as political campaigns had embraced sickle cell anemia as a fashionable cause. Preparations began for a new motion picture, *A Warm December*, in which Sidney Poitier would play a widowed American doctor in London who had fallen in love with a mysterious young African woman afflicted with sickle cell anemia. The doctor — renowned for establishing neighborhood clinics throughout a "world dangerously close to having too few doctors in too many places" — remained unaware of her condition and was confused by her enigmatic disappearances and her resistance to his advances. What begins as a film of love and intrigue turns into a film on health awareness as the doctor discovers her true condition. He explains to his young daughter that "one in five hundred American blacks have it. . . . It is a black disease." There is no cure, he continues, only "ways to treat the crises," and though "there are those who go into their thirties," many die earlier. Even as *A Warm December* went into production, national television specials were already dramatizing the disease. The local *Memphis Press-Scimitar* pointed to "two popular nighttime programs, *Marcus Welby, MD*, and a special movie starring Bill Cosby [that] dramatized the tragic impact of the disease."[77] Writers at the *Tri-State Defender*, however, were not impressed with these portraits. One article criticized the ways in which both Cosby's made-for-television movie and the episode of *Marcus Welby, M.D.* perpetuated false beliefs about the inability of sickle cell patients to "hold down jobs," as well as myths about their unreliability and their fragility. The analysis concluded, "Now it seems that the honest efforts of many will backfire if this kind of irresponsible dramatism and loose interpretation [of] medical facts is permitted to continue."[78] But loose interpretation — that is, bending the disease experience to suit the format of love stories, social dramas, or political commentary — was as inevitable in television and Hollywood as it was in politics.

By mid-1972, sickle cell anemia was being transformed by celebrity and becoming a well-known focus for black pride — and hence a potent political issue.[79] In cities like Oakland, Chicago, and Kansas City, it became a Black Panther political cause. Since the late 1960s, the Black Panther Party had advocated a radical, community-based self-sufficiency — brandishing weapons in the name of self-defense and engaging in armed standoffs with police in Oakland, where the national movement had a significant base. But as the Black Panthers came under legal and political attack amidst accusations of being more symbol than substance, they also took up the cause of building sickle cell disease awareness in organized health centers across the country.[80] This radical politics came to Memphis in June 1972, when the *Tri-State Defender* reported that hundreds of people attended a "black panther survival conference in Memphis," billed as "a means of unifying members of the oppressed communities around their own survival."[81]

Yet Black Panther Party politics in Memphis was decidedly less confrontational than in Oakland. For one thing, the *Defender* noted, "Dr. Alfred Kraus of the University of Tennessee . . . was there to carry out a Sickle Cell Anemia workshop," and also attending was the secretary of the regional sickle cell anemia council.[82] Such survival conferences appropriated sickle cell disease — a malady that had been often seen as a symbol of inherited black weakness — and turned it into a focus of community pride, strength, and self-sufficiency, uplift for the oppressed, and coalition-building for revolutionary social change. From this perspective, one local writer insisted that "finally sickle cell anemia is getting the attention it deserves, and black power is the reason why." Rudolph Jackson, the sickle cell researcher hired by St. Jude in the late 1960s (who had since moved to the National Institutes of Health), warned that in their efforts to gain legitimacy in black communities "some of the most militant groups, such as the Black Panthers, are now working against sickle cell disease."[83]

As different groups across the political spectrum placed their own meanings on the disease, it came to embody the social, political, and ideological tensions of the early 1970s. It could speak to the question of liberal government and federal race policy, and it could be molded to a conservative concern about drug addiction and excessive liberalism or to militant appeals for revolutionary change. For militants, moderates, liberals, and conservatives, there seemed to be many uses for sickle cell anemia. One Memphis newspaper, for example, commented that a case of a child with sickle cell disease shed new light on school integration and the busing crisis.[84] In the early 1970s, as a consequence of the disease's celebrity status, it came to stand for more than the patients' physical experience with pain or their struggle to be understood in society. Sickle cell disease could also stand apart from the patients themselves, a linchpin in many other political discourses. Any particular patient's experience — in the air force, on a school bus, in a classroom, or in a doctor's office seeking pain relief — could be read for its social and political meanings. As the disease became visible in this way, its utility in public discourse expanded greatly. Across the country, the disease took on meanings that would have been unimaginable in the 1930s (in the period of its deep obscurity) or in the 1950s (as it rose in local prominence as a matter associated with racial accommodation, civic pride, and faith in research).[85] In the early 1970s, the disease had come to bear the promise, and the enormous burden, of many political agendas.

Moreover, in the context of Washington's pork-barrel politics, the disease also grew in significance as a cash nexus. Cities like Memphis stood to gain from this national attention. On March 23, 1972, the House passed its version of sickle cell disease legislation. In May the House and Senate bills were reconciled and moved to the president's desk; on May 18 Nixon signed the Sickle Cell Anemia Control Act into law. After the event, Kuykendall seized the stage in Memphis, proudly announcing that the University of Tennessee's sickle cell clinic would become one of ten nationally funded centers — receiving nearly $500,000 in research aid. The only other southern city to become a center would be Augusta, Georgia.[86] As the *Press-Scimitar* reported, "Kuykendall (R-Tenn), whose congressional district was recently changed by the Democrats to include large numbers of blacks, made the grant announcement yesterday during a press conference at University of Tennessee."[87] Kuykendall's announcement could be read in many ways throughout the city. The congressman hoped that his own supporters would appreciate the economic windfall for Memphis health care. (Kuykendall had announced his successful lobbying for St. Jude federal funding at the same time.) The sickle cell story was also a major event for many black Memphians, but in the pages of the *Tri-State Defender*, Kuykendall was not the focus of attention. Rather, the newspaper praised "a group of Memphians of diverse political, racial, social and cultural backgrounds [who] worked hard to obtain the grant."[88] Few Memphians could be angry about the legislation, and no one could dispute that this was good for the health care business in the city. But some Memphians were cynical about Kuykendall's opportunism — especially as the details of the Control Act became more widely discussed.

The False Promise of Disease Celebrity

The Sickle Cell Anemia Control Act of 1972 created a wider knowledge of the malady, but it also provoked many new controversies. Throughout the legislative history of the Control Act, the Nixon administration had lobbied to show that new research could be undertaken by shifting funds within NIH's existing budget. It encouraged high profile gestures, including NIH's hiring of Rudolph Jackson from St. Jude in April 1972.[89] The Democratic Congress constantly pressed, however, for more funds for research than the administration had requested, and the final legislation also called for genetic counseling programs aimed at carriers of the trait. All of these areas — research, counseling, and the allocation of funds — had already stirred controversy, and the implementation of new initiatives would create even more. Before 1972, sickle cell anemia had become a symbol of neglect, but in the aftermath of legislation it would become a useful focal point for debates on many new topics — among them reproductive freedom in the black community.

During the congressional hearings, genetic counseling had emerged as a promising new method for identifying carriers and informing would-be parents of their status, so that if both were carriers they might either choose to avoid the 25 percent chance of having a child with sickle cell anemia or have children knowing the risks. Genetic counseling was presented as an efficient method of raising public awareness and of disease prevention, a new focus of health care that was especially promising in hereditary diseases (such as cystic fibrosis and Tay-Sachs disease) where the risk for two carriers having a child with the malady was quantifiable at 25 percent, or one in four. It was also a field fraught with controversy, however, even being described by some as the "new eugenics." Many states had passed, or were considering passing, laws for mandatory screening for sickle cell anemia and trait. The prospect of mandatory screening in schools, hospitals, and clinics reinforced the idea that genetic counseling had the capacity to deprive people of the basic right to make their own decisions about health care and reproduction.[90] The advent of reproductive counseling — in the era of abortion rights, *Roe v. Wade*, the first publication of *Our Bodies, Our Selves*, and broad struggles over women's reproductive rights — only aggravated the fears of many African Americans that counseling was a hidden form of population control.[91] In this context, participants in a national conference at Meharry Medical College in June 1972 attacked such laws for failing to protect patients' rights, insisting that "screening for the disease . . . should only be on a voluntary and confidential basis."[92] In promoting genetic counseling, surprisingly few legislators — black or white — foresaw the popular backlash against this perceived effort to "control" the reproduction of parents with sickle cell trait.

Another flash point was the question of whether the disease was evidence of hereditary African American inferiority. The argument over racial inferiority stretched back decades in the case of sickle cell disease — and centuries in other cases of race and diseases — but it reemerged suddenly in the late 1960s when physicist William Shockley and psychologist Arthur Jensen claimed that lower IQ test scores among African Americans was evidence of hereditary deficits in intelligence. Their arguments were intended as criticism of the "welfare state," and particularly of the liberal ideals that supported welfare spending. Shockley and Jensen argued that no amount of money or social engineering could change the racial differences in IQ and social achievement, which they believed were created by nature and sustained through inheritance.[93] These malicious assertions quickly became attached to the case of sickle cell anemia. In a March issue of the *Memphis Commercial Appeal*, one author (referring to two recent television movies) praised the shows for disputing that the sickle cell malady was "considered a 'racial disease' and, in some quarters, a mark of inferiority."[94] As Kuykendall himself noted in congressional hearings, "We have found in our attempts in demonstration projects in the city of Memphis, which has one of the largest concentrations of black people in the nation, that if this problem is not properly presented to the people, there appears to be a stigma which makes the citizenry reluctant to submit to a screening test."[95] Against the backdrop of the Shockley/Jensen assertions, the image of sickle cell anemia as an inherited black disease would inevitably carry connotations of inferiority. The popularity of Shockley's and Jensen's statements reinforced the perception that blacks and whites were indeed biologically different; the celebrity status of sickle cell disease suggested that there was merit in debating racial difference and inferiority.

Linus Pauling, now a Nobel laureate, had contributed to the "inferiority" label and to public anxiety about trait testing. Well known for his pathbreaking research on the role of hemoglobin in sickling, he now advocated extraordinary measures to prevent people with sickle cell trait — defined as heterozygotes in the language of biology — from having children. "Should not all young people be tested for heterozygosity in this gene?" he wondered in a 1968 *UCLA Law Review* article. "I have suggested that there should be tattooed on the forehead of every young person a symbol showing possession of the sickle-cell gene or whatever other similar gene . . . that he has been found to possess in a single dose."[96] To Pauling, this public marker could help these people identify one another. "If this were done, two young people carrying the same seriously defective gene in single dose would recognize this situation at first sight, and would refrain from falling in love with one another." In his view, the scheme would require "compulsory testing for defective genes before marriage, and some form of public or semi-public display of this possession, should be adopted."[97] Legislation in 1972 stopped far short of Pauling's outrageous scheme, but the damage had been done. The notion of publicly labeling carriers and controlling their childbearing in the name of "public health" had become respectable.

Memphis's Lemuel Diggs sought to limit the damage caused by the inferiority debates. In a letter to the *New England Journal of Medicine*, Diggs reminded fellow physicians not to make hasty generalizations about all African Americans and disease based on this single pathology. "It is to be remembered that 90 per cent or more of blacks in the United States and in the Caribbean area do not have sickle cell disease, and that the statistical chance that both parents will have the trait is approximately 1 percent."[98] On the other hand, Diggs sought the middle ground in the screening and counseling controversies, objecting to the characterization of genetic counseling as "black genocide." In the local Memphis press, he struggled to explain that white people also had cases of sickle cell anemia — as well as other comparable hemoglobin disorders. Indeed, Diggs noted, new theories suggested that the original sickle cell genetic defect probably did not even originate in Africa. Going farther back in evolutionary time, researchers now speculated that the genetic anomaly had probably migrated there from Asia. Using this array of data, Diggs insisted "that sickle cell is found among whites" and was "not a racial inferiority disease."[99]

By early 1972, these questions of "inferiority" had begun to overwhelm public discussions of the sickle cell experience. The prominence of a black "hereditary disease," if not the actual prevalence, gave a concrete example to those who wished to emphasize the existence of biological racial differences. The disorder could be coupled with IQ assertions to conveniently support arguments for innate racial inferiority. It was in this context that a former Memphis schoolteacher, Ernestine Flowers, began working with Diggs to address the actual problems of school performance in children with sickle cell anemia. Appealing for social understanding, Flowers acknowledged that "sickle cell children tend to achieve at lower levels educationally than their peers." But this was not because of their intelligence, and certainly not because of inherited deficits in intelligence. "It's not that they have lower intelligence but because they're so tired all the time that they can't listen and learn."[100] Such pleas for accurate understanding of the child's experience with sickle cell disease highlight the degree to which the ideological IQ controversy had overshadowed the discourse of illness experience, further revealing the downside of disease celebrity. The issues of

busing, education, inferiority, and genetic testing all tended to draw attention away from what it actually meant to live with the malady. The public
and professional debate had suddenly shifted, and the sweeping allegations
of biological inferiority supported many African Americans in their beliefs
that the black community was under assault — that genetic counselors and
disease screening programs secretly hoped to control and limit the reproduction of a "tainted" people.

Alfred Kraus (like Ernestine Flowers and others) struggled to maintain
the public's focus on clinical issues. For them, problems of school performance for sicklers was best understood through the clinical lens — for the
sickle cells flowing through the arteries, veins, and organs of sickle cell
patients tended to become trapped in minute places, clogging organs and
also causing brain infarcts and strokes, which had obvious implications for
slowing the mental capacity. Yet even these clinical assertions fostered the
stigma of inferiority.[101] Through these years, any discussions of the mental
status of children with sickle cell disease — no matter how well-meaning —
remained a sensitive issue. It was all too easy for those who wished to
promote black inferiority to use defensive, even compassionate, clinical
statements to support their sweeping claims about heredity and racial intelligence. By the early 1970s, this was one among the many controversies
spinning out from the disease's newfound celebrity. Medical authors found
themselves thrust into debates on inferiority, constantly attempting to set
the record straight. In 1973, for example, one writer in the *New England
Journal of Medicine* felt compelled to defend the intelligence of even the
carriers, insisting that "black children who carry one of the genes that
produce sickle cell anemia are healthy and normal, contrary to earlier reports that found them mentally and physically deficient."[102]

The disease experience was overshadowed as these issues revolved around
the status of the carrier, the question of black inferiority, and the defense
of reproductive freedom. Hoping to address these disturbing tendencies,
Kuykendall himself had focused on carriers in his congressional testimony.
He explained to his peers and the public that "the best way to explain the
disease is to give the true historical background. Being a carrier of the sickle
cell trait is not a weakness. It is not a stigma. Actually, it is a historical
strength. The sickle cell trait is a historical protection from malaria."[103]
Putting his best interpretation on this "historical strength," Kuykendall
speculated that the trait, rather than limiting employment opportunities, in
fact fostered new career options for black Americans. In a perverse use of
evolutionary theory, Kuykendall claimed that "an individual who has sickle

cell trait and desires to become a missionary in Africa would never have to worry about malaria. He is stronger there than any other people are."[104] Blacks might not be allowed to enter the air force, but they could become missionaries in Africa, for here, in their original homeland, their weakness was transformed into strength! Kuykendall's appeal to black biological strength demonstrated the extent to which the discourse on inferiority swelled around carriers and sicklers, drawing the entire "disease family" into debates about employment, opportunity, biological identity, and racial advancement in American society.

Thus, in the midst of rising celebrity, active political campaigning, and ideological posturing, sickle cell experts, patients, and advocates found themselves walking a tightrope, wavering in the spotlight between educating the public on one side and over-dramatizing the malady on the other. One Yale University pediatric hematologist, Howard Pearson, suggested that the problem with all this hype was that "education has been sorely neglected in the rush to run out and stick somebody and take his blood."[105] Screening and counseling programs had been hastily devised, and many were administered without regard to privacy and without awareness of the "eugenic implications" of genetic counseling. Writing in late 1972, Pearson concluded, "Perhaps we should wait until we have more to offer these people before we go around handing out such information [of sickle cell trait status] so casually."[106]

Ghanaian researcher Felix Konotey-Ahulu arrived in Memphis to speak on sickle cell anemia at the height of the disease's national celebrity in May 1972, giving Memphis researchers yet another opportunity to shape public opinion. Only a month earlier, Lemuel Diggs had traveled to Philadelphia to receive the Martin Luther King Medical Achievement Award as a "leading pioneer in the study and identification of sickle cell anemia" and for his lifelong dedication to the disease.[107] The event could be interpreted as a gesture of symbolic reconciliation between the King family and one accomplished citizen of the city where King was killed. Similarly, Konotey-Ahulu's arrival in Memphis a month later represented another symbolic moment — the arrival of an African perspective on the disorder. The Ghanaian researcher was pictured in the local papers standing alongside Diggs — two internationally renowned experts on the controversial disease. Sensitive to the stereotypes being generated about sickle cell anemia, Konotey-Ahulu spoke to his audience at the University of Tennessee about the pathology "in blacks and Caucasians."[108] In interviews during the visit, Diggs elaborated on his own belief that family planning should not be confused with population control. "It has nothing to do with racial genocide," he insisted.[109]

Because researchers were increasingly challenged to offer findings that were relevant to public debate, to social policy, and also to patient care, many of them began to turn toward the aggressive testing of purported cures in the early 1970s. Alfred Kraus's career, so closely linked to hemoglobin and the sickle cell crisis in the 1960s, would turn abruptly to the investigation of promising new desickling agents — chemical compounds that might prevent hemoglobin molecules from layering, thereby preventing sickling altogether. The shift reflected a new emphasis on bringing science into the clinic.

In the rush to find cures, however, other controversies arose. The pursuit of innovative treatments thrust the boldest researchers — and the most dramatic claims — into the intense media and political spotlight. Robert Nalbandian of the University of Michigan, for example, seized the moment. His claims about the benefits of urea in sickle cell disease had attracted optimistic media attention in 1971, despite their receiving no more than a "frosty assessment" from hematologists who bemoaned the fact that clinical studies supporting such optimism were insufficient. In practice, urea *was* an effective desickling agent, but it "worked" with rather severe side effects. Urea caused extensive dehydration, and its other effects had yet to be fully documented. Nalbandian, moreover, had administered urea to only two patients with sickle cell disease before declaring in a 1971 press conference that the new therapy was a success. Hematologists were immediately thrown into public debate. Many disputed outright the usefulness of the treatment, and they disagreed with Nalbandian's methods of seizing the media spotlight. As the *Medical World News* noted, "Charges of irresponsibility and sensationalism met with countercharges of scientific ignorance and illiteracy." As one Nalbandian critic explained, the hype around urea put patients in danger, for "as a result of the widespread publicity, I am afraid that some people are trying this therapy without proper guidance."[110] Others were more strident in their criticism, labeling Nalbandian's press statements as "terribly premature" and even "disgraceful." His defenders noted that the news briefing was "held primarily to find support for further urea trials," not to make therapeutic claims.[111] Clearly, researchers themselves were unsure how to proceed as they sought to be relevant, and as they turned directly into the glare of disease politics, racial controversies, and media attention.[112] Nalbandian had discovered an enormous public appetite for the promise — however remote and fleeting — of a cure.

The controversies over urea would produce a flurry of new clinical research activity promising dramatic "cures," but delivering few results. A new research agenda emerged that focused attention on the discovery and evaluation of a flood of potential new desickling agents, none of which would find their way into clinics. Some studies explored the possibilities of zinc and carbamyl phosphate, while others looked more closely at Nalbandian's claims about urea. Asked about urea in early 1972 after follow-up clinical studies had been done, Alfred Kraus noted that "the drug has a considerable drawback because it is a powerful diuretic, which means the patient must have large quantities of water because dehydration can cause a crisis." Urea therefore actually increased the likelihood of painful episodes. "Other drugs," noted Kraus, "may have the same benefits without the dangers."[113] Indeed, Kraus would participate in further studies of urea and other such agents, and in 1974 he took part in the powerful professional refutation of Nalbandian's claims about urea.[114] Kraus would pour his own effort into studying carbamyl phosphate, another promising—but ultimately ineffective—desickling agent. As head of a growing and productive research team, he would write some thirty-three professional articles on this and other compounds from 1970 to 1979.[115]

Public attention to sickle cell anemia thus came at a cost as popular and professional attitudes diverged dramatically in the early 1970s, shifting away from patients and reflecting diverse political positions. The atmosphere of sympathy for the patient's experience had been quickly transformed by new trends in research and social controversy about genetic counseling and black reproductive rights. Among physicians, scholars, and policymakers, questions of inferiority, addiction, and mental capacity came to symbolize the "real" problems inherent in sickle cell disease. For many black Americans, the disease now signified not pain and suffering per se, but the dangers of state-sponsored coercion and the loss of reproductive rights. By late 1972, many Memphians were also convinced that African Americans could be denied jobs or health insurance because they carried the trait.[116] For others, a new, hopeful era in aggressive therapeutic research had begun—but this boldness in research also posed many dangers to patients with the malady.

The Political Economy of Race Disease
In Memphis health care, however, the disease led to an economic infusion for the University of Tennessee—and here a few final ironies of disease celebrity emerge. The Sickle Cell Anemia Control Act was another brick in

the expansion of Memphis's health care infrastructure. Partly because of Kuykendall's influence, the University of Tennessee at Memphis had been selected as one of ten national locations for a federally financed comprehensive sickle cell center. As Kraus and others had successfully argued, Memphis was an ideal location. The notion of a comprehensive center was innovative, for it reflected the complexity of the disease experience. Patients with sickle cell disease suffered from a wide range of problems — infections, pain, blood clots — and they needed frequent transfusions as well as social support and guidance. To Kraus, "The idea [was to focus] the research activities of the entire University — all the various disciplines, basic sciences, and clinical — on sickle cell disease and trying to better delineate the disease itself and work out, if possible, means of management of the disorder."[117] By the early 1980s, federal funding for this center would be lost to other cities whose medical facilities defined more appealing research programs. But the University of Tennessee center had come a long way from its beginning as a small, one-man clinic — to earning national grants in the 1960s and becoming a national model for comprehensive care and integrated research in the early 1970s. Congressman Kuykendall would promote these accomplishments widely in his bid for reelection in 1972.[118]

But the politicization of sickle cell disease in the early 1970s only heightened competition among institutions for sickle cell funding and intensified the struggle for funding among other disease constituencies seeking relief for "their disease." Sensing the possible windfall in federal research dollars, for example, even St. Jude had climbed aboard the therapeutic bandwagon, "establishing a formal program for children with sickle cell anemia [and] a study . . . in 1971 to determine the effect of periodic blood transfusion on the frequency of crises, infections, hospitalizations, growth and development."[119] Nixon's targeting of disease fostered competition, but it also sowed seeds of resentment. Indeed, even black Americans wondered why sickle cell disease should be assigned a special status among pathologies when other health problems were even more important in black communities. In April 1972, for example, the Congressional Black Caucus embraced sickle cell legislation but also insisted that "the twisted priorities of government and grant-seeking institutes for concentrating on sickle cell anemia should be condemned, when essentially hypertension kills more Blacks in one year than Sickle Cell in twenty."[120] The caucus of black House members objected to the ways in which politicians and the research establishment capitalized on sickle cell disease, supporting instead the creation of a national sickle cell anemia center operated by the historically black schools of medicine at Howard and Meharry.[121]

Viewed from Memphis, the legislative process offered plenty of material to feed further cynicism about government and the role of disease as a commodity in federal research politics. According to Kraus, for example, "Nixon passed the legislation, but . . . it got funded in a backhanded way. . . . They took [research dollars] away from other things which made the other investigators very unhappy." "Cardiovascular disease [which saw its research funding drop in order to pay for sickle cell anemia programs] never got over it."[122] This tension among researchers, after all, was the obvious endpoint of Nixon's targeting specific diseases while reducing overall NIH spending. Compelled to find dollars to carry out the legislative mandate without specific new congressional appropriations, "the NIH was forced to take money from other things that they were supporting and put it into sickle cell."[123] The disease became a divisive issue, not only in society but also within the biomedical research establishment.

As one Memphis editorialist in late 1971 noted with obvious sarcasm, "It can be taken as an axiom of American life, that whenever a good cause comes along, those who would exploit it for their own advantage are never far behind. A case in point is sickle cell anemia."[124] To this writer, the administration's proposal to shift NIH research priorities was deeply troubling. "The best information is that the five million came out of research into hypertension (high blood pressure)." "Ironically," the author noted, "hypertension is a far worse killer of blacks than sickle cell anemia, and so in the long run Mr. Nixon has done black America no great favor with his little instance of robbing Peter to pay Paul for Dick's benefit."[125] The politics of health funding benefited not only Dick Nixon but also Dan Kuykendall. Both men won reelection in November 1972, Nixon by a landslide and Kuykendall — who gained about 11 percent of Memphis's black vote — with relative ease. (Two years later, however, he was defeated by Harold Ford, the first black person from Tennessee to serve as U.S. congressman in the twentieth century.)

In response to the cynicism about hypertension, a counselor at the Memphis sickle cell anemia center defended the allocation of dollars but also cautioned against the practice of pitting one disorder against another in the competition for public attention and research dollars. She bemoaned the competition for attention, noting that "the nation's effort to save people from hypertension and sickle cell anemia should be continued but not compared. We are dealing with human beings and not politics." Yet she also noted that the crucial difference between hypertension and sickle cell anemia was that "as sickle cell anemia is a hereditary disease, the danger of generations to come, to intermarry, and to transmit this disease, is growing."[126] The year 1972 had initiated an intense competition among disease constituencies — patients, families, advocacy groups, politicians, and researchers — for political appeal and funding.

The Cooley's anemia constituency, for example, had a powerful appeal, especially in the immediate wake of the legislative success of sickle cell anemia. Cooley's anemia, also known as thalassemia, was another hemoglobin-based, hereditary disorder with striking pathological similarities to sickle cell anemia. The disease also had an ethnic character, for it was more prevalent in Americans of Greek and Italian ancestry, and these patients and their advocates had an obvious question: Why was their disorder not given equal attention by Congress and the president? Members of Congress were compelled to respond for fear of being labeled as hypocrites. As Cooley's anemia legislation was crafted, the case struck many observers as "the epitome of the politicization of a disease." It seemed to reflect the "me-too-ism" that would come to define modern disease politics.[127] As *Science* magazine reported in November 1972, this political movement had its roots in cities with large concentrations of Greek and Italian Americans, cities like New Haven, Connecticut, where Congressman Robert Giaimo had taken up the cause. "A large number of his constituents are of Mediterranean ancestry and so is he," noted *Science*. Giaimo had insisted that "the federal government has been derelict in providing funds for research on this disease, which has certain similarities with sickle cell anemia," and his appeal had been heard.[128] A coalition of Cooley's anemia advocacy groups had quickly formed across the country, helping to increase pressure for legislation.[129] By late 1972, some observers believed that this was just the latest "ethnic disease of the month" — a phrase reflecting a distaste for the new disease politics and the competition for research funds on Capitol Hill.[130]

It would be wrong to conclude, however, that race and ethnicity were the only compelling forces shaping national disease politics in the early 1970s. Perhaps the most dramatic case of special disease funding in 1972 was the kidney disease legislation that passed Congress and was signed into law on October 30, 1972 — only a few days before the elections. The legislation — which ensured that all patients with kidney failure would receive Medicare funding for life-saving dialysis — was the epitome of that year's disease politics. Representatives of the National Association of Patients on Hemodialysis had explained their dilemma to the House Ways and Means Committee. The most dramatic moment of those hearings — an event that gained wide publicity — came when Shep Glazer, vice president of the group and a dialysis patient, underwent dialysis treatment before the committee.[131] Such staging highlighted the fact that members of Congress held life and death power over thousands of patients. The dialysis legislation dramatized the uneven distribution of medical care and underscored the role of the federal government in restoring equality to the free market in medical care.[132] In the broader context of liberal pressure for national health insurance, kidney dialysis — along with cancer and sickle cell disease — stood the best chance of legislative success, for these causes could be embraced by conservatives and moderates hoping to avoid more sweeping reforms. By the early 1970s, then, the story of sickle cell anemia was but one high-profile example among many of the ways in which patients' advocates, physicians and researchers, and consumer groups organized specific disease campaigns, put diseases on stage, and shaped federal health policy.

In the case of kidney disease, the new Medicare entitlement for kidney dialysis would lead to a dramatic expansion of Medicare costs — and its passage would only accelerate future drives for fiscal conservatism in health policy. In the case of sickle cell anemia, Nixon's initiative was also a mixed bag. It made the disease a divisive issue within society and within the biomedical research community, and there were many other ironies in this war on a "new" disease. The passage of mandatory screening initiatives stigmatized some children who were pulled from classes to be tested for the disease; confusion mounted over the differences between trait and disease; and directive counseling for carriers became associated with a "new eugenics." As we have seen, the passage of the Sickle Cell Anemia Control Act resulted in demands for "equal attention" to other ethnically specific, hereditary diseases — first from Greek and Italian Americans for Cooley's anemia, but later for people with Tay-Sachs disease.[133] Legislation that had emerged out of a political concern for African American pain had helped to give rise to a focus on "tainted" identities and helped to bring a new identity politics to the discourse of health care funding.

The focus on the patient's experience had given way to a new focus on the carrier, on reproductive decision-making, and on the social problems associated with the malady. Positive portrayals of African American pain and suffering gave way to defensive statements about the "fallacious theory that only blacks are victim of this peculiar disease" and insistence that "whites do indeed suffer from the disease." Other experts argued that "the black population has been subjected to so many myths that people don't realize this is a well researched disease."[134] Stigma and discrimination, it seemed, followed the disease as it rose to celebrity status. Its public image became a tangled mixture of clinical descriptions, scientific theories, and racial ideologies. How would this flood of information be sorted through and used? One author in the *Tri-State Defender* asserted that "employers who don't understand the sickle cell trait have in some instances fired employees who had it. Insurance companies have refused health insurance, and other have raised premiums."[135] Celebrity, in this telling, had put black consumers at increased risk.

Such concerns were intensified by yet another national controversy, for it was in this very year that the Tuskegee syphilis experiment scandal first attracted national press attention. In August 1972 details of the decades-long study of untreated syphilis in black men from rural Alabama became public. News stories documented how the U.S. Public Health Service had studied the progress of untreated syphilis in these men since the 1930s, and how the study had continued even after treatments became available. Characterized in the *Tri-State Defender* as a heinous act of "planned neglect," the experiment only fed suspicions about medical research among black Americans.[136] But if the Tuskegee study reflected a historical abuse of poor blacks that had only just been uncovered and was now mercifully ended, then sickle cell anemia opened another disturbing chapter in race and health in America. The new disease reflected a contemporary crisis at the intersection of black culture and American health care politics.

This was an environment where the politics of the carrier overwhelmed clinical descriptions and individual experiences of disease, in which the story of the now visible pathology reflected the continuing search for African American political power. The story of sickle cell disease in the early 1970s also revealed the ways in which the political process both channeled and deflected the popular activism of the time. It was a time of grudging recognition of the black experience, but it proved difficult to translate that awareness directly into health policy without creating enormous new stigmatizing burdens for black Americans and without fostering growing cynicism about racial politics.

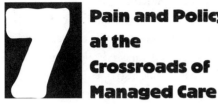

7 Pain and Policy at the Crossroads of Managed Care

In the 1930s, in juke joints throughout the Mid-South, blues musician Robert Johnson was heard singing the "Crossroads Blues." His words told of a fateful intersection where he struck a deal that changed his life. Johnson sang of how he went down to the crossroads and how he had sold his soul to the devil in exchange for uncommon speed and agility on the guitar. As blues scholar Francis Davis speculated, "Maybe the notion that a performer was evil incarnate . . . amounted to an insurance policy against some of the rough customers who assembled in the backwoods gambling dens."[1] Whether the song reflected authentic life experience or a stage persona invented as insurance against harm, Johnson's "Crossroads Blues" showed how chance encounters and dark exchanges could transform lives in the Delta.

Similarly checkered trade-offs have characterized the city of Memphis, its health care system, and, indeed, the evolution of sickle cell disease throughout the twentieth century. The crossroads city has been a place where perverse bargains were struck. Here men, women, and children migrated in the early twentieth century hoping to gain a new lease on life, making new arrangements — if not with the devil, with employers, city leaders, and the local political order — and reaping new rewards in the bargain.[2] Being a patient at the general hospital in the 1920s, 1930s, and 1940s, for example, meant that in exchange for access to free care and a chance for relief you also became a focus of medical education, or a potential subject for research. Even in the 1990s, in a municipal economy driven by new forces — Federal Express and tourism at Elvis's Graceland and the Civil Rights Museum — the city remained an important intersection of commercial and cultural exchange.

The rise of "managed care" in the form of a new initiative named Tenn-

Care brought Memphis medicine to its own crossroads — promising to redefine once again the economics of municipal medicine and bring speed and efficiency to a large, aging, economically ailing medical system.[3] In contrast to the 1960s and 1970s, when federal health care programs expanded precisely to remedy the exclusion of patients from a system defined by market forces and regional racial bias, the popular initiatives of the 1980s and 1990s turned this argument on its head. In the minds of many critics, TennCare, a state program that rejected the federal Medicaid program and committed to covering all poor Memphians while also opening their care to market competition and strict medical care guidelines, constituted another deal with dark, impersonal economic forces.

In early 1990s, Memphis children with sickle cell anemia encountered this new political and economic environment. How would their pain and the other dimensions of their experience be regarded in the context of managed care? Across the nation, many other patients and patient advocates wondered what the rise of an aggressive, market-oriented medicine spouting a tough fiscal ideology (embodied by hospital giants like Nashville's Columbia / HCA) would mean for their treatment.[4] The managed care model promised to remake the old health care system. It promoted the marketplace's supposed efficiencies and touted its ability to control costs, as opposed to the rising expenses and supposed waste of federal health care programs. Along with other trends, the rise of managed care would undermine those very urban academic medical centers that had flourished with the decades-long expansion of federal programs.[5] Sickle cell patients — beneficiaries of this expansion and of improvements in therapeutics — had also profited from health care activism and gained a higher but increasingly controversial public profile. Their care had improved further with the federal funding of comprehensive sickle cell centers. But these patients looked to the managed care trends of the 1990s and the early twenty-first century with some concern. Standing at the crossroads of managed care, they found themselves in a new political and economic climate that threatened to render their pain invisible once again.

To understand the recent history of sickle cell anemia we must examine the political forces and new economic ideologies that have brought people with the disorder to this new crossroads — including the declining sympathy for the pain and suffering of sickle cell anemia and the rise of market-oriented medicine. How would these issues resonate in Memphis and in the politics of regional health care? By the 1990s, new political realities had taken shape — most notably, Memphis's markedly diminished power within the state since the days of Boss Crump. Thus new dilemmas emerged for the sickle cell patient in the context of therapeutic innovation, marketing hype, and private medicine, amidst a growing crisis in urban academic health care and a rising tide of fiscal and social conservatism in medicine and society.

The Decline of Sympathy and the Threat of Invisibility

The contrast between the popular images of sickle cell anemia in the 1970s and in the 1990s offers a glimpse into the new health care environment — and into the threat of invisibility. In the early 1970s, sickle cell anemia had appeared on the national political scene as a case in point of long-ignored "pain and suffering" among African Americans. For liberals, moderates, and conservatives alike, the history of neglect and the disease's chronic, painful character seemed to reflect white America's neglect and misunderstanding of black health concerns — and demanded attention. The disease became a multipurpose metaphor, a proxy in social, economic, and political debates about a wide range of seemingly unrelated issues.[6] By 1971, it seemed to be relevant to debates about black intelligence and inferiority, reproduction and population control, busing and school integration, addiction and inner city pathology, and the aims and limitations of social liberalism. For some, sickle cell discourse also reflected the focus on the patients' experience of illness. Others would use the disease to highlight the need for a federal investment in research. "Research is being done all the time," said actor Sidney Poitier in his role as a physician in the 1973 sickle cell disease film, *A Warm December*. "Something can always break." For many, this investment in cures promised to restore equality in America.

Between the 1970s and the 1990s, these images changed significantly. Public commentators, for example, retreated strikingly from professing their unwavering social and professional sympathy for the painful experience of the sickler. At the peak of the disease's prominence in 1971, this image of authentic, often-ignored pain had become a dominant theme in the public discourse. One article in the pages of *Ebony* magazine, for example, highlighted the authenticity and gravity of pain for each individual sickler. "Go to any hospital frequented by blacks, and you will see them," the author wrote. "The one thing they will all have in common is the memory of excruciating pain."[7] Such stark and tragic descriptions of acute suffering could be found in mainstream magazines as well as in professional journals. Patients' bodies were "cramped and contorted with pain until, mercifully, they have perhaps lost consciousness."[8] In tracing the life of an elderly man with sickle cell anemia who had fought to become an accomplished physician, another author wrote of "the loneliness of his teen years," his struggles in a "life of chronic pain," and the frustration of "cradle-to-grave [medical] care to avoid crises."[9] In the early 1970s, hematological researchers like Johns Hopkins's Samuel Charache stressed that biomedicine had enormous difficulties measuring pain, but sympathetic professionals also emphasized the importance of believing in the authenticity of the patient's experience. Charache noted that "there is no diagnostic test that can rule out a crisis; unless there is concrete evidence to the contrary, the patient's statements [about pain] must be taken at face value."[10]

By contrast, some twenty years later, in a 1993 issue of *Discover* physician Elisabeth Rosenthal portrayed a new environment in which skepticism about this pain had not only appeared but also flourished (see illustrations). In her telling, many doctors had become frustrated by the constant persistent needs of the chronic illness, and their sense of sympathy for patients had been eroded. To dramatize her point, Rosenthal presented the case of Livinia Johnson, a woman whom Rosenthal had treated for over seven years. Johnson appeared in the clinic one day (as she often did) seeking pain medication. "We give lots of fluids to keep the blood thin and flowing as freely as possible and to prevent dehydration," noted Rosenthal. In pain management, however, the problem of narcotic painkillers had become controversial. "All sicklers . . . know by heart the pain cocktail that works best for them," said Rosenthal, but many health care practitioners doubted the need for pain medication. " 'You're giving her 125 milligrams of Demerol?' one doctor asks as he peers over my shoulder. 'I don't know. She sure looks good to me.' 'I think she's faking,' a nurse weighs in. 'Out in the waiting room she was writhing in pain, but I just passed by her room and she was *reading*.' "[11] Where in the 1970s the acknowledgment of pain had been deeply intertwined with rising respect for the patient's experience as a clinical and political issue, the question that emerges from Rosenthal's disturbing account is what cultural concerns and issues informed this growing skepticism about pain in the 1990s, and what does it reflect about the new crossroads of managed care?[12]

The seeds of skepticism were already being sown in the early 1970s, at the peak of sickle cell disease's own celebrity. For some observers, the disease's prominence symbolized a disturbing special-interest, "ethnic disease politics," in which national research priorities were being reshaped by consumer demand, political activism, pressure groups, and celebrities rallying around illnesses, favoring particular sufferers as more worthy than others. To many researchers in the 1970s (even to those sympathetic with the goals of civil rights and racial advancement), the shift in research funding to sickle cell disease and away from cardiovascular disease represented a disturbing trend.[13] The politics of funding for sickle cell anemia, cancer, Cooley's anemia, and end-stage renal disease was a harbinger of a spirited disease politics driven by patients' constituencies and their allies in the research community; this is a politics that was also reflected in the 1980s and 1990s in the history of AIDS, breast cancer, prostate cancer, and other disorders.[14] This kind of disease politics rode the waves of high expectations that new research initiatives could solve disease problems — if only enough dollars were devoted to the effort. Yet beneath the waves of optimism were powerful undercurrents of skepticism — about preferential disease targeting, about the scope and cost of such government programs, and about whether researchers could really deliver on their therapeutic promises. Even among black Americans, for example, the Sickle Cell Anemia Control Act had represented an overextension of federal power into delicate matters of family and reproductive freedom.

The early 1970s also saw the emergence of fiscal anxieties about the rising cost of health care and witnessed the legislative birth of health maintenance organizations (HMOs). These fiscal concerns would build steadily toward TennCare, toward privatization, and toward managed care in the 1990s. Within a year of signing sickle cell anemia legislation, President Nixon also signed into law the Health Maintenance Organization Act of 1973, seeking to accomplish through the market what Democrat Edward Kennedy's national health insurance proposal sought, in part, to accomplish — to limit the rising cost of health care.[15] Decades later, this goal would be a key appeal of managed care — using market competition to discipline consumer demand, to restrict health care providers from ordering too many tests, and to take over the administration of programs like Medicaid in an effort to limit their growth. In the conservative environment of the 1980s and 1990s, critics of federal health care programs increasingly heralded the notion that "free-market discipline" was an effective tool for controlling cost, for scaling back the expensive ideals of the 1960s, and for subsuming these ideals to the greater good of fiscal conservatism. Over the last two decades of the twentieth century, even as sickle cell disease continued to attract headlines, the very meaning of the ailment was changing again.

Perhaps most notably, fear of drug addiction had also intensified, providing a powerful backdrop for skepticism about the patient's pain in sickle cell anemia. As Elisabeth Rosenthal noted, "In this emergency room, because of both the nature of the disease and the nature of the neighborhood we're in, [sickle cell anemia] is seen most often in young, poor blacks — the very same population in which we most worry about narcotic addiction in the first place." "Add all this up," she concluded, "and it becomes way too easy for jaded doctors and nurses to dismiss a young sickle-cell patient as a faker just out to get drugs."[16] Amidst fears of addiction, drug abuse, and "fakers" duping the system (recalling, for example, Ronald Reagan's campaign indictment of "welfare queens driving Cadillacs"), it is not surprising that skepticism of patients' pain experience could be found in numerous other settings.[17] One New York patient recalled being told by an unsympathetic nurse, "I'm going to continue to bring your medicine late, and I'm going to do it on purpose because I know that you do not require this medication. You should just get out of bed right now because you're not sick, you're just faking it. You just want this drug like the rest of them."[18] A New York hematologist acknowledged that anxieties about race and frustrations with the management of chronic illness informed all of these therapeutic encounters in the 1990s. "There is a racial undertone to it," commented Ronald Nagel. "They become known as repeaters, so they get really bad medical care. They're left to the last."[19] As another author said, "Fear of addiction persists among providers despite facts that addiction resulting solely from hospital medication is rare, and that sickle cell disease patients are [themselves] deeply concerned over the side-effects of analgesics."[20] Thus, to some clinicians in the 1990s, the fear of addiction (however unwarranted and even irrational) persisted, sustained by a larger matrix of racial stereotypes and urban anxieties regarding drug abuse. These were reflections of disturbing general trends, for other medical studies confirmed that pain experienced by African Americans and ethnic minorities frequently went undertreated whatever its origin.[21]

In cities like Memphis with large populations of poor African Americans, according to local testimony the question of pain management was shaped by a deep-seated moral conservatism regarding drug abuse.[22] In Memphis, pain management in sickle cell disease had always been approached with trepidation. Alfred Kraus had commented on the local fear of using narcotics therapeutically and "creating addicts," but these fears reflected more the cultural climate than clinical observations. Kraus himself contended that the link between narcotic pain management and addiction was a weak one. "All these people that have painful episodes over and over again are given narcotics . . . [but] you can figure the ones with narcotic addiction on the fingers of one hand. I can think of two at the moment."[23] Kraus argued that "it takes the psychology of a drug addict" rather than frequent medication alone to create actual addiction behavior; addiction, he contended, was rarely the case in sickle cell anemia. In contrast to Kraus, Lemuel Diggs often gave more weight to his own (and his community's) fear of sickle cell addiction.[24] In the 1980s he stated that "what we recommend to do at home in the first place is to keep warm, and to drink plenty of water and to take simple pain remedies like aspirin and Tylenol — that type of thing, rather than go into the narcotics which they may become addicted to."[25] Recommendations on pain management varied by individual caregiver and by context. Other medical centers, depending on their locale and cultural environment, perhaps could afford to be more liberal and sympathetic.

Even as pain management attracted public and professional attention, skepticism blossomed (even in clinical discussions) about the authenticity of pain.[26] The transformation of pain discourse reflected the crisis of liberalism and the rising skepticism in mainstream white America about the authenticity of African Americans' presentations of their plight — a hallmark of late-twentieth-century conservatism. Clinical observations and decisions in the 1990s (as throughout the twentieth century) continued to be influenced by these political crises and anxieties, and by stereotypes about race and poverty. At work in these discussions were deeply rooted notions about black people, their inner city pathologies, and drug-seeking in urban America. In assessing pain, still sympathetic physicians found themselves struggling against the shifting tide to highlight the obstacles faced by sufferers, the immeasurable intensity of their pain, and the need for proper clinical recognition. As Charache stated in 1982, "Sickle cell anemia . . . occurs in black patients who still face obstacles that whites don't appreciate. . . . Treatable complaints must be recognized, painful episodes must be managed with knowledge that no type of pain is exclusively physical or mental."[27] Others, however, could only see the issue of pain management against the backdrop of the rising cost of liberal treatments for such chronic illnesses, an especially important issue for Medicaid patients (most of whom were white, but a disproportionate number of whom were black). As a sign of the growing tendency to rethink pain management in precisely this group, two authors in 1993 bemoaned the fact that "Medicaid patients [in hematology/oncology practices] received the most expensive class of pain medications at a significantly higher rate than other patients."[28] The treatment of sickle cell pain became a metaphor for the fact that the rising cost of liberal sympathy was paid by all American taxpayers.

The new image of sickle cell disease — as an expensive, inner city, chronic illness in which too-liberal pain management might actually *produce* drug addicts — reflected the changing political landscape. For one researcher writing in 1989, the treatment of the sickle cell "crisis" itself reflected a crisis of patient credibility. In the face of clinical inability to measure pain and to verify it in medicine's own objective terms, "the physician has only the patient's report of pain on which to base treatment and diagnosis decisions."[29] While this author confessed that there were some legitimate "risks of iatrogenic addiction," he insisted that addiction behaviors — involving hording, theft, self-administration, and solicitation — were rarely evident among patients with sickle cell anemia. Yet the question of their credibility and of the authenticity of self-reporting pain persisted. Some physicians felt compelled to insist that ignoring pain was dangerous in itself — for pain was a clinical "harbinger of potential catastrophe," correlating with lack of oxygen, stroke, and even death.[30]

In the 1970s sympathy for pain had been rooted in a pervasive cultural endorsement of the principle of restorative justice — a powerful motif embracing activism in the righting of past wrongs. Increasingly in the 1970s and into 1980s and 1990s, sickle cell physicians had good reasons to ally themselves with these ideals, and to identify with the experiences of their patients, since they shared a mutual interest in making the plight of sickle cell victims more visible. But in the increasingly conservative environment of the 1990s, many such specialists realized that they needed to explain their sympathies in other ways. Boston hematologist Orah Platt, for example, pointed to history, reminding her peers that "pain is such a regular feature of sickle cell anemia that in some African languages the disease is referred to as 'a state of suffering.'"[31] Others would compare the experience of the sickler with other familiar cases of ignored pain in chronic disease such as cancer, terminal illness, and in emergency room care.[32]

The crucial problem with pain in medicine, of course, was that it was invisible within the culture of clinical measurement. The reliable measurement of pain had always eluded medicine. Medical scientists had evolved no routine methods for transforming the patient's experience to graphical representation. Thus pain continued to exist in the realm of the subjective — and because of it, medical professionals regarded self-reporting of pain with suspicion. This was as true in new diseases fighting to establish themselves in the 1980s, such as chronic fatigue syndrome, as it was in established diseases like sickle cell anemia.[33] Medical practitioners' very inability to speak "objectively" on the topic merely accentuated the power of cultural assumptions in their clinical practices.[34]

But even as the principles and values underlying pain management were loudly debated, the economic and political context of these discussions was changing. In conducting their studies and writing articles on pain management in sickle cell anemia, researchers in the 1990s — whether they acknowledged it or not — were shedding light on the late-twentieth-century political economy of race and health care. To many observers, liberal, compassionate relief from pain seemed increasingly inconsistent with political trends and also with dominant fiscal concerns. Many researchers and physicians now asked, Can we afford therapeutic compassion? Is medicine's compassion misplaced? How are we best to study and understand the phenomenon of pain in sickle cell anemia? Against this backdrop, some pediatricians and hematologists bemoaned the fact that "the gatekeeper model used by many managed care plans poses a major barrier to appropriate care of children and adolescents with sickle cell disease."[35] As this writer also noted, patients turned to the courts more and more to protest these trends: "It is probably no coincidence that in this decade, as managed care has made enormous inroads, malpractice litigation for sickle cell disease has jumped 10-fold."[36]

The political shaping of therapy was also evident in the way that doctors, researchers, and policymakers talked about other clinical dilemmas surrounding sickle cell disease — including infection management, bone marrow transplantation, and the continuing search for innovative treatments. Before exploring how these dramas played out in Memphis, we will look at how these other therapeutic discourses overlapped with and informed images of race and the inner city, and what they reveal about the changing medical marketplace in the 1980s and 1990s.

The Patient and the Medical Marketplace

Amidst these discussions about pain, parallel discussions emerged around other therapies as innovation marched on, producing several "breakthroughs" in sickle cell anemia — many of which fell short of their promise. But whether successful or not, each innovation illuminates how economic trends in corporate, market-driven medicine drove patients along different trajectories.[37] Some of these breakthroughs could be characterized as public relations ploys, some of them resulted in only partially effective treatments, and some of them were authentic cures that unfortunately fell within the reach of only a few patients. Considered together, they exemplify how late-twentieth-century health care marketing could promote each development as a cure when it was, at best, a small therapeutic improvement. Moreover, market medicine — which imposed its own rationing logic — put most of these "cures" well beyond the reach of most consumers and posed different kinds of problems for patients.[38]

A good example of hype and undelivered promise was the story of a drug called 5-azacytidine. In 1982 *Newsweek* reported that the cancer drug had resulted in "a sharp rise in hemoglobin levels and . . . improvement in symptoms" not only in sickle cell anemia but also in beta-thalassemia.[39] In particular, the drug stimulated the production of fetal hemoglobin — a form of hemoglobin that did not sickle as readily as adult hemoglobin in sickle cell disease and that the body usually ceased producing shortly after infancy. At the same time, the public was quick to note that the drug appeared to work in a unique way, for it seemed "to reactivate apparently intact genes that had been dormant since birth." Statements such as these envisioned the new drugs as harbingers of a future of genetic medicine. This was to be an era in which "doctors hope[d] eventually to use recombinant DNA techniques to cut out 'bad' genes and substitute 'good' ones."[40] Echoing wide professional enthusiasm, such popular press articles embraced the forward-looking, optimistic interpretation of the 5-azacytidine findings. Researchers themselves proclaimed, as they had in the case of urea, that "a major new step in treating disease [has demonstrated] beyond doubt that genetic manipulation has come to the bedside."[41]

But by the late 1980s, the promise of 5-azacytidine had crumbled. It had produced no actual benefits for patients and, indeed, had subjected them to increased risks of contracting cancer.[42] Still, the vision of hemoglobin manipulation was widely embraced, and other researchers championed the "long-term goal of gene therapy for sickle cell disease . . . [which seemed to] only await additional technical advances for increasing the efficiency of gene transfer and the level of gene expression."[43] In general, the mid-1980s saw an upsurge of interest in the genetic manipulation of disease and in a variety of "gene therapies" for intractable disorders like sickle cell anemia. Other long-time sickle cell anemia researchers endorsed the vision, agreeing that "replacing defective genes with normal ones [would be] 'the ultimate therapy,'" for it would represent the culmination of Pauling's pioneering work, as well as the final manifestation of a search for a usable desickling agent.[44]

The advent of Bristol-Myers's cancer drug hydroxyurea (HU) in the 1990s was part of this turn toward the use of recombinant DNA techniques in drug production. For some, the emergence of HU represented a culmination of this "genetic" therapy research program — manipulating the body to alter the way it produced a protein, without direct manipulation of the genetic material of patients. This agent was one of a new class of drugs that held "dazzling promises," just as urea had in the 1970s and 5-azacytidine had in the 1980s. Marketed by Bristol-Myers, HU had been used first to treat leukemia, but in the early 1990s clinical trials of the new drug on sickle cell anemia had begun. The *Wall Street Journal*, other news media, and professionals greeted these trials with a modest amount of fanfare. HU was seen as the long sought after "genetic switch" for regulating sickle cell anemia.[45] Just like 5-azacytidine, it triggered the production of fetal hemoglobin. The drug showed promise not only for stimulating fetal hemoglobin (HbF), but also for decreasing the number of painful crises, thereby accomplishing several goals. It mitigated the patient's pain, and it could reduce hospitalization—thus saving money in a society increasingly obsessed with the rising costs of health care. HU appeared to be a perfect drug for addressing the biological, experiential, and social problems represented by sickle cell anemia patients in the early 1990s.

But the question of the safety of the new agent remained unresolved. Similar to the history of knee-jerk enthusiasm for urea and 5-azacytidine, the question of side effects remained peripheral amidst the growing HU fanfare. As researchers had begun clinical trials on 5-azacytidine, they had learned that it was carcinogenic in laboratory animals. Against the backdrop of urea and 5-azacytidine, then, researchers greeted hydroxyurea with a mixture of optimism and caution. One well-established sickle cell anemia researcher, Hopkins's Samuel Charache, noted that although early studies revealed that the number of crises had clearly decreased with administration of HU, the agent was still considered a "dangerous drug." Its side effects remained unstudied. Moreover, the question of how to use HU to address pain would continue to pose obstacles. As Charache noted in 1990, "We have never precisely defined what crises are[,] and placebo effects are very powerful, so even though [preliminary studies of HU] came out the way we'd like, this doesn't really mean anything. We have to do a controlled trial before anyone is going to believe that HU does anything for these patients."[46]

In their rapid embrace of the latest "breakthrough cure," popular and professional discussions ignored many of these limitations. Widespread endorsement for the Bristol-Myers drug catapulted it into the mainstream media. Even though HU's only therapeutic promise lay in its potential for reducing crises (rather than eliminating them altogether), some professionals spoke of this "genetic switch" in exalted terms. "For the first time," stated NIH researcher Griffin Rodgers, "we're treating the underlying disease, instead of simply the complications."[47] In fact, however, HU only treated pain—a complication of the disorder—and it did so incompletely. But as researcher Howard Pearson commented, "Effective pharmacologic therapy for the hemoglobinopathies has been a Holy Grail sought by several generations of clinical investigators."[48] Their enthusiasm for the latest "cure" highlighted that fact, but it also highlighted the central place that "pain" had taken in the public and professional image of sickle cell anemia. Such enthusiasm also pointed to the appeal of the idea of genetic manipulation—regardless of its actual benefits for patients. Rodgers and others were careful to warn doctors, however, that research enthusiasm should not be interpreted as endorsement of the drug, for "at the current time, treatment with such agents such as HU and/or recombinant human erythropoetin should be considered *experimental*, and efforts should be made to enroll eligible patients into ongoing clinical trials, where possible."[49]

The breakthrough, it seems, was still in its experimental stage. According to standard regulatory practice, such drugs, though promising, had to pass the hurdle of proof—Food and Drug Administration (FDA) evaluation and approval. Clinical trials had to establish their value, so patients were encouraged to enroll *as research subjects* in trials—in which they were given a 50-50 chance of being assigned a placebo or HU. Even as HU trials began, researchers cautioned that "several issues of hydroxyurea therapy remain unresolved, including differences in patients' drug clearance, predictability of drug response, reversibility of sickle cell disease–related organ damage by hydroxyurea, and the efficacy of elevated HbF."[50] Late in 1994 Charache noted that problems of interpreting preliminary results persisted; in many cases "crises decreased during treatment, but this decrease was noted before the HbF levels increased."[51] Into late 1994, then, the potential clinical value and side effects of hydroxyurea remained unproven to the satisfaction of researchers, the FDA, or the sickle cell patient.

Validation of the benefits of HU came in early 1995, when Charache announced that the Bristol-Myers drug was judged to be so effective in reducing crises that the multicenter clinical trials were halted.[52] Despite the drama of the announcement, Charache himself remained cautious. In a field given to hyperbole and inflated rhetoric of "breakthroughs" and "cures," he emphasized that "hydroxyurea is a *treatment* for the disease and not a *cure*."[53] The trials confirmed that HU had "reduced by 50 percent the number of pain episodes, hospitalizations, situations requiring blood transfusion and incidents of a life-threatening complication called acute chest syndrome, which is characterized by fever and severe chest pain."[54] Such findings, although quite positive, could never live up to the initial inflated promise. The trials also raised questions about adverse effects that would not be answered for several years. In 1995, however, the only adverse effects discussed publicly were "that high dose hydroxyurea caused the suppression of bone marrow, which makes blood cells . . . [and that] the drug might increase the risk of a type of leukemia."[55] Such concerns, though noted, were again brushed aside.

The halting of the HU trials exemplified two important features of 1990s research: the powerful role of pharmaceutical companies in speeding new drugs through the FDA drug approval process and to the market, and the role of academic medical research in studying, judging, and ultimately validating the claims of pharmaceutical companies. Though academic researchers like Charache were not themselves the drug innovators, they played a crucial role in shaping public understanding about these treatments and "cures." Not only drug companies and researchers, but insurance companies, patients and their families, and regulatory agencies like the Food and Drug Administration watched attentively as such innovative products made headlines and then passed through trials. Some of these drugs would become routinely used in clinics, but many would not.

Indeed, it is no coincidence that such drugs moved quickly through the trials process, for beginning in the 1980s this goal had come to be a focal issue at the FDA. In the Reagan and Bush administrations, with their promotion of free market–based solutions to social problems, FDA oversight of drugs was altered dramatically. Under attack for being too concerned with patient protection and putting too much "red tape" in the way of both desperate patients and of drug innovators, the FDA was pushed to work more closely with industry to facilitate drug production. Certainly the advent of AIDS and aggressive lobbying for new AIDS drugs increased pressure for accelerated drug approval.[56] New rules promoting "accelerated approval" in 1987 even changed the way drug effectiveness was judged. Before the 1987 rule, drugs were evaluated for effectiveness only "according to their effect on the illness or patient's length of survival." But the new rule "allowed FDA to approve drugs based on a reasonable 'surrogate endpoint'"—such as CD4 counts in AIDS, or reducing the number of crises in sickle cell disease—regardless of the overall effect on the illness.[57]

After the HU trials were halted in January 1995, the *Wall Street Journal* noted that FDA approval was only one of the obstacles standing between Bristol-Myers's financial gains and the patient's relief from pain. Another obstacle was the insurance industry. "Until it is approved," the *Journal* pointed out, "Bristol-Myers is forbidden from marketing the drug for the malady, but yesterday's announcement is expected — indeed, intended — to encourage doctors treating patients with severe forms of the disease to prescribe it."[58] Asked for his opinion, Samuel Charache hoped that the FDA would approve the drug as soon as possible. FDA approval, he suggested, would convince reluctant insurance companies to reimburse physicians who chose to prescribe HU, and this would speed pain relief to patients. "If a third-party payer says he's not going to pay until the drug is approved, it will leave a lot of patients out in the cold," Charache stated.[59]

Thus, as in the case of narcotic pain relief, the case of HU exposed the ways in which various social interests mediated the relief of pain in sickle cell anemia in the 1990s. HU, however, was a method of pain relief without the social baggage of narcotic pain medication; it was an innovation that all could embrace. It was not controversial, partly because it was market friendly and it raised no complex political conundrums similar to narcotics. For the academic scientists, the trial could be celebrated as a crucial validation of their search for the "Holy Grail."[60] It was also a crucial development for Bristol-Myers. At the same time, third parties (insurance companies, Medicare, and Medicaid) would now negotiate whether patients would have access to these drugs. All of these stakeholders stood at the crossroads of medicine in the 1990s, and all of them stood to profit from pain relief via HU.

Even as these negotiations took place, HU quickly became integrated into the care of sickle cell anemia patients. But by late 1996, adverse consequences began to emerge. As in the previous "breakthroughs" in sickle cell anemia treatment, optimism gave way to caution. Writing in the pages of *Hematology/Oncology Clinics of North America* in 1996, Charache suggested that the "long-term risks are worrisome. . . . In a large study [of patients with another disease, polycythemia vera] . . . development of leukemia was more common in patients treated with hydroxyurea, but the difference in incidence from that in . . . [a control group] was not significant."[61] With the new agent on the market, physicians and patients stood by its ability to reduce painful crises but worried about the prospect of developing leukemia later in life. By the end of the decade, the long-term safety of HU therapy was still in doubt.

The rhetoric surrounding HU was narrowly focused, for many public and professional discussions defined efficacy in terms of pain reduction and cost reduction. The story of HU therefore reveals what the market, in conjunction with academic medicine, could and could not offer. Corporate interests and consumer pressures, along with academic clinical trials and the FDA, sped HU to the clinic. By their nature, insurance companies, HMOS, and third-party payers would attempt to limit that flow and to control costs, either by finding cost-saving drugs or by limiting consumption of drugs and services. And despite the outpouring of optimism about HU, the drug could not be considered a "cure" and the long-term dangers of its frequent use remained unclear, as Samuel Charache had noted.

Race and the Therapeutic Lottery

If HU represented the free market's ability to deliver innovative pain relief to sickle cell anemia patients, bone marrow transplantation (BMT) represented the ability of another recent innovation to deliver actual cures. BMT was a booming industry in the 1980s, as a rising number of private centers offered the service for cancer patients and others. These centers posed new dilemmas for people with sickle cell disease. Because BMT was classified as a medical "procedure," rather than a drug per se, its regulation did not fall within the purview of the FDA. Since BMT had been employed successfully in the treatment of some leukemias in the 1970s, practitioners expanded its applications to other disease in the 1980s. In the case of breast cancer, for example, BMT "entered the medical marketplace in the 1980s before studies to test its effectiveness had even begun."[62] Though unproven by clinical trials, it was popular with consumers as an alternative to standard radiation and chemotherapy. The success of BMT in the private sector spurred academic health centers to compete for patients by opening centers of their own.

In the 1980s and 1990s, therefore, even as academic medical centers sat in judgment of Bristol-Myers's therapeutic claims, they also developed their own innovations. In late 1984 a study at St. Jude Children's Hospital in Memphis dramatically revealed that "doctors have cured a case of sickle cell anemia with a bone marrow transplant."[63] The case was one of an eight-year-old girl with leukemia and sickle cell disease who, after bone marrow transplantation, appeared to see a remission in both disorders.[64] Her recovery from the transplantation had been tortuous, and reports cautioned that "this life-saving therapy will be suitable for only a small minority of victims of the disease . . . the transplants [were] fatal about 30 percent of the time."[65] Moreover, not all patients with sickle cell anemia could be candidates for BMT because transplantation required the availability of donors with matching bone marrow (usually siblings or close relatives). Even if matching donors could be found (using a test for the substance HLA), it was clear to researchers that this transplantation amounted to a high-stakes lottery. For those patients who found matched donors, there were several possible outcomes — unambiguous "cure," sudden death, continuing with unchanged sickle cell anemia, or trading the old disorder for a new disease.

One long-term consequence was the "major immunological complications, particularly graft-vs.-host disease, which currently limit[s] the more widespread use of marrow transplantation in the therapy of sickle cell anemia."[66] Graft-versus-host disease (GVHD) was an immunological "attack" upon the patient by the grafted marrow — and thus a profound and devastating failure of BMT. GVHD could be fatal, but it also could become a chronic disease, thereby replacing one chronic condition (sickle cell anemia) with another (GVHD). For all of these reasons, although public accounts greeted BMT as a "cure" and rarely delved into these ambiguities, professional opinion remained deeply divided. Noted two researchers in 1989, "The use of this technique at its present stage of development for the treatment of . . . sickle cell anemia . . . is controversial, raises serious ethical issues, and cannot be recommended routinely at this time."[67] From the outset, researchers greeted the reports on bone marrow transplantation and sickle cell anemia with cautious optimism along with an awareness of the moral and ethical entailments of such advances in therapy.[68]

If HU represented a limited treatment for pain, BMT was another partial "cure" — with a more profound set of risks — within one of academic medicine's own expanding cottage industries. Entering the 1990s, academic hematologist/oncologists began a vigorous debate about the use of BMT in sickle cell anemia.[69] In a 1990 conference at Seattle's Fred Hutchinson Cancer Research Center, the debate exposed a deeper tension between those who believed that small therapeutic advances were most appropriate for this multidimensional disease and those who advocated bold risk-taking in the pursuit of dramatic breakthroughs. One specific question was how these issues should be discussed with patients, with subjects in clinical trials, and with their families, and how the choices and risks should be weighed and regulated.

In a real sense, the key questions were to whom researchers owed their allegiance and who would bear the burden of risks in the pursuit of therapeutic innovation. A significant group of researchers voiced caution about all of these therapeutic uncertainties, allying themselves with patients. Speaking of the effects of BMT in Cooley's anemia, one researcher noted that "bone marrow transplantation was associated with as much as 25% mortality and the event-free survival was as low as 65% . . . one has to be selective of the type of patient that can be transplanted, rather than transplant all patients indiscriminately."[70] Ronald Nagel agreed, stating that "it is clear to me that the level of mortality, for a procedure intended to cure a disease that manifests such diverse patient-to-patient phenotypic expression, is clearly unacceptable if marrow transplantation is intended as an across-the-board recommendation."[71]

For Nagel, the BMT dilemma merely made explicit some of the problems that were latent with other therapeutic innovations. First, he highlighted how research findings were limited in their general applicability because of researchers' imprecise knowledge of variations from patient to patient (in pain, anemia, or other clinical problems). A second problem made evident by BMT was the role of innovative therapies in "trading one disease for another." As Ernest Beutler summarized the situation, "Little would be gained by sickle cell disease patients if they merely traded the morbidity associated with their primary disorder for a new set of disabling symptoms resulting from their treatment."[72]

By contrast with this cautious appraisal of BMT, others like E. Donnall Thomas (Nobel laureate for his use of BMT on leukemia, who himself had faced similar criticism early in his leukemia research) spoke in favor of some degree of risk-taking by researcher and patient in the use of BMT, allying themselves with long-term progress and with patients in the distant future. "We heard an argument that a 10% mortality with transplantation may not be acceptable. On the other hand, we have heard that the quality of the life for sickle cell patients in many instances is perhaps worse than death. This is going to be a very subjective decision. . . . Some physicians would demand that marrow grafting have almost a zero risk before it should be undertaken in sickle cell disease. I think that is an excessive requirement."[73]

The BMT dilemma also prompted researchers to discuss the broader social contexts in which these choices were made — and to tackle the problem of who would be making the choices. Ronald Nagel stated clearly that "it is not the physician but the patient who should be making the final decision. Unfortunately, because the patient usually tends to be very young, this decision will fall on the parent or guardian. The role of the physician . . . is to provide the most objective, dispassionate, and informed counseling in which the available data are presented in clear terms, and with the appropriate caveats as to their application to individual cases."[74] Moreover, Nagel wondered how the socioeconomic circumstances and options of such families might influence their therapeutic decisions — sometimes for the worse.

"Is there not room for [parents] taking risk for the wrong reasons?" he wondered. "What if some parents or guardians decide on marrow transplantation because they believe they cannot provide appropriate support to their child for socioeconomic reasons?"[75] Indeed, for some researchers the question was not how to weigh the statistics, but the pros and cons of presenting this option at all to families, especially those under desperate social circumstances and perhaps looking for a one-time fix, wary of the long-term costs of caring for a child with chronic sickle cell anemia. (In fact, some studies of BMT on the African continent justified the "therapeutic" use of the technology by explaining that patients had no access to conventional therapies.)

But to what extent could drawing sickle cell patients and their socioeconomically vulnerable families into the lottery of BMT be considered ethical, or exploitative, or merely normal medicine? This question underlay the discussion of BMT and its regulation in the 1990s. Relying on "consumer demand" as the primary guide to using a dangerous therapy posed significant problems for ethicists and regulators alike. And to what extent did academic medical centers' economic interest in transplant centers inform their discussions about the BMT lottery? As Renée Fox and Judith Swazey have shown in their study *Spare Parts: Organ Replacement in American Society*, it was in the 1980s and 1990s that organ transplants became large income-producing ventures for academic medicine.[76] The development of organ transplant centers was only loosely regulated by hospital ethics committees and institutional review boards (in some instances) and was not regulated at all by the FDA. It was left to the professional norms and values of particular research communities to dictate how transplantation would be discussed with patients.

In the context of this expansion, several researchers at the University of Chicago (a large regional center of transplant activity) launched a subtle critique of the idea that medical paternalism was necessary to protect vulnerable patients from the consequences of their own consumer decisions. The researchers announced that they had been denied the right to do BMT experiments by their institutional review board and voiced their frustration with the standard ways of regulating this research. Their solution to an impasse with the institutional review board was to try to hand the decision over to parents (and thus to the marketplace of consumers). In a study of the opinions of a wide range of parents whose children had sickle cell anemia, the researchers asked the parents to explain what they perceived to be an acceptable risk. They found that "at least 13 percent of parents might be expected to consent . . . given current rates of morbidity and mortality [and that these parents] weighed the risks and benefits of bone marrow transplantation . . . in a different way from members of our institutional review board."[77] The families in this 13 percent had similar profiles—they tended to have female children with sickle cell anemia, and they tended to have greater formal education. In the thinking of the researchers, the dilemma could be best resolved by deferring to these risk-taking families, even though these families shared specific profiles that others might see as problematic or disqualifying.[78] Here was an argument for by-passing the regulators and letting "the marketplace" speak for itself.

In the mid-1990s researchers remained divided on these issues, even as they held tightly to the reins of decision-making. Noted two Boston researchers in 1996, "Clinicians must now weigh the pros and cons . . . the irrefutable advantage of transplantation is that a successful outcome is definitive, and unless severe, chronic graft-versus-host disease occurs, the procedure is curative. But the potential for cure comes at a considerable risk, most of which is incurred at the time of the procedure."[79] Weighed against this tragic calculus, HU at least had a more "humble goal" of pain relief and "could be discontinued" if complications appeared, and narcotic pain management was as controversial but not as therapeutically satisfying—nor as potentially fatal.[80] By the mid-1990s, then, most hematologists/oncologists involved with the care of sickle cell anemia had grown quite adept at debating the practice, ethics, and socioeconomic problems associated with various treatments and weighing one mode of therapy against another, even if they did not agree with their proper uses.[81]

In the case of BMT, cost and access also played a role in researchers' evaluations. As one popular news account pointed out, "The transplant costs about $150,000 and is typically covered by insurers. Conventional treatment [by comparison] . . . runs roughly $30,000 to $50,000 a year and can only relieve symptoms."[82] Writing about this economic calculus in late 1996, Samuel Charache stated that "there is no debate over the [greater] cost-efficacy of transplantation in the patient who has disease-free survival."[83] These patients, however, constituted (as in 1990) only a tiny percentage of all sickle cell anemia patients—those who qualified for BMT by finding a matched donor, and those within that group who survived and prospered after the operation.[84] Yet Charache noted that, for most sicklers, "over the lifetime of a . . . patient with moderately severe disease, medical expenses alone are several fold greater than the cost of transplant."[85] The key questions for researchers were which patients could find an HLA-matched donor marrow, which would have insurance to approve the procedure, and which of this tiny percentage of patients would then survive the dangerous "experimental therapy" in order to benefit from this economic trade-off.[86] Thus BMT invited patients and their families to take a high-stakes therapeutic gamble that offered the chance of long-term freedom from disease and costly medical care, but also the possibility of trading one chronic disease for another, or death.

The stories of HU and BMT reflect much about the advent of for-profit, market-oriented perspectives in medicine in the 1990s, and the costs of these developments to patients with sickle cell anemia. Rather than curing sickle cell anemia, these innovative therapies were associated with a multiplying of therapeutic options. The growing importance of cost control in American health care only highlighted that hematology-oncology was one of the high-cost specialties that needed greater fiscal discipline. Thus therapeutic discussions about pain management and bone marrow transplantation could never be very far removed from the more highly charged issues of the 1980s and 1990s — inner city drug addiction, the rising cost of medical care for the poor, and the benefits and drawbacks of the marketplace in solving America's health care problems.

Memphis's Lingering Conservatism

How did such national therapeutic dramas play on the Memphis stage — if at all? Throughout the city's history, even its so-called liberal reformers often took what others in the nation might call moderate or conservative positions. They were always careful not to violate social norms, lest they be accused of uprooting traditional values.[87] These realities informed their politics as well as the local trajectory of sickle cell anemia.

In clear contrast to researchers like Samuel Charache, Orah Platt, Ronald Nagel, and Elliot Vichinsky, Memphis's leading sickle cell researchers struck a conservative pose in these decades on many of the contentious social issues surrounding sickle cell anemia. By the 1970s, Lemuel Diggs was credited with giving the disease greater visibility in the city and nationally, and with dismissing the frequent characterization of sickle cell anemia as a "racial inferiority disease."[88] Yet, by comparison to other experts on the disease in the 1980s and 1990s, Diggs was a conservative voice — particularly in his ideas about whether women with sickle cell anemia should have children and whether people with sickle cell trait should undertake military service. Diggs confronted all of these issues as a pathologist who had dedicated his life to studying specific anatomical features of the disease. From his viewpoint both as a Memphian and as a student of the body, he weighed in on two of the more social (rather than therapeutic) controversies of the 1980s.[89]

The exclusion of people with sickle cell trait from the United States military services was an issue that Diggs took up in the 1980s and continued to champion until his death in 1995. In World War II, Diggs had been part of the first study to examine this question. Two researchers at the time argued that "the potential danger involved is by no means negligible, particularly as our armed forces are concerned. . . . Having sickle cell trait . . . [the person] may become the victim of his constitutional biological inferiority and succumb under circumstances which are innocuous to average normal people."[90] Despite the heated rhetoric, such disease discussions had little impact on the general policy of integration in the 1940s. But with sickle cell anemia's more central role in American culture and politics in the early 1970s, the U.S. Air Force had decided to act. People with sickle cell trait were barred from flying based on studies suggesting that these otherwise "normal" people might possibly fall into "crisis" caused by sickling blood cells when they were deprived of oxygen at high altitude. The policy meshed neatly with the common view that "people who have sickle cell anemia [were] stricken with 'crises' [particularly] under stressful situations."[91] What was presumably true for sickle cell anemia seemed, according to common sense, to be true for sickle cell trait as well. While many researchers objected that there was little scientific consensus to support this ban, Diggs supported the move.

In 1976 Diggs expanded the argument by suggesting that some high school athletes with trait were also at risk.[92] His concerns flew in the face of the personal testimony of men like Pittsburgh Pirates star pitcher "Doc" Ellis.[93] Diggs's concerns were not those of a man committed to reforming the image of sickle cell trait, but those of a pathologist who, throughout his fifty-year career, remained fascinated with the ways in which context and environmental circumstances might induce the "benign" trait to become pathological. In the 1970s and early 1980s, the resolution of such public policy questions depended in part upon Diggs's opinions — and the air force upheld its ban.

In 1984, however, public policy shifted when the air force rescinded its ban. Diggs, now approaching his mid-eighties, responded with a series of articles in *Aviation Space and Environmental Medicine* in which he argued vigorously that "the main purpose of the military services is the defense of the country, at time of war, the maintenance of an aggressive, efficient, and effecting offense."[94] Admitting men and women with sickle cell trait to the military, he insisted, was contrary to these goals. "Military services," he stated, "cannot afford to take preventable risks . . . [and] based on the facts that are now known, the author believes that individuals with sickle cell trait (HbS) are at greater risk than those without the trait when engaged in military activities that regularly expose them to hypoxic environments or that require maximum stamina."[95] Yet Diggs was increasingly in the minority on this holdover issue from the 1970s. Responding to his claims in 1988, several other researchers set out to determine "if sickle cell trait represents an inherent adverse effect on response to training," and they observed "no statistically significant differences . . . between the sickle cell trait and the control groups at the end of basic training for any of the measured variables at peak exercise."[96] Another holdover issue from the 1970s in which Diggs took a conservative position was the question of whether women with sickle cell anemia should have children. Diggs remained convinced that the likelihood of complications in pregnancy did not justify the risks.[97]

In an atmosphere of lingering national concern about discrimination in employment, access to services, and citizenship, to many observers Diggs's positions on both military service and pregnancy seemed to support discrimination and extend inequality. His opinions, however, fit into a growing trend in the corporate uses of sickle cell trait testing. In the 1980s and 1990s, the designation of having sickle cell trait did bring with it the possibility of loss of employment or loss of health insurance. What had begun as a test to be used by individuals to enable informed decisions about their own reproduction had migrated into corporate venues. Employers like DuPont were accused of using sickle cell trait testing in job placement because of the assertion that people with the trait were "hypersusceptible" in the chemical workplace (see illustrations).[98] By the mid-1990s, one study noted that out of a sample of 300 people with a range of genetic problems, half had faced some form of discrimination.[99] (Of course, the challenge of obtaining insurance to cover the cost of therapy continued to constrain the therapeutic options of parents with sickle cell trait who had children with sickle cell anemia.)[100]

Most notably, it was the research questions Diggs took on and the character of the studies coming from Memphis that suggested a more conservative stance on the disease. Lemuel Diggs continued to be ambivalent, for example, about the special attention given to sickle cell anemia, and he argued that "the ideal will be to merge sickle cell anemia care into the care of other diseases, not to have separate, permanent facilities."[101] Diggs's views were those of a southerner concerned about the consequences of ongoing "special treatment" for the African American malady, but other researchers in other locales in the 1990s were quite certain that separate, comprehensive care facilities were the only means of continuing to keep visible, and to treat effectively, the plight of these children. But all of these views were expressed amidst a much more ominous set of developments in Tennessee health care. With the advent of the TennCare program, managed care innovations in health care for poor Tennesseans promised to overwhelm both the voice of academic medicine and the visibility of the patient with sickle cell anemia.

The Crossroads: TennCare and the New Politics of Patienthood

In one sense, the cities of Memphis and Nashville represented two polar opposite approaches to health care—one rooted in the aging urban academic medical center like Memphis's University of Tennessee, the other rooted in newfangled private, for-profit health care corporations like Nashville's Columbia/Hospital Corporation of America (HCA). The 1990s brought to light the growing tension between these two cultures, and the failure of the Clinton administration's national health care reform in 1993 set the stage for an aggressive push by market-oriented enthusiasts to seize the health care initiative.

Increasingly in the 1980s and 1990s, the fate of welfare recipients, poor patients, and many of the more vulnerable people with sickle cell anemia would be decided in the "laboratories of the states." Because Medicaid depended upon states to provide their own funds to match federal grants, changes in the financing of health care for the poor throughout America was becoming an economic necessity for state governors as well as for national politicians. The costs of financing the Medicaid program were rising faster than all other state costs in the 1980s and 1990s. In the period from 1985 to 1994, for example, Tennessee's Medicaid eligibility grew from 694,000 to 1.1 million, and half of Tennessee's children were on Medicaid by 1994.[102] Pressure built for controlling these and other rising costs of health care. In the early 1990s state governments across America sought and obtained greater flexibility in running these programs—including passing new initiatives mandating their privatization.

In early 1994 Tennessee sprinted into the lead among states aggressively reforming their Medicaid programs. In his final year as governor, conservative Democrat Ned McWherter of Tennessee was able to enact a dramatic transformation in Medicaid known as TennCare. Fiscal conservatism had become one of the new political and economic realities of the 1990s, and this viewpoint was embodied in state programs like TennCare. The program was driven, in many regards, by the desire to bring down rising costs by embracing government partnerships with health care companies spouting aggressive Columbia/HCA-style free market ideology.[103] TennCare was also an expression of the declining significance and power of Memphis and of the conservative turn in state politics. These political forces — along with pharmaceutical innovation — would have a lasting impact on sickle cell anemia.

In 1995 Tennessee elected Republican governor Don Sundquist, a Shelby County resident who was also a supporter of TennCare. One Memphis news organization noted that Sundquist was "the first governor in a generation to be elected from what was once, in the long-gone days of Boss Ed Crump, the state's politically dominant area."[104] Still the most populous area of the state, in the 1990s West Tennessee was portrayed as "fallen, economically and politically, into the shadows of metropolitan Nashville, not only the seat of state government but a rapidly ascendant business-entertainment center."[105] The location of health care giant Columbia/HCA in Nashville was only one of the indicators of that city's ascent and the shifting fortunes of Memphis. As one medical journal noted in 1996, "Just up the river from Chattanooga, the Hospital Corporation of America (HCA, now part of the behemoth Columbia/HCA) advanced the trend of interesting Wall Street in health care. And TennCare, the state's revolutionary Medicaid waiver program, has been credited with accelerating the incursion of managed care into areas that might otherwise have remained HMO-free for years to come."[106] Meanwhile, in a racially polarized election in 1991, Memphis had elected its first African American mayor, W. W. Herenton.[107] The Bluff City now joined New York, Los Angeles, Chicago, and others in achieving black representation at this level of city government. It was a heavily African American and still strongly Democratic city in an increasingly Republican and fiscally conservative state whose economic center had shifted toward Nashville.

In Sundquist's Tennessee, TennCare became an exemplar of the efficiency and cost-containment potential of for-profit health care and its ability to widen insurance coverage to over 90 percent of the uninsured. Such programs also became lightning rods for critics, for as with the new therapies like HU and BMT, these market innovations would fail to deliver on the hype, and they too could have their own disastrous consequences for some patients. In a state with high poverty rates among African Americans, the TennCare reform had important implications for many black Tennesseans as well as for citizens of west Arkansas, north Mississippi, and north Alabama.

Among the first casualties of TennCare were the academic medical centers like University of Tennessee (now named the UT Health Science Center). Their vulnerability exposed the ways in which such centers had depended upon the bodies of poor sick people as educational and research material since the early twentieth century, and as a cash nexus since the 1960s. The ascendance of such institutions in power and prestige in the late twentieth century had paralleled and nurtured the rising profile of diseases like sickle cell anemia. But as two authors wrote in 1996, "TennCare, implemented virtually overnight . . . enrolled 25 percent of the state's population [1.2 million] into managed care plans. Academic health centers in Tennessee have experienced long-term fallout from the transition. As large providers of Medicaid services, they are dependent on the program for clinical patients, revenues, and supplemental payments to offset the costs of charity and graduate medical education."[108] As these authors pointed out, the TennCare model had enormous appeal in an era of federalism and "returning power to the states." But this shift to the states also coincided with a rising regard for the marketplace model of medicine and a shift away from an appreciation of academic health centers — the very institutions that had helped to place sickle cell anemia and other obscure diseases in the national spotlight in the 1950s and 1960s.

It soon became clear that TennCare, while broadening insurance coverage and slowing the expanding cost of Medicaid, was a devastating innovation for Memphis hospitals and for the visibility of a range of chronic childhood diseases.[109] As Gregg Meyer and David Blumenthal found in one study, "Patients most likely to stay with academic health centers (AHCs) . . . are those most dependent upon its services. As a result, AHCs find it easy to retain their sickest patients but find other providers wooing their healthier ones."[110] Managed Medicaid, in short, would leave academic health centers caring for the sickest and most costly patients. "Vanderbilt Health Plan has documented [the] adverse selection for a number of costly conditions including AIDS, cystic fibrosis, and low birthweight babies."[111] These trends imposed particularly harsh penalties for Memphis because of its unchanging "geographically-based adverse selection" based on its bordering Mississippi and Arkansas.[112] Memphis's academic hospitals, in this climate, were caught in a bind, for uninsured patients were "still going to [the] Memphis safety-net hospital, which saw revenue drop $42 million when TennCare arrived. To survive, the hospital has slashed staff, cut services, and begun to turn away some indigent patients."[113] Patients themselves criticized the dramatic decline in the quality of their care after TennCare.[114]

By 1996, a popular and professional backlash against these developments had begun, but it was strong enough only to modify some of the proposals, not reverse them. First, it became clear that private health care organizations were not as efficient as advertised. Falling behind in their payments to Tennessee doctors and hospitals, numerous managed-care organizations came under fire for their own inefficiencies.[115] Governor Sundquist's decision to shift mental health services into a managed-care network called TennCare Partners also prompted accusations that the companies cut needed services to mentally ill patients.[116] Prodded by Memphis's U.S. congressman, Harold Ford Jr. (who had been elected to his father's former seat in late 1996), the federal Health Care Financing Administration sent inspectors to check on the TennCare program's operation.[117] One year later, Columbia/HCA itself came under attack from the U.S. Justice Department for "systemic" fraud in billing practices, while the American media and national and state politicians began to consider a variety of ad hoc proposals to regulate the perceived excesses of privatization and managed care.[118]

Against this backdrop of political and economic anxieties about both the old health care system and the new one, sickle cell anemia inevitably became characterized as a "costly" childhood disease, a disorder prevalent in a group of people often labeled as dependent on federal funding for treatment. It was perceived as a disease in which the liberal style of therapy (especially as carried out in academic research institutions) warranted close fiscal scrutiny, and one in which marketplace innovation opened up new life-saving possibilities and deadly dilemmas. The story of the disease in the 1980s and 1990s highlights the social and political underpinning of these therapeutic discourses. Discussions about the disease's proper therapy and its social implications were undertaken in a skeptical, and sometimes hostile, social context.[119] Therapeutic practices would be evaluated in terms of cost, while the very notion of the centralized urban academic health center where research, patient care, and education occurred in tandem became anathema to the free market enthusiasts of the 1990s. Therapeutic discourse on such topics as pain, pain management, and addiction encoded debates about the limits of patients' rights and the role of free-market forces and managed care in medicine.

The rise of managed care provoked two disturbing trends in the care of sickle cell patients: the dumping of the extremely ill and costly patients into the more comprehensive academic health centers, and the pressure to place other sickle cell patients in clinics set apart from academic health centers in the name of reducing costs. At a 1997 national meeting of sickle cell anemia experts, Elliot Vichinsky noted that sickle cell patients were part of a costly and vulnerable group taken care of by a specialty group under intense fiscal scrutiny since "hematology-oncology patients cost about 63 times the cost of the average child needing medical care." Faced with such costs, insurers and HMOs were pushing for "rationing care to sickle cell sufferers, reducing access to specialized care."[120] The push to remove sickle cell anemia care from centralized facilities into community settings meant, for Vichinsky, a dangerous shift since community-based doctors had been shown to be ill-equipped for handling the clinical complexity of the disease.[121] Referring to a study of sickle cell anemia in Alabama, Vichinsky insisted that the disease was one in which it was impossible and unwise to separate the primary care aspects that could be handled by community-based doctors from the tertiary care aspects that were best managed in comprehensive academic health centers.[122]

Indeed, in July 1996 Vichinsky would tell *New York Times* columnist Bob Herbert the story of a young girl with sickle cell disease he had once cared for at the Children's Hospital in Oakland. When her mother changed jobs and enrolled in an HMO, "they told her she had to get care in a suburban hospital" because it was more cost-effective. But as columnist Herbert wrote, "First-class treatment requires a team approach . . . usually to be found in urban centers." A controversy soon emerged around the practice of giving frequent blood transfusions to prevent strokes. "The treatment was turned over to a hematologist who had little experience treating sickle-cell patients," wrote Herbert. "The new doctor decided that there was not enough evidence that the frequent transfusions were necessary. He stopped them." The story of this black child's care, "hijacked by inflexible, cold-hearted, corporate types whose interests are in profits, not patients," ended tragically. "The kid," said Vichinsky, "went on to have a stroke and died."[123]

Such writings on therapeutics and sickle cell disease followed the current of broader discussions about the plight of the urban academic center and its comprehensive care model, about the decentralization of care, and about the adverse consequences of saving money by reducing health care consumption. Such controversies informed other therapeutic debates. Looking critically at the use of antibiotics in the treatment of sickle cell crises, for example, St. Jude researcher J. A. Wilimas argued in 1993 that "outpatient treatment saved a mean $1,195 per febrile episode." Wilimas also argued that "with the use of conservative eligibility criteria, at least half the febrile episodes in children with sickle cell disease can be treated safely on an outpatient basis, with substantial reductions in cost."[124] Left unanswered was the question of what these developments would mean for the patients themselves.

TennCare represented an outgrowth of these national economic and political trends in health care. In its wake came the decline of the academic medical centers, robbed of the very commodities and resources that had contributed to their expansion in the post–World War II era—sick patients, federal research grants, and federal reimbursement for the care of the poor. At the same time, hematology-oncology also suffered as a field, for it was increasingly characterized as a problem area, an exemplar of high-cost medicine within the bloated academic medical center. With these multiple shifts in the political economy of 1990s medicine, such experts feared that the visibility of sickle cell anemia would decline as the care of patients was decentralized, and that the social significance of their suffering would diminish.

By the end of the twentieth century, people with sickle cell disease in Memphis had arrived at another crossroads. The road at the end of the century was a far busier intersection than in earlier decades—a place where health care commerce was heavy, where the flow of funds from the federal and state governments was overwhelming, and where the traffic in disease commodities and health care services was intense. The cost of traveling the road by oneself had risen sharply, and in choosing which path they would take, sickle cell patients were compelled to decide whether to accept the promises of government, pharmaceutical companies, academic researchers, insurers, or managed care companies.

Conclusion
Race against Disease

Studies of the past can yield many different lessons that vary depending upon who recalls the past and what purpose is served by their recollections. In the preceding pages, some clear lessons flow from the history of sickle cell disease. The malady's emergence from invisibility into clinical and wide political significance provides a window on the changing health care system in twentieth-century America. The development of knowledge about the disorder has itself served diverse ideological and social agendas. In the preceding chapters, I have explored the political uses of this knowledge. I have also examined the evolving economic significance of disease in American society, and the ways in which racial politics has influenced the recognition of sicklers, their medical treatment, and the very symbolic meaning of their disorder. This telling produces a history that differs markedly from traditional accounts of the malady, for the previous pages focus primarily on the transformation of the meaning of the disorder and on the implications for patients, medicine, and society.

Traditional accounts of the malady offer much that is of value, but they can also replicate and reinforce disturbing stereotypes or perpetuate scientific or social ideologies without fully analyzing these stereotypes and ideologies as part of an evolving problem of race and disease. Some historians, for example, have taken up the story of the disease's evolutionary identity—its role in the defense against *falciparum* malaria in Africa. This understanding of the disease's past emerged in the 1950s and countered an older image of the disorder as a hereditary blemish. Based on the evolutionary model, sickle cell disease (or any hereditary disorder, for that matter) was redeemed. Through the lens of evolutionary biology, the disease is portrayed merely as the unfortunate consequence of two doses of a "good" gene that was meant to protect against malaria. Using the theoretical claims

of evolutionary biology, modern observers now insist that only the ignorant could regard sickle cell disease as evidence of a tainted identity. Evolution, it is said, teaches that the abnormal gene has a power to protect, and
that this protective power was fully manifested in the African homeland
where malaria prevailed.

This theory is invoked today as an instantiation of a biological rule that
is often used to make an important moral claim — that separating "good
genes" from "bad genes" is difficult, if not impossible. The evaluation of the
"goodness" or "badness" of genes or traits depends upon the environment
in which those genes and traits function. The moral lesson of sickle cell
disease is clear. To speak of the malady as a genetic taint (or as evidence of
inferiority) is to be culturally ignorant and to ignore how context deter-
mines the function and value of genes.

The *falciparum* malaria theory — first generated in the 1950s and 1960s —
has had continuing symbolic and moral significance in an era of rapidly
advancing knowledge of genetics and disease. As a theory, it contains important moral truths about the complexity of human traits and of identity itself.
The theory also supports particular ideas about black people in America. It
exemplifies a complex inheritance. It testifies, if implicitly, to the formidable
adaptive capacity of black Americans in their original lands. It highlights the
paradoxes of black survival in adverse environments.[1] For black Americans,
the disease (springing from a proud, strong African past) becomes an
existential metaphor demonstrating how a people with a unique ancestry
were uprooted, how their unique strength became exclusively a mortal
burden, and how this complex ancestry has been profoundly misunderstood
in American society.[2] Refracted through the powerful lens of evolutionary
biology, the painful sickle cell disease could thus be used to exemplify
African American experience. In this history, evolutionary biology testifies
to, and authenticates, black experience and black identity.

Some authors have looked to more recent events in the story of disease
to frame an understanding of the African American experience. They focus
on the genetic counseling controversies of the 1970s, which offer important
historical lessons about the dangers implicit in translating knowledge about
race and biology into coercive reproductive policies. Unlike the eugenic
targeting of the "mentally retarded" and the "unfit" for sterilization in the
1910s, 1920s, and 1930s, genetic counseling in the 1960s and 1970s offered
sickle cell carriers information on their chances of producing a child with
the disease. In an era where patients' rights and informed consent emerged
as key concepts in health care, many counselors and policymakers believed

that a parent—knowing the odds of producing a child with sickle cell disease—would choose to forego having children with another carrier. But many others did not embrace free choice, choosing instead to promote mandatory screening and a more directive approach to genetic counseling for people with sickle cell trait, and this introduced coercion and eugenic overtones into counseling.

Few proponents of applied genetics in the 1970s were prepared for the angry backlash from African Americans concerning overzealous genetic screening. Few anticipated that many black people would resent intrusive reproductive guidance in the name of eradicating a "black disease." Moreover, even fewer saw that many African Americans had come to identify with the pain and suffering of sicklers—especially as the patients' experiences emerged into public view and their lives, extended by medical care, became open books for public interpretation. Despite their pain, sicklers were living longer than ever. Against this backdrop, the goal of preventing the birth of other sicklers would seem drastic, culturally insensitive, and even genocidal. Looking back at this controversy, geneticists and health policymakers frequently recall the backlash as a warning that the use of hereditary knowledge can pose unforeseen dangers to individual self-determination, promote discrimination, and (when directed at a single minority group) feed legitimate fears of a return to eugenics and genocide.[3]

These two often-cited cautionary lessons from the history of sickle cell disease—that even "bad" genes can have "good" functions, and that applications of genetic knowledge in the name of public health can trample individual self-determination and group identity—have powerful resonance in our time. For we live in an era of rapidly advancing knowledge about the role of genetic mechanisms in many diseases like Alzheimer's, scientific forays into the genetic origins of behaviors like homosexuality, and wild speculation about the possibilities of genetic manipulation and therapy.[4] The case of sickle cell anemia reinforces our sensitivity to the fact that governments, insurance companies, HMOs, drug companies, and employers all have interests in genetic disease testing, manipulation, and eradication and that these interests do not necessarily coincide with those of the individual with disease. In the era of the Human Genome Project, the story of sickle cell disease's political history in the 1970s is often recalled precisely because it contains a warning for other groups of sufferers as we produce more information on the genetics of their maladies. It highlights the problem of translating genetic expertise into policies that support rather than erode autonomy, self-determination, and individual/group identity.

A third historical lesson about sickle cell disease, often told somewhat self-servingly by professional researchers, offers a positive model for the future—a road map for how a cure will one day emerge and how our society can avoid these ethical entanglements. Biomedical scientists often fondly recall the pioneering work of Linus Pauling, whose midcentury research on the role of hemoglobin in sickle cell disease helped transform the disorder into the "first molecular disease." The discovery also spurred the growth of molecular biology. These same scientists have forgotten (or perhaps never knew) Pauling's later bizarre public health suggestion of tattooing sickle cell carriers on the forehead in order that they might recognize each other early in life and "avoid falling in love," thereby reducing the incidence of the disease. Instead, today's clinical scientists recall Pauling as the primary author of the pathbreaking 1949 treatise, the paper that helped move medicine down the modern road toward molecular analysis of disease and molecular cures.

Since then, clinical scientists working on sickle cell disease have constantly claimed to be part of Pauling's legacy. Writing in 1970, for example, Robert Nalbandian could present his urea treatment as a testament to the continuing significance of Pauling's molecular understanding of the disease. Nalbandian (and Pauling himself) saw this treatment as "chemically rational" because it manipulated the disorder at the molecular level. Urea appealed at this scientific level because, in theory, it showed that "the sickling tendency can be reversed and the misshapen cells returned to normal."[5] At the level of the patient and the clinic, however, urea was an abject failure — it had far too many terrible side effects for any patient to ingest it. A quarter-century later, in 1995, researchers would hail yet other breakthroughs, such as the drug hydroxyurea, as the realization of Pauling's vision.[6] For generations of clinical scientists, then, Pauling's insight has remained a crucial historical touchstone. Despite the profound failure of Nalbandian's urea treatment, and though hydroxyurea is useful only in reducing pain and is in no sense a cure, researchers continue to invoke Pauling's work in order to refresh molecular medicine's sense of purpose and to suggest to the public that biomedicine marches rationally along a great lineage.

These three snapshots of the disease's past — its evolutionary history, the genetic counseling controversies, and Pauling's legacy — carry very different messages. One historical recollection endorses a complex African American identity, a second warns against the excesses of applied genetics, and a third situates modern biomedicine in its own proud and productive past. The first speaks to patients and to African Americans trying to shape a sense of themselves and their history; the second tells policymakers to be cautious in trying to translate hereditary knowledge into workable public health programs; and the third speaks to clinical scientists seeking to craft, sustain, and legitimate their research agendas.

But if we look over the history of sickle cell disease as presented in the preceding pages, and if we see the malady against the backdrop of racial politics in the South, several other lessons emerge that move beyond the perpetuation of ideologies and examine the often problematic relationships between ideology and patients' experiences. Attention to the disease's early obscurity, its changing clinical identity and popular visibility, and its increasing celebrity status provides a more complex cultural understanding of the past.

Celebrity status was a mixed blessing for sicklers. "Celebrity status," writes P. David Marshall in his *Celebrity and Power*, "confers discursive power: within society, the celebrity is a voice above others, a voice that is channeled into the media systems as being legitimately significant."[7] But celebrity status not only engenders power, it also exposes the celebrity to derision as an idol, a false icon. "In one sense, the celebrity represents success and achievement within the social world," continues Marshall. "[But] the sign of the celebrity is ridiculed and derided because it represents the center of false value . . . the success expressed in the celebrity posture is seen as a success without the requisite association with work."[8] The same can be said of popular symbols such as disease. Celebrity status for sickle cell anemia opened into public debate problems of authenticity, false value, and unearned and unwarranted recognition. Coping with these issues has since become important in the lives of sickle cell patients, even as new diseases, particularly breast cancer and AIDS, have taken over the celebrity spotlight.[9]

The disorder's history in a particular city, Memphis, Tennessee, draws our attention to the local social relations and ideologies that made the once-invisible disease both visible and celebrated. How did the malady influence — like syphilis and tuberculosis in earlier times — the politics of racial health in Memphis and in America? Answering this question required examining not only the biological evolution of disease, but also the social evolution of Memphis's health care system — defined by citizens and elected officials, by the declining status of cotton and the rising significance of health care in the city's economy, and by political trade-offs as African Americans negotiated for power and influence in the Bluff City. The rise and fall of clinical awareness of people with the disorder, the recognition of their plight as culturally legitimate, and ongoing debates about their medical treatment must be understood in terms of this local political economy.

A Crossroads City on the Health Care Margins

For more than 100 years, Memphis, like Chicago, New York, Philadelphia and other American cities, has been a haven for African Americans seeking better lives.[10] Yet heavy mortality in crowded ghettos has also made the city an enemy of the people. Health in Memphis reflected this paradox of urbanization. The city's politicians constantly voiced their ambivalence about being a regional center for health care and other services; even as the city drew its economic strength and cultural identity from the Deep South, its leaders sought to keep neighboring people at arm's length, especially when they were ill. Memphis remained a deeply ambivalent city, in part because of its position at the confluence of urban and rural cultures and as a collision point for divergent regional attitudes. Sickle cell anemia's early trajectory was defined by this small world — obscured by the prevalence of malaria and by diagnostic conservatism, entangled with racial ideologies, and circumscribed by finger-pointing over who was to blame for infant mortality. Any new understanding of the disease had to contend with this ideological reality before it could gain legitimacy.

By the 1950s, federal and philanthropic money pouring into the city's medical system had produced a new urban landscape. An academic research center blossomed around the University of Tennessee and expanded in cultural significance through the 1960s. Specialized new facilities like St. Jude's Children's Research Hospital appeared. A civic culture emerged that was now proud to advertise its place on the frontlines in the fight against disease. Memphis dedicated itself to building a civic image rivaling Chicago, New York, Boston, and Atlanta. Gone was the city's historical ambivalence about the influx of sick people from the rural hinterlands. The changing political economy of health care resulted, slowly, in the perception of sickle cell disease as a cutting-edge disorder and as a disease with increasing ability to mobilize civic sentiment.

As a novel illness experience was framed, dramatizing a hidden legacy of black pain and suffering, a potent cultural appeal took shape.[11] The disease's appearance — in scientific journals as a "molecular" puzzle, in popular media as a mysterious "painful, new disorder," and, later, in political hearings as a "neglected" experience of a long-suffering people — transmuted an obscure pathology into a usable resource. Disease became a commodity, an entity traded in public and private markets, used by scientists to attract research grants, by physicians and health centers to earn clinical income, and by sufferers and their advocates to make demands for resources or more compassionate care.

In 1950s Memphis, recognition of sickle cell disease represented a liberal hope that attention to pain and suffering in children might help Memphians move toward racial accommodation and compassion, even as more angry struggles raged over segregation. But as African Americans gained higher visibility and political power in the 1960s, and as whites fled to the suburbs and into the Republican Party, sickle cell disease came to symbolize more than ever the experience, identity, and concerns of blacks. With the rise of federal research and health care funding, the disease became an economic boon for researchers, the university, and the city as a whole. In the late 1960s, the former staunchly Democratic city found itself represented by Republican congressman Dan Kuykendall, for whom the disease became a poster case for moderate compassion mixed with fiscal sobriety, a platform for expressing his fears about drug addiction, and a cash cow. The disease experience represented an existential crisis that could be harnessed to the endeavors of scientists and activists, patients and politicians, to give the air of humaneness to their endeavors. The pain and suffering of sicklers endowed medicine with a moral and social dimension. The rising profile of chronic pain shifted the sights of scientists away from "sickled cells" per se, redefining the relationship of black Americans to a health care system that was blind to their experience. By the 1970s, the plight of sicklers was the stuff of political consciousness-raising and medical liberalism, as well as cynical campaign oratory. For Americans, the disease would soon come to represent issues of group survival and neglect, as well as the limits of both compassion and social control.

By the end of the twentieth century (some eighty years after the disease's "discovery" and some fifty years after Pauling's molecular insight), the urgency of these meanings has diminished, and the attention paid to sickle cell disease has receded noticeably. Over time, the plight of sicklers had been dragged into a broad spectrum of clinical and social debates. Sickle cell disease was used to comment on the logic of busing to achieve school integration, on black intelligence, on the psychology of drug addiction, and (in the 1990s) on the vagaries of managed care. Wherever there was a racial controversy, sickle cell anemia might be evoked. Into the last decade of the century, sickle cell legislation still stirred resentment as a case in point of "special interests politics."[12] It also helped to open a controversial new stage in the influence of identity politics in the research funding process.[13] In the wake of sickle cell's popularity, commentators expressed concern about all of these developments, and about the excesses of liberalism in pain management. In all of these debates, the disease was the proxy for a wide range of "race issues" in American society. The association between disease and African American social identity had been solidified, and this very association made sickle cell anemia into a cultural signpost.

In the meantime, the urban academic medical center that blossomed in the 1950s and helped fuel a new awareness of sickle cell disease was weakened by economic and political trends in 1990s health care. In the 1950s, the Memphis academic medical center's growing prosperity dramatically refashioned the city's economy. By contrast, the late twentieth century saw cutbacks in the federal support for research and for patient care at the city's medical centers. The shift in power from the urban academic medical center to the health care corporations, and the creation of TennCare and the privatization of Medicaid, further undermined Memphis's institutions, drawing former Medicaid patients — who had become an economic centerpiece of academic medicine — out of the university hospitals. In the 1990s, as the fight against disease was rapidly transformed into the fight to lower health care costs, cities like Memphis were no longer on the frontlines. Cities like Nashville, the state capital and home to the health care corporation Columbia / HCA — one of the largest in the country — had become central to this new fight to manage health care costs. By the 1990s, Memphis was an African American–controlled city in a white southern state. It was also a Democratic city in an increasingly Republican state, and its health care system represented a costly, declining model of health care in the age of privatized medicine. The city at the crossroads of southern culture, economics, and politics was a city on the margins.

How the late-twentieth-century shift in the political economy of health care will define the fate of people with sickle cell disease in the twenty-first century is not yet clear. But numerous observers agree that the new system has not been kind to teaching hospitals, that it is not kind to many patients, and that "in the worst predicament of all are children with major chronic diseases struggling to fit into the capitated, gatekeeper system of managed care."[14] Managed care TennCare-style threatens to bring a new kind of invisibility to people with sickle cell disease.

Visibility, Celebrity, and the Problem of Pain
This transformation in perceptions conjures forth Ralph Ellison's *Invisible Man* — the chronicle of a nameless man who escaped the invisibility of

the South only to find himself transformed into a visible racial stereotype in the minds of northerners. The nameless narrator concluded that his own invisibility was not inherent in his being but "occurs because of a peculiar disposition of the eyes of those with whom I come in contact." Journeying from anonymous beginnings in the rural South through the world of college educators, social reformers, and political activists, he found that at each stage his identity was defined by the agenda of others, his invisibility becoming "a matter of the construction of their inner eyes." In the end, the narrator reflected that "I was pulled this way and that for longer than I can remember. And my problem was that I always tried to go in everybody's way but my own. I have also been called one thing and then another while no one really wished to hear what I called myself."[15] Sicklers have traveled a similar path. The eyes of others — evolutionary biologists looking back to Africa, clinical scientists seeking breakthrough cures, liberal reformers endorsing compassion and pain relief, and conservative ideologues fearful of drug addiction — have structured the interpretation of their experience. Sicklers too have "come a long way and returned and boomeranged a long way from the point in society toward which [they] originally aspired."[16] They emerged slowly into the limelight of post–World War II American biology, medicine, and politics, and yet they hover, like the Invisible Man, on the precipice between celebrity and invisibility.

The question of pain management in the clinic exposes this dilemma, for it highlights both conservative fears of drug addiction and the difficulties of practicing liberal, compassionate medicine in inner city America. Where in the 1930s sickle cell disease blurred into the politics of malaria and infant death, today it is often entangled with the politics of pain — its symbolism, its alleviation, and its contested authenticity in medicine and society. In moving beyond narratives of disease evolution, beyond the 1970s screening controversies, and beyond debating Pauling's legacy, this book has revolved around the problems of pain, experience, and recognition.

In seeking lessons from the past, there can be no better place to end than with the problem of pain in sickle cell disease, for it reveals that the disease has many other dimensions — and one of my concerns in this book has been how this distinctive kind of pain was translated, at a particular historical moment, into a measure of power.[17] The path from neglect to recognition of pain — and toward celebrity — has not been without problems. Certainly the disease's distinctive pain and suffering mobilized compassion, generated resources, and raised consciousness about the plight of African Americans in the 1960s, 1970s, and even today. But the public discourse of pain in the 1970s also suggested that what was actually at stake in each patient's experience were *feelings* and long-standing historical slights in the black community at large. Such characterizations of the illness experience fostered a view of sickle cell anemia as an experience writ large upon the black population, and this generalization also invited popular skepticism and resentment about the privileging and uses of that experience.[18] Yet the power of pain produced cultural recognition and pain relief protocols. The story of pain in sickle cell disease highlights the ways in which even this single, vital aspect of the disease experience has continually been culturally reconstructed for a variety of ends.

The problem of pain pushes us to ask new questions about race relations, biological understanding, and medicine. Indeed, the problem of pain in sickle cell disease — its meaning, alleviation, proper management, problematic measurement, and cultural significance — moves us considerably forward in understanding the contemporary politics of race and health. Where some would have us still debating questions of whether race is a biological concept, or whether sickle cell anemia proves that African Americans are biologically different from whites, this study has attempted to move beyond these debates, to situate these discourses themselves in historical contexts, and to move on to the problem of the patients' experiences and the evolving black experience. If we can comprehend this pain, its historical invisibility and its gradual emergence in the twentieth century, its existential meaning and its cultural manipulation — in the city of the blues and in America — we will gain valuable insight into the significance of sickle cell anemia and the politics of race and health in American society.

Notes

INTRODUCTION

1. Samuel Cartwright, "Report on the Diseases and Physical Peculiarities of the Negro Race," *New-Orleans Medical and Surgical Journal* 7 (1851). Quoted in Martin Pernick, *A Calculus of Suffering: Pain, Professionalism, and Anesthesia in Nineteenth-Century America* (New York: Columbia University Press, 1985), 155.

2. Memphis Minnie [Lizzie Douglas], "Memphis Minnie-jitis Blues," June 5, 1930, on *Memphis Minnie, Hot Stuff Collector's Edition (1930–1941)*, Peermusic (Magnum America) MCCD001.

3. Speaking on the topic of visible signs and diseases, Michel Foucault observed of early-nineteenth-century Paris medicine that "every manifestation of disease could . . . take on the value of sign, providing an informed medical reading could place it in the chronological totality of illness." Michel Foucault, *The Birth of the Clinic: An Archaeology of Medical Perception*, trans. A. M. Sheridan Smith (New York: Vintage, 1973), 159.

4. Todd Savitt and M. Goldberg, "Herrick's 1910 Report of Sickle Cell Anemia: The Rest of the Story," *Journal of the American Medical Association* 261 (January 13, 1989): 266–71.

5. Stuart B. Edelstein, *The Sickled Cell: From Myths to Molecules* (Cambridge, Mass.: Harvard University Press, 1986).

6. Felix I. D. Konotey-Ahulu, "Chwechweechwe: The African Rheumatic Syndrome That Came to Be Known as Sickle Cell Disease — A Personal Testimony" (1984), Box 18, Folder: "Konotey-Ahulu," Maxwell Myer Wintrobe Papers, Marriott Library Special Collections, University of Utah, Salt Lake City.

7. This distinction between illness and disease is adeptly explored by Arthur Kleinman, who writes, "By invoking the term illness, I mean to conjure up the innately human experience of symptoms and suffering. . . . Disease, however, is what the practitioner creates in the recasting of illness in terms of theories of

disorder." Arthur Kleinman, *The Illness Narratives: Suffering, Healing, and the Human Condition* (New York: Basic Books, 1988), 3, 5.

8. C. Lockhard Conley, "Sickle Cell Anemia: The First Molecular Disease," in *Blood, Pure and Eloquent: A Story of Discovery, of People, and of Ideas*, ed. Maxwell Wintrobe (New York: McGraw-Hill, 1980), 319–71.

9. Keith Wailoo, "Detecting 'Negro Blood': Black and White Identities and the Reconstruction of Sickle Cell Anemia," in *Drawing Blood: Technology and Disease Identity in Twentieth-Century America* (Baltimore: Johns Hopkins University Press, 1997), 134–61.

10. Anthony C. Allison, "Protection Afforded by Sickle-Cell Trait against Subtertian Malarial Infection," *British Medical Journal* 1 (1954): 290–94.

11. The ban was lifted in 1981.

12. Of course there are also several notable exceptions. See, for example, Charles Rosenberg, *The Cholera Years: The United States in 1832, 1849, and 1866* (Chicago: University of Chicago Press, 1962); Allan Brandt, *No Magic Bullet: A Social History of Venereal Disease in America since 1880* (New York: Oxford University Press, 1984); and, more recently, Steven Epstein, *Impure Science: AIDS, Activism, and the Politics of Knowledge* (Berkeley: University of California Press, 1996).

13. Kleinman, *Illness Narratives*, 5.

14. For more on the character of southern cities, see David R. Goldfield, *Cotton Fields and Skyscrapers: Southern City and Region, 1607–1980* (Baton Rouge: Louisiana State University Press, 1982), and, more recently, David R. Goldfield, *Region, Race, and Cities: Interpreting the Urban South* (Baton Rouge: Louisiana State University Press, 1997). See also Blaine Brownell and David R. Goldfield, eds., *The City in Southern History: The Growth of Urban Civilization in the South* (Port Washington, N.Y.: Kennikat Press, 1977).

15. Thomas Childers, "Memphis," *American Heritage*, October 1998, 100.

16. Jack Temple Kirby, *Rural Worlds Lost: The American South, 1920–1960* (Baton Rouge: Louisiana State University Press, 1987).

17. James Jones, *Bad Blood: The Tuskegee Syphilis Experiment* (New York: Free Press, 1981).

18. "Physicians," Jones points out, "had come dangerously close to depicting the syphilitic black as the representative black . . . the result was a powerful rationale for inactivity in the face of disease." Ibid., 28.

19. On this economy, see Eugene Genovese, *The Political Economy of Slavery: Studies in the Economy and Society of the Slave South* (New York: Vintage, 1967). See also Leslie Howard Owens, "Into the Fields — Life, Disease, and Labor in the Old South," in *This Species of Property: Slave Life and Culture in the Old South* (New York: Oxford University Press, 1976), 19–49, and Elliott Gorn, "Black Magic: Folk Beliefs of the Slave Community," in *Science and Medicine in the Old South*, ed. Ronald Numbers and Todd Savitt (Baton Rouge: Louisiana State University Press, 1989), 295–326.

20. Eric Foner, *Reconstruction: America's Unfinished Revolution, 1863–1877* (New York: Harper and Row, 1988), 37. See also Gavin Wright, *Old South, New South: Revolutions in the Southern Economy since the Civil War* (New York: Basic Books, 1986).

21. Thomas Murrell, "Syphilis and the American Negro: A Medico-Legal Study," *Journal of the American Medical Association* 54 (March 10, 1910): 848.

22. A study along these lines is George Fredrickson, *Black Image in the White Mind: The Debate on African-American Character and Destiny, 1817–1914* (New York: Harper and Row, 1971); see also, more recently, Darryl Michael Scott, *Contempt and Pity: Social Policy and the Image of the Damaged Black Psyche, 1880–1996* (Chapel Hill: University of North Carolina Press, 1997).

23. James Bardin, "Some Public Health Aspects of Race Relationships in the South," in *Lectures and Addresses on the Negro in the South* (Charlottesville, Va.: Michie Company, 1915), 77. As Bardin noted, where fifty years earlier tuberculosis was insignificant, it was now widely labeled a "scourge of the race."

24. For black pastor T. O. Fuller, for example, "Memphis being the principal city in this section of the delta and one of the largest inland cotton and lumber markets in the world, Negro labor has played a very large part in making Memphis a big industrial and financial center." T. O. Fuller, *The Story of Church Life among Negroes* (Memphis: T. O. Fuller, 1938), 1.

25. Thus did Virginia slave owner John Walker take an interest in the suffering of slave women, men, girls, and boys. When a slave girl, Ellen, had "taken sick," "Doc Henley was sent to for to see her." Walker reported that "[the Doctor] says her disease is the Rheumatism she has no use of her legs they are lifeless cant move them at all . . . when moved has very severe and excruciating pain in her arms and breast." Quoted in Todd Savitt, *Medicine and Slavery: The Diseases and Health Care of Blacks in Antebellum Virginia* (Urbana: University of Illinois Press, 1978), 54.

26. Ulrich Phillips, "Black-Belt Labor, Slave and Free," in *Lectures and Addresses on the Negro in the South* (Charlottesville, Va.: Michie Company, 1915), 32. Indeed, as one South Carolina minister, J. H. Thornwell, preached in 1850, the moral economy of slavery gave masters not only "a right to [the slave's] labor" but a concern for the slave's health and welfare. In this system, punishment was one of the "painful necessities" for reinforcing responsibility. Thornwell called on his listeners to understand that this kind of pain visited upon slaves ought not, as it did in the North, "awaken the indignation of loyal and faithful citizens," for it was consistent with the preservation of any state or society. Rev. J. H. Thornwell, *The Rights and Duties of Masters* (Charleston, S.C.: Steam Power Press of Walker and James, 1850), 25.

27. Quoted in James Cobb, *The Most Southern Place on Earth: The Mississippi Delta and the Roots of Regional Identity* (New York: Oxford University Press, 1992), 84.

28. Ibid., 103.

29. Foner, *Reconstruction*, 37.

30. Gaines Foster, "The Limitations of Federal Health Care for Freedmen, 1860–1868," *Journal of Southern History* 48 (1982): 349–72.

31. The literature on nineteenth-century African American health care and institutions is small. See Mitchell Rice, *Health of Black Americans from Post Reconstruction to Integration, 1871–1960: An Annotated Bibliography of Contemporary Sources* (New York: Greenwood Press, 1990). By contrast, the literature on African American health care, hospitals, and medical institutions in the twentieth century has been growing in recent decades. See, for example, Vanessa Gamble, *Making a Place for Ourselves: The Black Hospital Movement, 1920–1945* (New York: Oxford University Press, 1995); David McBride, *Integrating the City of Medicine: Blacks in Philadelphia Health Care, 1910–1965* (Philadelphia: Temple University Press, 1989); Darlene Clark Hine, *Black Women in White: Racial Conflict and Cooperation in the Nursing Profession, 1890–1950* (Bloomington: Indiana University Press, 1989); and Edward Beardsley, *A History of Neglect: Health Care for Blacks and Mill Workers in the Twentieth-Century South* (Knoxville: University of Tennessee Press, 1987).

32. Andrew Cunningham and Perry Williams, eds., *The Laboratory Revolution in Medicine* (Cambridge: Cambridge University Press, 1992). For insight into the bacteriological laboratory's implications for public health, see George Rosen, *A History of Public Health* (Baltimore: Johns Hopkins University Press, 1958). See also Judith Walzer Leavitt, *The Healthiest City: Milwaukee and the Politics of Health Reform* (Princeton: Princeton University Press, 1982).

33. On Lynk, see Todd Savitt, "'A Journal of Our Own': The Medical and Surgical Observer at the Beginnings of an African-American Medical Profession in the Late Nineteenth Century," part 1, *Journal of the National Medical Association* 88 (1996): 52–60. Part 2 appears in *Journal of the National Medical Association* 88 (1996): 115–22.

34. Indeed, for many philanthropists, entrepreneurs, religious activists, and others, the South — "industrially underdeveloped," racially divided, and "lagging" in urban growth, education, and professional expertise — became a special cause. John D. Rockefeller and, later, merchants like Chicago's Julius Rosenwald promoted science as part of a vision of health uplift, financing regional campaigns against diseases like hookworm and syphilis. Philanthropy financed the efforts, for example, of Charles Wardell Stiles, a lone evangelist in the battle against hookworm who introduced thousands of rural folk to microscopes and uncinariasis through tent revivals and public demonstrations. An excellent study of the hookworm campaigns of this era is John Ettling, *The Germ of Laziness: Rockefeller Philanthropy and Public Health in the New South* (Cambridge, Mass.: Harvard University Press, 1981).

35. The *National Negro Health News* reflected these themes. See, for example, Mrs. M. M. Hubert Jackson, "Club Women's View of National Negro Health Week,"

National Negro Health News 3 (April–June 1935): 3; and "A Suggested Year-Round Program," *National Negro Health News* 4 (January–March 1936): 5.

36. See Barbara Rosenkrantz, *Public Health and the State: Changing Views in Massachusetts, 1842–1936* (Cambridge, Mass.: Harvard University Press, 1972). This was not a new concern; indeed, this trend had begun in the mid-nineteenth century. See Rosenberg, *Cholera Years*; Leavitt, *Healthiest City*; and Stuart Galishoff, *Newark: The Nation's Unhealthiest City, 1832–1895* (New Brunswick: Rutgers University Press, 1988).

37. Frank Smythe, "A Golden Opportunity for the University of Tennessee Medical College," *Memphis Medical Journal* (October 1924): 214–18.

38. This commodity value (which has posed an important problem in the history of clinical medicine) has been discussed by other historians, among them Ruth Richardson, *Death, Dissection, and the Destitute* (New York: Routledge and Kegan Paul, 1987), and Robert Blakely and Judith Harrington, eds., *Bones in the Basement: Postmortem Racism in Nineteenth-Century Medical Training* (Washington, D.C.: Smithsonian Institution Press, 1997). See also Russell Maulitz, *Morbid Appearances: The Anatomy of Pathology in the Early Nineteenth Century* (New York: Cambridge University Press, 1987).

39. As historian Owsei Temkin has put it, in this century it has become increasingly possible to speak of health as a "purchasable commodity" and, as a consequence, as a political right. Owsei Temkin, "Health and Disease," in *The Double Face of Janus and Other Essays in the History of Medicine* (Baltimore: Johns Hopkins University Press, 1977), 437.

40. See, for example, Arjun Appadurai, ed., *The Social Life of Things: Commodities in Cultural Perspective* (New York: Cambridge University Press, 1986); Meredith Turshen, *The Political Ecology of Disease in Tanzania* (New Brunswick: Rutgers University Press, 1984); and Randall Packard, *White Plague, Black Labor: Tuberculosis and the Political Economy of Health and Disease in South Africa* (Berkeley: University of California Press, 1989).

41. Jean-Christophe Agnew, "The Consuming Vision of Henry James," in *The Culture of Consumption: Critical Essays in American History, 1880–1980*, ed. T. J. Jackson Lears and Richard Wightman (New York: Pantheon, 1983), 67.

42. René Dubos, *Mirage of Health: Utopias, Progress, and Biological Change* (New York: Harper and Row, 1959).

43. Ernst Boas, *The Unseen Plague: Chronic Disease* (New York: J. J. Augustin, 1940), x.

44. James H. Robinson noted in the 1930s: "This difference in geographical features causes Memphis to stand out in singular contrast to the three other large cities, Nashville, Chattanooga, and Knoxville[,] in commercial interests and industrial pursuits, in topographical layout and structural appearance." James H. Robinson, "A Social History of the Negro in Memphis and in Shelby County" (Ph.D. diss., Yale University, 1934), 23.

45. Ibid., 24. See also Cobb, *Most Southern Place*, and Robert Sigafoos, *From Cotton Row to Beale Street: A Business History of Memphis* (Memphis: Memphis State University Press, 1979).

46. In 1900 some 80 percent of Memphis's residents had come originally from Mississippi and the Tennessee countryside. David Goldfield, "A Regional Framework for the Urban South," in his *Region, Race, and Cities*, 51. For Mencken's quote on Memphis, see Charles Reagan Wilson and William Ferris, eds., *Encyclopedia of Southern Culture* (Chapel Hill: University of North Carolina Press, 1989), 1460.

47. David Cohn, *God Shakes Creation*, 2d ed. (New York: Harper and Brothers, 1935), 14.

48. James W. Silver, *Mississippi: The Closed Society* (New York: Harcourt, Brace, and World, 1964).

49. Blaine Brownell, "The Urban South Comes of Age, 1900–1940," in Brownell and Goldfield, *The City in Southern History*, 138.

50. Quoted in Dewey Grantham, *The South in Modern America: A Region at Odds* (New York: HarperCollins, 1994), 28.

51. See Richard Powell, "The Blues Aesthetic: Black Culture and Modernism," in *The Blues Aesthetic: Black Culture and Modernism*, ed. Richard Powell (Washington, D.C.: Washington Project for the Arts, 1989), 21–23.

52. See Richard Wright's introduction to the three-album set *Southern Exposure: The Blues of Josh White*, Mercury Records (October 1940), 2. Quoted and cited in Clyde Woods, *Development Arrested: The Blues and Plantation Power in the Mississippi Delta* (New York: Verso, 1998), 33. As Wright continues, "Common everyday life, the background of our national life is to be seen through the blues: trains, ships, trade unions, planes, the Army, the Navy, the White House, plantations, elections, poll tax, the boll weevil, landlords, epidemics, bosses, Jim Crow, lynching . . . their very titles indicate the mood and state of mind in which they were written."

53. Michael Harris, *The Rise of the Gospel Blues: The Music of Thomas Andrew Dorsey in the Urban Church* (New York: Oxford University Press, 1992).

54. George Washington Lee, *Beale Street: Where the Blues Began* (New York: Ballou, 1934), 133. See also Margaret McKee and Fred Chisenhall, *Beale, Black, and Blue: Life and Music on America's Main Street* (Baton Rouge: Louisiana State University Press, 1981).

55. Lee, *Beale Street*, 134. These lyrics are also discussed in Randolph Meade Walker, "The Role of the Black Clergy in Memphis during the Crump Era" (thesis, Memphis State University, 1975), 3. See also the discussion in Gloria Brown Melton, "Blacks in Memphis, Tennessee, 1920–1955: A Historical Study" (Ph.D. diss., Washington State University, 1982), 36–37.

56. Beale Street became the center of black business, including the health business and funeral parlors, as well as the music business. Novelist and businessman

George Lee described it as the most bustling street in the South. It was home, as well, to a few black doctors and white entrepreneurs like drugstore owner Abe Plough. Memphis was certainly an alluring hub for rural blacks and whites because of its services, entertainment, and anonymity—but it was also a dangerous city known as the "murder capital of the nation" in the 1920s, a city where police, gangsters, and unhealthy slum conditions posed their own risks. George Lee believed that this penchant for violence had rural origins. George Washington Lee, *River George* (New York: Macaulay, 1937).

57. Frankie Winchester, *Oral History of Lemuel Diggs* (Memphis: Memphis State University Press, 1980), 16. But, as Diggs noted, "the Dean more or less said 'we are mainly interested in you teaching' and running a good program for these patients. Research is not a major effort here" (ibid.).

58. Lemuel Diggs, "Organization of St. Jude Research Hospital," *ALSAC News*, April 14, 1961, 4, in Box 13, Folder: "Lemuel Diggs," Wintrobe Papers. The national expansion of university research ushered into existence new institutions in Memphis—St. Jude Children's Research Hospital, LeBonheur Hospital, the E. H. Crump Hospital—and initiated new research agendas in existing hospitals.

59. The use of blood plasma and penicillin to save soldiers' lives convinced many Americans that good health was—or should be—within everyone's reach, and these rising expectations stimulated federally financed hospital construction, boosted enrollments in health insurance plans, and challenged the legitimacy of the South's segregated urban health care system.

60. For a useful analysis of the social meaning of suffering across cultures, see Arthur Kleinman, Veena Das, and Margaret Lock, eds., *Social Suffering* (Berkeley: University of California Press, 1997).

61. Richard Nixon, "Health Message," February 18, 1971, *Congressional Quarterly Almanac* 27 (February 1971): 37A–38A.

62. See, for example, Sander Gilman, *The Visibility of the Jew in the Diaspora: Body Imagery and Its Cultural Context*, B. G. Rudolph Lectures in Judaic Studies (Syracuse, N.Y.: Syracuse University, 1992), 29.

CHAPTER 1

1. John Dollard, *Caste and Class in a Southern Town* (New Haven: Yale University Press, 1937). See also Carter Godwin Woodson, *The Negro Professional Man and the Community* (Washington: Association for the Study of Negro Life and History, 1934), and Herbert Morais, *The History of the Negro in Medicine* (New York: Publisher's Company, 1967).

2. Maceo Walker, Oral History, in George Washington Lee Collection, Memphis and Shelby County Public Library, Memphis.

3. William D. Miller, *Memphis during the Progressive Era, 1900–1917* (Memphis: Memphis State University Press, 1957), 118. Whether in search of economic

opportunities or in flight from the threat of violence and lynching, migrants— both the marginally prosperous and the poor—looked to Memphis as an urban promised land. From 1900 through the booming 1920s, the Great Depression, and into the 1950s, they came in ebbs and flows from the Deep South, working against the current of the Mississippi River. Some newcomers would linger and then journey farther north to St. Louis, Chicago, or even New York. But many remained in Memphis. For Walker, the city on the high ground along the bluffs, with its towering new constructions, offered a freer hand in the business of medicine and the prospect of uplifting the lives of black people.

4. Walker's son Maceo recalled that although his father was a physician by training, he was also a businessman, and "one [of the careers] had to go because both were growing so he chose the business career." Maceo Walker, Oral History.

5. Until the 1960s, Fuller would be remembered as the last African American elected to the state legislature. Walter B. Weare, *Black Business in the New South: A Social History of the North Carolina Mutual Insurance Company* (Urbana: University of Illinois Press, 1973; reprint, Durham, N.C.: Duke University Press, 1993).

6. Blaine Brownell, "The Urban South Comes of Age, 1900–1940," in *The City in Southern History: The Growth of Urban Civilization in the South*, ed. Blaine Brownell and David R. Goldfield (Port Washington, N.Y.: Kennikat Press, 1977), 128.

7. Blair Hunt, Oral History, Memphis and Shelby County Public Library, Memphis.

8. David Tucker, *Black Pastors and Leaders: The Memphis Clergy, 1819–1972* (Memphis: Memphis State University Press, 1975), 133. Tucker notes that Hunt's "eloquent sermons urged his congregation to set their thoughts on the joy of knowing Jesus, to prepare for the future, and to wait for God to change the white man" (132).

9. Ibid., 55.

10. After publishing strong antilynching tracts, Ida Wells had been forced to leave the city in the 1890s, run out of town by white supremacists with her office burned to the ground. A year after Fuller's arrival, a mob lynching of Ell Person in Memphis made national headlines. James Weldon Johnson, "The Lynching at Memphis," *Crisis* 14 (1917): 185–88, reprinted in *The Selected Writings of James Weldon Johnson*, vol. 2, *Social, Political, and Literary Essays*, ed. Sondra Kathryn Wilson (New York: Oxford University Press, 1995), 23–29.

11. William Ivy Hair, *Carnival of Fury: Robert Charles and the New Orleans Race Riot of 1900* (Baton Rouge: Louisiana State University Press, 1976); Roberta Senechal, *The Sociogenesis of a Race Riot: Springfield, Illinois, in 1908* (Urbana: University of Illinois Press, 1990); Elliot Rudwick, *Race Riot of East St. Louis, July 2, 1917* (Carbondale: Southern Illinois University Press, 1964); Lee Williams, *Anatomy of Four Face Riots: Racial Conflict in Knoxville, Elaine (Arkansas),*

Tulsa, and Chicago, 1919–1921 (Hattiesburg: University and College Press of Mississippi, 1972); and William Tuttle, *Race Riot: Chicago in the Red Summer of 1919* (New York: Atheneum, 1970; reprint, Urbana: University of Illinois Press, 1996).

12. Rev. Calvin Mims of Cedar Grove Baptist Church, quoted in Randolph Meade Walker, "The Role of the Black Clergy in Memphis during the Crump Era" (thesis, Memphis State University, 1975), 16.

13. On Robert Church Sr., see George Lee, *River George* (New York: Macaulay Company, 1937); see also "The Most Representative, Wealthiest and Popular Man of His Race in the South (Robert R. Church Sr.)," *Planters Journal* (Memphis) 15 (September 15, 1906): 1, and A. E. Church, *The Robert R. Churches of Memphis: A Father and Son Who Achieved in Spite of Race* (Memphis: A. E. Church, 1974).

14. Patricia LaPointe, *From Saddlebags to Science: A Century of Health Care in Memphis, 1830–1930* (Memphis: The Foundation, 1984), 46. Lynk's modest school had graduated some 216 black doctors since its founding. Several of its graduates set up practices in Memphis. On Lynk's early years as editor of a regional black medical journal, see Todd Savitt, "'A Journal of Our Own': The Medical and Surgical Observer at the Beginnings of an African-American Medical Profession in the Late Nineteenth Century," part 1, *Journal of the National Medical Association* 88 (1996): 52–60. See also Miles Vandahurst Lynk, *Sixty Years of Medicine: Or the Life and Times of Dr. Miles V. Lynk* (Memphis: Twentieth Century Press, 1951), and Blair Hunt, Oral History.

15. One study of a key black institution of this era is E. Franklin Frazier, *The Negro Church in America* (New York: Schocken Books, 1964), 53. For a description of Memphis in this period, see Gerald Mortimer Capers Jr., *The Biography of a River Town: Memphis, Its Heroic Age* (Chapel Hill: University of North Carolina Press, 1939; reprint, New Orleans: Gerald Capers Jr., Tulane University, 1966). On the New South, see C. Vann Woodward, *Origins of the New South, 1877–1913* (Baton Rouge: Louisiana State University Press, 1951), and George Tindall, *The Emergence of the New South, 1913–1945* (Baton Rouge: Louisiana State University Press, 1967). See also Gavin Wright, *Old South, New South: Revolutions in the Southern Economy since the Civil War* (New York: Basic Books, 1986), and Hollis R. Lynch, *The Black Urban Condition: A Documentary History, 1866–1971* (New York: Crowell, 1973).

16. Gloria Brown Melton, "Blacks in Memphis, Tennessee, 1920–1955: A Historical Study" (Ph.D. diss., Washington State University, 1982), 25–26. Melton notes, "In 1920, 82 percent of the employed black women held jobs primarily as laundresses and domestic servants. Ten percent worked as seamstresses or as semi-skilled factory operatives, and 4 percent were included among the professions as teachers, nurses, or musicians" (ibid.).

17. Ibid., 120. In 1900 the city's population stood at 102,320, 48.8 percent of which

was nonwhite (mostly African American). In 1910, of a total population of 131,105, some 40.1 percent was nonwhite. In 1920 the nonwhite population had dropped slightly, to 37.7 percent of a total of 162,351. In 1930, following a decade of tremendous growth, about 38.2 percent of a total population of 253,143 was nonwhite. In 1940 the figure had climbed to 41.1 percent nonwhite among a total population of 292,942. Based on U.S. Department of Commerce, Bureau of the Census, *The Negro in the United States, 1920–1932* (Washington, D.C.: U.S. Government Printing Office, 1935), 33.

18. Thomas Woofter, *Negro Problems in Cities* (Garden City, N.Y.: Doubleday, Doran, 1928), charts on page 60. See also Leigh Fraser, *A Demographic Analysis of Memphis and Shelby County, Tennessee, 1820–1972* (master's thesis, Memphis State University, 1974). For a recent analysis of urban development in another New South city, see Thomas Hanchett, *Sorting Out the New South: Race, Class, and Urban Development in Charlotte, 1875–1975* (Chapel Hill: University of North Carolina Press, 1998).

19. Woofter, *Negro Problems in Cities*, 28.

20. Ibid., 79, 83. See also Melton, "Blacks in Memphis," 23. For comparison, see Allan Spear, *Black Chicago: The Making of a Negro Ghetto, 1890–1920* (Chicago: University of Chicago Press, 1967); Joe Trotter, *Black Milwaukee: The Making of an Industrial Proletariat, 1915–1945* (Urbana: University of Illinois Press, 1985); and Gilbert Osofsky, *Harlem: The Making of a Ghetto* (New York: Harper and Row, 1966).

21. Michael Honey, *Southern Labor and Black Civil Rights: Organizing Memphis Workers* (Urbana: University of Illinois Press, 1933), 30. Information drawn from the U.S. Department of Commerce, Bureau of the Census, *Classified Index of Occupations, Fifteenth Census of the United States* (Washington, D.C.: U.S. Government Printing Office, 1930).

22. Christopher Silver, "The Changing Face of Neighborhoods in Memphis and Richmond, 1940–1985," in *Shades of the Sunbelt: Essays on Ethnicity, Race, and the Urban South*, ed. Randall Miller and George Pozzetta (New York: Greenwood Press, 1988), 102. As Silver notes, by 1950 socioeconomic differentiation was also evident in the fact that of all black residential units in North Memphis, owners of homes comprised 53 percent of all residents (2,120 of 3,991), while in the more populous South Memphis, owners comprised only 29 percent (4,822 of 16,414). Ibid.

23. This regional account of the emerging medical and public health system, taking into account politics, race, and urban culture, contrasts with accounts that focus on the emergence of laboratory and research medicine as the center of the new system. For other works on the social transformation of medicine as portrayed in the education- and philanthropy-centered analysis, see Howard Berliner, *A System of Scientific Medicine: Philanthropic Foundations in the Flexner Era* (New York: Tavistock, 1985), and Richard Brown, *Rockefeller Medicine Men: Medicine*

and Capitalism in America (Berkeley: University of California Press, 1979). While not ignoring the significance of laboratory medicine, the account presented here explores the ways in which a particular urban-rural politics, an ambivalence to "outsiders," and the rise of the federal government contributed to the shape of the unfolding health care system in the urban South.

24. For a comparison with similar health discourse in northern contexts, see Alan Kraut, *Silent Travelers: Germs, Genes, and the "Immigrant Menace"* (New York: Basic Books, 1994).

25. Eric Foner, *A Short History of Reconstruction, 1863–1877* (New York: Harper and Row, 1990), 37.

26. See Robert Wiebe, *The Search for Order, 1877–1920* (New York: Hill and Wang, 1967).

27. With names like Mt. Sinai, Lutheran, St. Francis, and Baptist Memorial, these hospitals reflected the ideals of religious denominations and ethnic groups in every American city. George Rosen, *The Structure of American Medical Practice, 1875–1941*, ed. Charles Rosenberg (Philadelphia: University of Pennsylvania Press, 1983), 23.

28. An important study of American society in this era is Wiebe, *Search for Order*. See also Ellis Hawley, *The Great War and the Search for a Modern Order: A History of the American People and Their Institutions, 1917–1933* (New York: St. Martin's Press, 1979), and Oscar Handlin, *The Uprooted* (Boston: Little, Brown, 1973).

29. Frazier, *Negro Church in America*.

30. T. O. Fuller, *The Story of Church Life among Negroes* (Memphis: T. O. Fuller, 1938), 16.

31. Ibid.

32. See, for example, N. N. Puckett, *Folk Beliefs of the Southern Negro* (Chapel Hill: University of North Carolina Press, 1926).

33. See Nancy Tomes, *The Gospel of Germs: Men, Women, and the Microbe in American Life* (Cambridge, Mass.: Harvard University Press, 1998).

34. On schools, see Vincent Franklin, *The Education of Black Philadelphia: The Social and Educational History of a Minority Community, 1900–1950* (Philadelphia: University of Pennsylvania Press, 1979). See also James Anderson, *The Education of Blacks in the South, 1860–1935* (Chapel Hill: University of North Carolina Press, 1988), and James Leloudis, *Schooling the New South: Pedagogy, Self, and Society in North Carolina, 1880–1920* (Chapel Hill: University of North Carolina Press, 1996). The varied evolution of Jim Crow arrangements in housing, schools, and worship has been well documented by American historians. See C. Vann Woodward, *The Strange Career of Jim Crow*, 3d rev. ed. (New York: Oxford University Press, 1974). On housing segregation, see Christopher Silver and John V. Moeser, *The Separate City: Black Communities in the Urban South, 1940–1968* (Lexington: University Press of Kentucky, 1995); on segregation in religion, see Paul Harvey, *Redeeming the South: Religious Cultures and Racial Identities among*

Southern Baptists, 1865–1925 (Chapel Hill: University of North Carolina Press, 1997), and Hans A. Baer and Merrill Singer, *African-American Religion in the Twentieth Century: Varieties of Protest and Accommodation* (Knoxville: University of Tennessee Press, 1992).

35. From the standpoint of black women's history, this argument is made cogently and powerfully in Evelyn Brooks Higginbotham, *Righteous Discontent: The Women's Movement in the Black Baptist Church, 1880–1920* (Cambridge, Mass.: Harvard University Press, 1993).

36. Connie Wolff to James S. Robinson, June 4, 1928, Unit 50, Folder 2, James Robinson Papers, Southern Historical Collection, University of North Carolina at Chapel Hill.

37. Indeed, from glancing at a map of regional cotton production, one might suppose that Memphis was not primarily connected to the state of Tennessee at all, but rather that it was attached to a wide swath of territory stretching thousands of miles through the cotton-growing, cotton-producing belt, from central Georgia through Alabama, Mississippi, and Arkansas, and touching the western edge of Tennessee only at Memphis. Dewey Grantham, *The South in Modern America: A Region at Odds* (New York: HarperCollins, 1994), 29.

38. Paul Preble, "A Review of Public Health Administration in Memphis, Tennessee," *Public Health Bulletin* 113 (Washington, D.C.: U.S. Government Printing Office, 1921), 17.

39. Richard Hepler, "Bovine Tuberculosis and the Battle for Pure Milk in Memphis, 1910–1911," *West Tennessee Historical Society Papers* 40 (December 1986): 6–23.

40. Preble, "Public Health Administration," 82.

41. W. F. Walker, *Survey of the Health Problems and Facilities in Memphis and Shelby County, Tennessee from the Year 1929* (Memphis: Committee on Administrative Practice of the American Public Health Association, 1930), 108.

42. Similar tensions emerged in all major cities. See, for example, Morris Vogel, *The Invention of the Modern Hospital: Boston, 1870–1930* (Chicago: University of Chicago Press, 1980). See also Rosemary Stevens, *In Sickness and in Wealth: American Hospitals in the Twentieth Century* (New York: Basic Books, 1989), and David Rosner, *A Once Charitable Enterprise: Hospitals and Health Care in Brooklyn and New York, 1885–1915* (New York: Cambridge University Press, 1982). For discussions of corporate trends in America, see Alfred Chandler, *The Visible Hand: The Managerial Revolution in American Business* (Cambridge, Mass.: Belknap Press, 1977); Hawley, *The Great War*; and Alan Trachtenberg, *Incorporation of America: Culture and Society in the Gilded Age* (New York: Hill and Wang, 1982).

43. For overviews and case studies of these institutional developments, see, for example, Vanessa Gamble, *Making a Place for Ourselves: The Black Hospital Movement, 1920–1945* (New York: Oxford University Press, 1995). See also Edward

Beardsley, *A History of Neglect: Health Care for Blacks and Mill Workers in the Twentieth-Century South* (Knoxville: University of Tennessee Press, 1987); David McBride, *Integrating the City of Medicine: Blacks in Philadelphia Health Care, 1910–1965* (Philadelphia: Temple University Press, 1989); Darlene Clark Hine, *Black Women in White: Racial Conflict and Cooperation in the Nursing Profession, 1890–1950* (Bloomington: University of Indiana Press, 1989); and Susan Smith, *Sick and Tired of Being Sick and Tired: Black Women's Health Activism in America, 1890–1950* (Philadelphia: University of Pennsylvania Press, 1995).

44. A useful analysis of black physicians' perceptions of segregation is Edward Beardsley, "Making Separate Equal: Black Physicians and the Problems of Medical Segregation in the Pre World War II South," *Bulletin of the History of Medicine* 57 (1983): 382–96.

45. Abraham Flexner, *Medical Education in the United States and Canada* (New York: Carnegie Foundation for the Advancement of Teaching, 1910), 180. See also Marvin Graves, "The Negro as a Menace to the White Race," *Southern Medical Journal* 9 (1916): 407–13.

46. Flexner, *Medical Education*, 180.

47. The violence of Jim Crow in Memphis was perhaps most evident to working-class African Americans. See Kenneth Goings and Gerald Smith, "'Unhidden Transcripts': Memphis and African-American Agency, 1862–1920," *Journal of Urban History* 21 (March 1995): 372–94.

48. For regional cotton planters, insurance provided a safeguard from the vagaries of bad weather, the boll weevil, a poor crop, or bad health. For Americans and citizens of other industrializing nations, the search for national "sickness insurance" became a significant political issue. See Ronald Numbers, *Almost Persuaded: American Physicians and Compulsory Health Insurance, 1912–1920* (Baltimore: Johns Hopkins University Press, 1978).

49. Frederick Hoffman, *History of the Prudential Life Insurance Company of America, 1875–1900* (Newark, N.J.: Prudential Press, 1900); Frederick Hoffman, "Race Traits and Tendencies of the American Negro," American Economic Association, *Publications* 11 (August 1896): 6.

50. Burial signified one of the important passages of life, and for many southern blacks it was an event with deep otherworldly significance. As Charles Joyner has noted, funerals could have "considerable pageantry and display . . . as elaborate a part of the slave life cycle . . . as weddings." Charles Joyner, *Down by the Riverside: A South Carolina Slave Community* (Urbana: University of Illinois Press, 1984), 138. On funeral insurance in the early twentieth century, see Weare, *Black Business*. See also Winfred Octavus Bryson Jr., "Negro Life Insurance Companies: A Comparative Analysis of the Operating and Financial Experience of Negro Legal Reserve Life Insurance Companies" (Ph.D. diss., University of Pennsylvania, 1948); Morton Keller, *The Life Insurance Enterprise, 1885–*

1910: A Study of the Limits of Corporate Power (Cambridge, Mass.: Belknap Press, 1963); and M. S. Stuart, *An Economic Detour: A History of Insurance in the Lives of American Negroes* (New York: W. Mallie and Company, 1940).

51. Robert Sigafoos, *From Cotton Row to Beale Street: A Business History of Memphis* (Memphis: Memphis State University Press, 1979), 94.

52. See S. R. Bruesch, "Collins Chapel Hospital" and "Jane Terrell Baptist Hospital," in *History of Medicine in Memphis*, ed. Marcus Stewart and William Black (Jackson, Tenn.: McCowat-Mercer Press, 1971), 132, 178.

53. See Fuller, *Church Life among Negroes*, 28.

54. Otis S. Warr, "Medical Memphis: A Century of Progress, 1830–1930," pt. 2, *Memphis Medical Journal* (September 1931): 138.

55. One survey noted, without additional commentary, that colored patients were not received at the white Baptist Memorial Hospital. See U.S. Public Health Service Report, "Synopsis for the Guidance of Hospital Inspectors," August 19, 1920, Box 50, Entry 29, Folder: "Memphis, Tenn., Memphis General Hospital," Records of the U.S. Public Health Service, Record Group 443, National Archives and Records Administration, College Park, Maryland.

56. The Collins Chapel Connectional Hospital proudly and self-consciously promoted itself as "the only colored hospital serving all of Arkansas, all of Mississippi, Kentucky and West Tennessee." "A Hospital Project to Meet an Imperative Need" (Memphis: Collins Chapel Hospital, New Building Fund, 1945). See also Donald R. Harris, "A Hospital for the Negroes of Memphis: Collins Chapel Hospital, 1910–1970," Memphis and Shelby County Public Library, and LaPointe, *From Saddlebags to Science*, 46.

57. Among the new hospital facilities in this era were Baptist Memorial Hospital (1912), Crippled Children's Hospital (1919), Methodist Hospital (1921), Veterans Hospital (1921), and the Physicians and Surgeons Building at Baptist Hospital (1928). There were also smaller hospitals built in this period, including the black-run Mercy Hospital (1918) and Royal Circle Hospital (1921). From LaPointe, *From Saddlebags to Science*, 48.

58. Flexner, *Medical Education*, 181.

59. Lynk was a prominent layman in the CME Church. Fuller, *Church Life among Negroes*, 29.

60. Kenneth Ludmerer, *Learning to Heal: The Development of American Medical Education* (New York: Basic Books, 1985).

61. Berliner, *System of Scientific Medicine*. See Alan Trachtenberg, *The Incorporation of America: Culture and Society in the Gilded Age* (New York: Hill and Wang, 1982), and Wiebe, *Search for Order*.

62. Blair Hunt, Oral History, 6. The rhetoric of "great works" drawn from Protestant theology helped to legitimate and give meaning to medical institutions throughout the state. While Hunt praised Lynk's school for its great work, Otis Warr of Memphis later praised Lynk's college for "doing a great work during

her existence as a medical institution." See John M. Maury, "The Hospitals of Memphis," *Memphis Medical Journal* (June 1926): 137, and Warr, "Medical Memphis."

63. Flexner, *Medical Education*, 308.

64. Ibid.

65. On industrial capitalism and horizontal and vertical integration, see Alfred Chandler, *Scale and Scope: The Dynamics of Industrial Capitalism* (Cambridge, Mass.: Belknap Press, 1990); on corporate capitalism in the early twentieth century, see Gabriel Kolko, *The Triumph of Conservatism: A Reinterpretation of American History, 1900–1916* (New York: Free Press of Glencoe, 1963), and David Noble, *America By Design: Science, Technology, and the Rise of Corporate Capitalism* (New York: Knopf, 1977).

66. Smythe, "A Golden Opportunity," 214–18.

67. MGH promoted itself as a charity facility born out of municipal Christian stewardship. See Warr, "Medical Memphis," 138.

68. S. R. Bruesch, "City of Memphis Hospital," in Stewart and Black, *History of Medicine in Memphis*, 86.

69. Basil MacLean, *The City of Memphis, Tennessee, 1949: A Study of Negro Hospital Needs* (Rochester, N.Y.: Basil C. MacLean, George William Graham and Lloyd Mussells, Associates, 1949).

70. "Records of the General Inspection Service, August 19, 1920, Memphis General Hospital," Box 50, Entry 29: "Martinsville-Memphis," Records of the U.S. Public Health Service, Record Group 443, National Archives.

71. Stuart Galishoff, "Germs Know No Color Line: Black Health and Public Policy in Atlanta, 1900–1918," *Journal of the History of Medicine and Allied Sciences* 40 (January 1985): 29.

72. S. R. Bruesch, "Old Times in Memphis Medicine," *Memphis Medical Journal* (August 1951): 125.

73. This interaction between indigent patients and teaching physicians was not a new trend. A convergence between poverty, disease, and medical education had defined medical practice through previous centuries as well, taking particular form with urbanization, industrialization, and the availability of dying and dead bodies in almshouses in the late eighteenth and nineteenth centuries. Ruth Richardson has noted that by 1800, "in medical circles, market terminology was being applied to human corpses apparently without embarrassment." Such language highlighted the growing value of cadavers — particularly of the poor — for anatomical teaching. In the United States, physicians undertaking such teaching practices often did so illicitly because of legal or moral objections. By the late nineteenth and early twentieth centuries, however, this system of cadaver-based education was changing, especially with the increasing significance of the laboratory in medicine. The value of animal experiments and tests on living patients in medical education rose sharply in these years, gradually crowding out old-

style pathology teaching. Ruth Richardson, *Death, Dissection, and the Destitute* (New York: Routledge and Kegan Paul, 1987), 55.

74. James R. Reinberger, "Modern Prenatal Supervision," *Memphis Medical Journal* (February 1932): 29–30.

75. For an analysis of the history and politics of infant and maternal health, see Richard Meckel, *"Save the Babies": American Public Health Reform and the Prevention of Infant Mortality, 1850–1929* (Baltimore: Johns Hopkins University Press, 1990).

76. On uplift ideology and African Americans, see Kevin Gaines, *Uplifting the Race: Black Leadership, Politics, and Culture in the Twentieth Century* (Chapel Hill: University of North Carolina Press, 1996), and Tera Hunter, *To 'Joy My Freedom: Southern Black Women's Lives and Labors after the Civil War* (Cambridge, Mass.: Harvard University Press, 1997).

77. Inculcating poor patients with new health beliefs necessarily involved educating other black women about new notions and practices of health and new methods of health surveillance. See Hine, *Black Women in White*, 72–74. On black women in the South during this period, see Glenda Gilmore, *Gender and Jim Crow: Women and the Politics of White Supremacy in North Carolina, 1896–1920* (Chapel Hill: University of North Carolina Press, 1996).

78. Reinberger, "Modern Prenatal Supervision," 32.

79. Ibid.

80. W. F. Walker, *Survey of Health Problems*, 54.

81. Ibid., 33.

82. Reinberger, "Modern Prenatal Supervision."

83. Ibid.

84. For more on this politics and a critical look at the claims of obstetricians in their battles against midwifery in this era, see Charlotte Borst, *Catching Babies: The Professionalization of Childbirth, 1870–1920* (Cambridge, Mass.: Harvard University Press, 1995). See also Judith Walzer Leavitt, *Brought to Bed: Childbearing in America, 1750–1950* (New York: Oxford University Press, 1986). On infant mortality specifically in Memphis, see Preble, "Public Health Administration," 42–43.

85. Robert W. O'Brien, "Beale Street, A Study of Ecological Succession," *Sociological and Social Research* 26 (May–June 1942): 433.

86. Ibid.

87. "Magic Doctors of Harlem are Health Menace," *New York Telegram*, January 9, 1928, in *[L. S. Alexander] Gumby Collection of the American Negro, Scrapbooks* (New York: Columbia University Libraries, 1971–74), microfilm, reel 1.

88. For insight into conjure doctoring, see Paul Dunbar, *In Old Plantation Days* (New York: Dodd, Mead, 1903), especially "The Conjuring Contest." See also Charles Chesnutt, *The Conjure Woman and Other Conjure Tales* (1899; reprint, edited with an introduction by Richard Brodhead, Durham, N.C.: Duke Uni-

versity Press, 1993); Puckett, *Folk Beliefs of the Southern Negro*; Paula Hathaway Anderson-Green, "Folklore and Fiction in Nineteenth-Century North Carolina: Taliaferro's 'Fisher River' and Chesnutt's 'The Conjure Woman'" (Ph.D. diss., Georgia State University, 1980); and Theophus H. Smith, *Conjuring Culture: Biblical Formations of Black America* (New York: Oxford University Press, 1994), 167.

89. "Midwives Must Follow Strict Set of Rules," *Memphis Press-Scimitar*, June 21, 1935. For discussion of the urban economy in 1920s Memphis, see Robert Lanier, *Memphis in the Twenties: The Second Term of Mayor Rowlett Paine, 1924–1928* (Memphis: Zenda Press, 1979), particularly "Strong in Mind and Body," 12–15. See also William D. Miller, *Memphis during the Progressive Era*. For studies of the contrast between the urban and rural experience of black Americans, see Carter Godwin Woodson, *The Rural Negro* (Washington, D.C.: Association for the Study of Negro Life and History, 1930); Louise Venable Kennedy, *The Negro Peasant Turns Cityward; Effects of Recent Migrations to Northern Centers* (New York: Columbia University Press, 1930); and Woofter, *Negro Problems in Cities*, 60. For discussions of municipal politics in other cities, with some discussion of health politics, see Spear, *Black Chicago*; Osofsky, *Harlem*; and James Grossman, *Land of Hope: Chicago, Black Southerners, and the Great Migration* (Chicago: University of Chicago Press, 1989).

90. See Lawrence Levine, *Black Culture and Black Consciousness: Afro-American Folk Thought from Slavery to Freedom* (New York: Oxford University Press, 1977).

91. James Weldon Johnson, "Now We Have the Blues," *New York Amsterdam News*, July 7, 1926, reprinted in Wilson, *Selected Writings of James Weldon Johnson*, 2:388–91.

92. See Puckett, *Folk Beliefs of the Southern Negro*

93. Among its lyrics, "Memphis Minnie-jitis Blues" notes: "Mmmmmm, this meningitis killin' me. . . . My head and neck was failin' me, / feel like my back was breakin' two, / Lord I had such a mood that mornin', / I didn't know what in the world to do." Memphis Minnie [Lizzie Douglas], "Memphis Minnie-jitis Blues," June 5, 1930, on *Memphis Minnie, Hot Stuff Collector's Edition (1930–1941)*, Peermusic (Magnum America) MCCD001.

94. Fuller, *Church Life among Negroes*, 46.

95. Ibid., 42. "Health," Fuller noted to his fellow ministers, "is absolutely essential to the spread of the gospel."

96. For Crump's role in labor politics, see Michael Honey, *Southern Labor and Black Civil Rights: Organizing Memphis Workers* (Urbana: University of Illinois Press, 1993).

97. William D. Miller, *Mr. Crump of Memphis* (Baton Rouge: Louisiana State University Press, 1964), 79.

98. Ibid., 92–96.

99. Alfred Steinberg, *The Bosses* (New York: Macmillan, 1972), 80.

100. One 1939 article noted that "in bringing in the vote, he has used the well-known methods used by political bosses in other American cities." Jonathan Daniels, "He Suits Memphis," *Saturday Evening Post*, June 10, 1939, 22. In having a "beloved" political boss, Memphis would stand apart from other southern cities like Nashville, Birmingham, and Atlanta and closer to northern cities of the time.

101. Preble, "Public Health Administration," 16.

102. David Tucker, "Black Pride and Negro Business in the 1920s: George Washington Lee of Memphis," *Business History Review* 43 (Winter 1969): 437.

103. George Washington Lee, quoted in Melton, "Blacks in Memphis," 80.

104. Founded in 1905, the City Federation of Colored Women's Clubs was a branch of the National Federation of Colored Women's Clubs. Ibid., 95.

105. James Weldon Johnson, "The Colored Woman Voter," *New York Age*, September 18, 1920, reprinted in *The Selected Writings of James Weldon Johnson*, vol. 1, *The New York Age Editorials, 1914–1923*, ed. Sondra Kathryn Wilson (New York: Oxford University Press, 1995), 82. For further discussion of gender, race, and voting in the South, see Gilmore, *Gender and Jim Crow*.

106. E. H. Crump to Hill McAllister, November 5, 1920, p. 2, Hill McAllister Papers, AC 75-118, Box 9, Folder 5, Tennessee State Library and Archives, Nashville.

107. E. H. Crump to Hill McAllister, June 28, 1919; Crump asked McAllister to give his support to placing a Vocational School for Negro Girls in Memphis in a letter of March 11, 1922. Both in McAllister Papers, ibid.

108. The contrast in perspectives is between Paul Lewinson, *Race, Class, and Party: A History of Negro Suffrage and White Politics in the South* (New York: Oxford University Press, 1932), 138, 162, and Ralph Bunche, *The Political Status of the Negro in the Age of FDR*, ed. Dewey Grantham (Chicago: University of Chicago Press, 1973), 73. See also V. O. Key, *Southern Politics in the State and Nation* (New York: Vintage Books, 1949); according to Key, "Crump sees that Memphis Negroes get a fairer break than usual in public services" (74). To compare Memphis's black politics with that of other cities, see Osofsky, *Harlem*, and Spear, *Black Chicago*. On San Antonio voting, see David R. Johnson, John A. Booth, and Richard J. Harris, eds., *The Politics of San Antonio: Community, Progress, and Power* (Lincoln: University of Nebraska Press, 1983).

109. The 1924 election is said to have been won by Crump's candidate, who defeated the Ku Klux Klan's candidate by some 4,000 votes, on the strengths of African American votes. Lanier, *Memphis in the Twenties*, 96.

110. See Michael L. Goldstein, "Black Power and the Rise of Bureaucratic Autonomy in New York City Politics: The Case of Harlem Hospital, 1917–1931," *Phylon* 41 (June 1980): 187–201; and "The Case of Harlem Hospital," *The Crisis* 23 (November 1921): 24–25. See also Guichard Parris and Lester Brooks,

Blacks in the City: A History of the National Urban League (Boston: Little, Brown, 1971), 131.

111. Goldstein, "Black Power."

112. From the perspective of one clergyman, it was the Baptist ministers who were most closely allied with Crump. The Methodists never became a significant force in city politics because of the frequency with which clergy were moved around by the bishop in a church organization that was more centralized than the Baptist church. See Randolph Meade Walker, "Role of the Black Clergy," 12.

113. Quoting Crump, Fuller wrote: "Negroes have to work for their living. Nobody goes out of their way to take care of them. . . . It is pitiful to see them hobbling around, deformed — forced to keep on going day after day." "Well said," interjected Fuller. In general, Fuller believed that Crump's sympathy for African American hardship was echoed in "the city of Memphis [which] takes pride in what it has done for the Negro population . . . [with its] three splendid parks, one playground, one swimming pool, two wading pools." T. O. Fuller, *Bridging the Racial Chasms: A Brief Survey of Inter-racial Attitudes and Relations* (Memphis: T. O. Fuller, 1937), 44. Similarly, historian William Miller, describing Crump's creation of a park for blacks in 1913, wrote that "Crump might have been thinking of Negro votes, but he could also just as well have considered it a matter of justice." William D. Miller, *Mr. Crump of Memphis*, 87.

114. According to local lore, just before the election Crump "sent dozens of teachers along Beale Street to teach the Negro population how to write." Steinberg, *The Bosses*, 82.

115. James H. Robinson, "A Social History of the Negro in Memphis and in Shelby County" (Ph.D. diss., Yale University, 1934), 23.

116. For first quote, see Malcolm Rice Patterson Papers, Box 12, Newsclippings, Tennessee State Library and Archives. For second quote, see Steinberg, *The Bosses*, 106.

117. Grantham, *The South in Modern America*, 48.

118. Ibid., 157.

119. James Weldon Johnson noted that "we have often said that if the Negro were suddenly taken out of the South, the white people would very soon realize how much less money there would be left in the public funds for public schools or any other purpose. The exodus from the South is in a large measure demonstrating the truth of that statement." James Weldon Johnson, "Southern Political Economy," *New York Age*, July 7, 1922, 102, reprinted in Wilson, *Selected Writings of James Weldon Johnson*, 1:49. See also James Weldon Johnson, "The Importance of the Negro to the South," *New York Age*, August 16, 1916, reprinted in ibid., 115. Sociologist Franklin Frazier perhaps overstated the im-

pact, noting that "the movement of Negroes to cities . . . uprooted the masses of Negroes from their customary way of life, destroying the social organization which represented both an accommodation to conditions in the rural South and an accommodation to their segregated and inferior status in Southern society." Frazier, *Negro Church in America*, 53.

120. Or they could stroll past the Mercy Hospital on Mississippi Avenue with its twenty-five beds. See LaPointe, *From Saddlebags to Science*, 46. Memphis in 1926 could proudly claim four such "colored" hospitals. John M. Maury, "The Hospitals of Memphis," *Memphis Medical Journal* (June 1926): 138.

121. Hine, *Black Women in White*.

122. Eric Foner, *Reconstruction: America's Unfinished Revolution, 1863–1877* (New York: Harper and Row, 1988).

123. LaPointe, *From Saddlebags to Science*, 48. As LaPointe noted, the Veterans Hospital purchased an old Methodist Hospital building to undertake this expansion. For more on the political economy of veterans' health and welfare, See Theda Skocpol, *Protecting Soldiers and Mothers: The Political Origins of Social Policy in the United States* (Cambridge, Mass.: Belknap Press, 1992).

124. Letter from "3462.27" to Hon. P. C. Harris, Adjutant General, U.S. Army, April 25, 1921, Box 196, Folder: "Colored Soldier 3462.27 Complaint Form," Records of the U.S. Public Health Service, Record Group 90, National Archives.

125. Ibid.

126. Pete Daniel, "Black Power in the 1920s: The Case of Tuskegee Veterans Hospital," *Journal of Southern History* 35 (1972): 368–88, quote at 377.

127. Ibid., quotes at 373 and 376; see also Raymond Wolters, "Major Moton Defeats the Klan: The Case of the Tuskegee Veterans Hospital," in *The New Negro on Campus: Black College Rebellions of the 1920s* (Princeton: Princeton University Press, 1993), 137–91.

128. Daniel, "Black Power in the 1920s," 370.

129. Ibid., 380.

130. The Tuskegee Veterans Hospital was but one example of health politics under the Harding administration. The president's public response to the findings of Joseph Goldberger on pellagra in the South drew unwanted attention to this disease problem and also angered defensive southerners. Goldberger's tour of orphanages, prisons, and hospitals from 1917 to 1921 had led him to conclude that pellagra was caused by the unvaried "southern diet" of meat, meal, and molasses. He characterized this diet as an outgrowth of regional poverty and of the single-minded dependence on the cotton crop. Many southerners regarded these suggestions as an insult to the region—a criticism of its institutions, its culture, and its values. Harding's public comments, drawing attention to "famine and plague" in the region, only heightened regional defensiveness. Eliza-

beth Etheridge, *The Butterfly Caste: A Social History of Pellagra in the South* (Westport, Conn.: Greenwood Press, 1972). See also Elizabeth Etheridge, "Pellagra: An Unappreciated Reminder of Southern Distinctiveness," in *Disease and Distinctiveness in the American South*, ed. Todd Savitt and James Harvey Young (Knoxville: University of Tennessee Press, 1988), 110–19. Noted one southerner sympathetic to Goldberger and Harding, "That there is an epidemic that is sapping the manhood and womanhood of the South no sensible observing man can doubt. . . . [But] the southern gentleman thinks he is being personally insulted when anybody charges that a considerable portion of the people of his county are in a starving condition. He takes it as a reflection on his generosity." Charles Stoll to President Harding, July 27, 1921, quoted in Etheridge, "Pellegra," 111.

131. In 1920, for example, one investigator reported, "I consider the [Memphis General] Hospital a good hospital and doing good work, even though the patients are charity and not of the high type, as ordinarily found in a private institution." The report recommended "that colored patients only be sent to this Hospital, as the Baptist Memorial Hospital, Memphis Tenn., does not receive them." U.S. Public Health Service Report, "Synopsis for the Guidance of Hospital Inspectors."

132. Preble, "Public Health Administration.

133. Ibid., 80. See also Stewart and Black, *History of Medicine in Memphis*. At the same time, the U.S. Children's Bureau, a division of the Department of Labor, was engaged in surveys of infant and maternal mortality throughout the Memphis region. Such federal agencies interested in health matters tended to provide only survey information, advice, and gentle criticism in the South. These self-conscious outside investigators into southern public health usually avoided anything that sounded like criticism or disdain.

134. See, for example, Preble's call for reorganization of the public health system in 1921. Preble, "Public Health Administration," 85.

135. Such foundations also supported education at Tuskegee and at Howard and Meharry Medical Colleges.

136. John Ettling, *The Germ of Laziness: Rockefeller Philanthropy and Public Health in the New South* (Cambridge, Mass.: Harvard University Press, 1981), 1.

137. Ibid.

138. James Jones, *Bad Blood: The Tuskegee Syphilis Experiment* (New York: Free Press, 1981). On Rosenwald, see Judith Sealander, *Private Wealth and Public Life: Foundation Philanthropy and the Reshaping of American Social Policy from the Progressive Era to the New Deal* (Baltimore: Johns Hopkins University Press, 1997). See also A. Gilbert Belles, "The Julius Rosenwald Fund: Efforts in Race Relations, 1928–1948" (Ph.D. diss., Vanderbilt University, 1972).

139. As Johnson saw it, "The Rosenwald Fund experiment in mass control of syphi-

lis was probably the most successful in bringing a large number of persons to have blood tests made than any similar venture." Charles Spurgeon Johnson, *Shadow of the Plantation* (Chicago: University of Chicago Press, 1934), 202.

140. Ibid.

141. At the time he wrote, Johnson was unaware of the shifting purpose of the study.

142. Memphis could claim some twenty-three "Rosenwald schools" that were either built or renovated by matching grants to community organizations and city governments. Statistics cited in Charles S. Johnson, *Shadow of the Plantation*, 136. The motivation and interest of Rosenwald continues to be a source of much debate among historians of medicine and education. See Jerry Wayne Woods, "The Julius Rosenwald Fund School Building Program: A Saga in the Growth and Development of African-American Education in Selected West Tennessee Counties" (Ph.D. diss., University of Mississippi, 1995).

143. George Washington Lee, *Beale Street: Where the Blues Began* (New York: Ballou, 1934), 197.

144. Ibid.

145. Ibid., 198.

146. Ibid., 197. Beale Street had already attracted a handful of eminent black physicians, but Lee noted that "with all the training and culture these doctors represent they have never been able to get together to accept the Rosenwald hospital offer or to request the city administration to carry out its promise to build a much-needed hospital for its community of ninety thousand people" (ibid.)

147. Ibid., 198.

148. As several historians have noted, Rosenwald helped to build many such institutions, but he required state control of them, which diminished local black control. George Lee, who made his living in insurance, had also proposed building a new black college in Memphis in the late 1920s. His efforts were defeated by the opposition of civic clubs and, again, by the city government. Neither saw any political or economic value in such an institution. As the failure revealed, Memphis was a city proud of its own institutions and defensive about its stature. City leaders proved to be wary of any outside influences that might reshape race relations. Wary and conservative businessmen and politicians looked skeptically at federal investigators as well as philanthropic bequests, even in the early years of the Depression when resources were scarce.

149. Meharry Medical College survived on support from foundations established by Andrew Carnegie, John D. Rockefeller, and Julius Rosenwald. See James Summerville, *Educating Black Doctors: A History of Meharry Medical College* (University: University of Alabama Press, 1983). When the financial collapse of this black medical college seemed imminent in 1919, it was the Carnegie Foundation and the Rockefeller General Education Board that contributed $300,000 for its continuation. The Carnegie-sponsored Flexner Report had labeled

Meharry "a most creditable institution" and the best hope for black health in the region. Flexner, *Medical Education*, 309.

150. As one report later noted, "Sixty percent of the colored physicians in Memphis are graduates of [Meharry] . . . but their numbers were still small because 'young Negro physicians are not attracted to Memphis because hospital facilities are not available to them.'" MacLean, *City of Memphis*, 21. C. A. Terrell, founder of the Terrell Hospital, was a product of Meharry. Tuskegee had obtained a prominent position in the national philanthropic mind-set for its production of undergraduates and agricultural workers. Finally, Atlanta institutions like Fisk University, where Charles Johnson and others conducted academic studies of black life in the region, attracted support for their scholarship, as well as for their production of black scholars.

151. A bequest by Baltimore philanthropist Johns Hopkins in the 1870s had converted that sleepy "southern" town in Maryland into a national exemplar of medical education and research within twenty years. This model had appealed to corporate giants like John D. Rockefeller and Andrew Carnegie and led to the creation of new medical institutions like the Rockefeller Institute for Medical Research in New York City. See Donald Fleming, *William H. Welch and the Rise of Modern Medicine* (Baltimore: Johns Hopkins University Press, 1954), and George Corner, *A History of the Rockefeller Institute, 1901–1953: Origins and Growth* (New York: Rockefeller Institute Press, 1964). Andrew Carnegie had supported the Tuskegee Institute in Alabama because of the modest vision of Booker T. Washington. See Louis Harlan, *Booker T. Washington: The Wizard of Tuskegee, 1901–1915* (New York: Oxford University Press, 1983). A generation of business-philanthropists followed the lead of Rockefeller and Carnegie. Julius Rosenwald, Chicago department store mogul, supported health care institutions in the North and, most notably, in the South. On Julius Rosenwald, see Sealander, *Private Wealth and Public Life*. See also M. R. Werner, *Julius Rosenwald: The Life of a Practical Humanitarian* (New York: Harper, 1939), particularly chapter 5, "The Negroes," 107–36.

152. James Buchanan Duke's bequest resulted in the transformation of Trinity College in Durham, North Carolina, into Duke University, and George Eastman's generous endowment created the University of Rochester. In addition, Michigan magnate Thomas Henry Simpson left $400,000 for the creation of an Ann Arbor medical research institute. All of this activity occurred in the 1920s. On Eastman, see George Corner, *George Hoyt Whipple and His Friends: The Life-Story of a Nobel Prize Pathologist* (Philadelphia: Lippincott, 1963).

153. "John Gaston, Citizen," in John Harkins, *Metropolis of the American Nile: Memphis and Shelby County, an Illustrated History* (Woodland Hills, Calif.: Windsor Publications, 1982), 87.

154. Otis S. Warr, "Medical Memphis: A Century of Progress, 1830–1930," pt. 1, *Memphis Medical Journal* (August 1931): 120.

155. A similar vision had, of course, informed the creation of Memphis's denominational hospitals, both black and white. In 1914, for example, the Methodist conferences of Memphis, North Mississippi, and North Arkansas had raised funds for the new hospital facility in Memphis. LaPointe, *From Saddlebags to Science*, 48.

156. Members of the South Memphis Business Men's Club, located near Gaston's neighborhood, lobbied unsuccessfully for six months to use the funds to bring the new hospital to their section of town. Lee, *Beale Street*, 194–97.

157. Roger Biles, "The Persistence of the Past: Memphis in the Great Depression," *Journal of Southern History* 52 (May 1986): 183–212. See especially pages 192–95.

158. Newspaper accounts of the conditions at MGH only generated further concern, as one 1934 headline portrayed poor patients living amidst vermin and fear. "Rats Romp under Beds and Scare Patients at Ancient City Hospital," proclaimed the anti-Crump, reform-oriented *Press-Scimitar*. The subtitle read, "One Sick Man in Crowded Ward Spends Time Watching Roaches Climb Up Walls — All Helpless as Lights Go Out." *Memphis Press-Scimitar*, 1934.

159. On the supreme court case, see "Clear Last Barrier from Hospital Path — Supreme Court Affirms . . . ," *Memphis Commercial Appeal*, June 24, 1934. The city obtained an additional loan from the Public Works Administration and raised another $400,000 from selling municipal bonds for what became Gaston Hospital. See "PWA Hospital Loan Approved," *Memphis Press-Scimitar*, June 28, 1934; "Gaston Bonds Yield Hospital $394,000," *Memphis Commercial Appeal*, August 15, 1934.

160. "Hospital Work Begins Today," *Memphis Press-Scimitar*, October 13, 1934.

161. In 1937, in an expression of the city's continuing ambivalence and hostility to migrating patients in its hospitals, officials again sought to raise the barriers to entry by nonresidents. "Hospital Tightens Up on Admissions Rules," *Memphis Commercial Appeal*, May 12, 1937.

162. MacLean, *City of Memphis*.

163. See Grantham, *The South in Modern America*, 125. Historian Roger Biles has argued that in Memphis "the New Deal was filtered through the Crump regime" and that progressive policies merely reinforced Crump's power, African Americans' subjugation, and the dominance of a rural mind-set. Roger Biles, *Memphis in the Great Depression* (Knoxville: University of Tennessee Press, 1986), 86–87. Biles also argues that "while the New Deal had altered the face of the city, in fact, the addition of new buildings, roads, sewers, and parks was essentially a cosmetic change. . . . Inadvertently, federal policy reinforced the essentially rural character of the city, as New Deal farm programs drove thousands of Mid-South sharecroppers and tenant farmers off the land into the region's major city. Once in Memphis, they continued to infuse the city with rural mores, ideas, and values" (211–12). Similarly, James Cobb, in his study

of the Mississippi Delta, has suggested that federal crop subsidies and agricultural programs did little to loosen white control of black labor. James Cobb, *The Most Southern Place on Earth: The Mississippi Delta and the Roots of Regional Identity* (New York: Oxford University Press, 1992). Such historians dispute the argument that blacks were the primary beneficiaries of federal largesse in these years. In areas of health care, federal dollars did build new facilities. See also Bruce Schulman, *From Cotton Belt to Sunbelt: Federal Policy, Economic Development, and the Transformation of the South, 1938–1980* (New York: Oxford University Press, 1991).

164. Biles, "Persistence of the Past," 202–3.

165. For example, slum clearance and public housing construction—framed by local officials as public health initiatives—effectively re-created the lines of segregation. "White-only" public housing (built by PWA funds) meant, in the words of Memphis's public health superintendent Lloyd Graves, that the nearby "50 dilapidated Negro shacks had to be torn down because of their objectionable character and location just across the street." Lloyd M. Graves and Alfred H. Fletcher, "Some Trends in Public Housing," *American Journal of Public Health* (January 1941): 70. These shacks were replaced, noted Graves, by a "new modernistic doctors' office." At the same time, Graves suggested that the construction of government housing was merely resulting in shacks elsewhere in the city, amounting to "100 percent slum shifting." Ibid.

166. Memphis wrapped itself symbolically in cotton, creating in these years the civic pageantry of the Cotton Carnival to celebrate and promote the declining crop. But the city's economy had also become more diverse, for Memphis was becoming a major distribution center for hardwood lumber and wood products.

167. The cotton economy, as social scientist Howard Odum wrote in 1936, was still "the most dominant and definitive factor of all the region's agrarian cultures." Howard Odum, *Southern Regions of the United States* (Chapel Hill: University of North Carolina Press, 1936), 59.

168. Biles, "Persistence of the Past," 199.

169. Julius Rosenwald Fund, *Negro Hospitals: A Compilation of Available Statistics* (Chicago: Julius Rosenwald Fund, 1931), 34.

170. O. W. Hyman, "The Influence of Recent Changes in the Distribution of Physicians upon the Conditions of Medical Practice in Tennessee," *Memphis Medical Journal* (May 1932): 93.

171. This continued a trend that had begun in the 1920s when U.S. Public Health Service officer Joseph Goldberger provoked regional controversy with his linking of cotton and pellagra (see note 130 above). Goldberger believed that a single-minded reliance on cotton had crowded out other dietary products. Moreover, his economic analysis traced the rise and fall of pellagra to fluctuations in cotton prices—when prices fell, wages fell, and when wages fell, diet suffered and incidence of pellagra rose. See Etheridge, *Butterfly Caste.*

172. Thus, when B. G. Olive, debit agent and state manager of Universal Life's Arkansas office, arrived in Memphis in 1932 to become agency director, his arrival was seen as evidence of "the rapid growth and development of Negro Insurance Companies," proof that the tentacles of Memphis-based insurance reached far into the countryside. T. A. Johnson, ed., *A Classified Directory of Negroes of Memphis and Shelby County* (Memphis: Negro Chamber of Commerce, 1941), 14. See also B. G. Olive Jr., "Looking Back at the Insurance Business," Universal Life Insurance Company, *The ULICO* 22 (Fall 1973): 36.

173. Charles Spurgeon Johnson, *The Collapse of Cotton Tenancy: Summary of Field Studies and Statistical Surveys, 1933–35* (Chapel Hill: University of North Carolina Press, 1935), 22. Loss of soil fertility, decline of world markets, and, most important, the mechanization of farming seemed to suggest that even if cotton survived as a viable crop, the system it supported would continue its decline. Yet planters would persist in portraying themselves as benevolent sponsors of an agrarian tradition that made them responsible for the religion, recreation, health care, and education of their workers. Donald Grubb, *Cry from the Cotton: The Southern Tenant Farmers' Union and the New Deal* (Chapel Hill: University of North Carolina Press, 1971), 11.

174. Charles S. Johnson, *Collapse of Cotton Tenancy*, 17. Johnson noted, moreover, that "in the first place, diseases are not adequately diagnosed because of the uncertain relation of doctors to sick persons, the rather general ignorance of disease, the reliance upon folk diagnosis and cures, and the exceedingly high rate of venereal infection in the population." Charles S. Johnson, *Shadow of the Plantation*, 187.

175. Charles S. Johnson, *Shadow of the Plantation*, 207.

176. Woodson, *The Rural Negro*, 2. Woodson also took up Goldberger's argument, noting that "in the sugar and cotton plantation districts, where the one crop idea has not yet been uprooted, the Negro tenants and laborers must live on such food as is supplied to them by the plantation commissary" (4). As he pointed out, "The soil is rich enough to produce vegetables in abundance, but the time of the laborers is required in the production of cotton or sugar, and these things must be imported or foregone. If brought in, the best vegetables would never reach these peasants, for such eatables would find a better market among persons of more favorable circumstances" (5).

177. Ibid., 6–7.

178. Johnson predicted that mechanization of cotton picking would "automatically release hundreds of thousands of cotton workers particularly in the Southeast, creating a new range of social problems." Charles S. Johnson, *Collapse of Cotton Tenancy*, 33.

179. Charles S. Johnson, *Shadow of the Plantation*, 209.

180. For a short, useful analysis of Memphis Minnie and of doctors and disease in

the blues, see Paul and Beth Garon, *Woman with Guitar: Memphis Minnie's Blues* (New York: Da Capo Press, 1992), 143–62.

181. The song was surely a symbol of the rising visibility of pain, anxiety, and despair. Memphis provided a stage for the dramatization of this plight. At the same time, the song reflected the national appeal, particularly among working-class African American consumers, of the musical form itself and Memphis's role as a crucible of these new expressions. Larry Nager, *Memphis Beat: The Lives and Times of America's Musical Crossroads* (New York: St. Martin's Press, 1998); see also W. C. Handy, *Father of the Blues: An Autobiography* (New York: Da Capo Press, 1941). On African American consumerism, see Robert Weems, *Desegregating the Dollar: African-American Consumerism in the Twentieth Century* (New York: New York University Press, 1998).

182. See, for example, "Clinical Pathological Conference, University of Tennessee — November 26, 1924," *Memphis Medical Journal* (December 1924): 277–79: "Case: D.B.B., colored female infant aged 22 months, admitted to the Memphis General Hospital . . . with a history of sudden onset, high fever, copious nasal discharge"; and Bruce Tinkler, "Amebic Abscess of the Liver; Report of Two Cases," *Memphis Medical Journal* (July 1926): 169–70: "Case 1. A negro man was admitted to the Memphis General Hospital . . . because of pain in the right upper quadrant of the abdomen."

183. Biles, "Persistence of the Past."

184. In his novel *River George*, black Memphian George W. Lee portrayed the city as a refuge for a hapless but proud black man unjustly accused of murder in his hometown in Mississippi.

CHAPTER 2

1. In some ways, this exploration of the invisibility of pain and suffering can be seen as an elaboration of Merleau-Ponty's statement that "bodily experience forces us to acknowledge an imposition of meaning which is not the work of a universal constituting consciousness, a meaning which clings to certain contents." Maurice Merleau-Ponty, *Phenomenology of Perception*, trans. Colin Smith (New York: Routledge, 1989), 147.

2. I have discussed this motif in American disease discourse elsewhere. See Keith Wailoo, "Detecting 'Negro Blood': Black and White Identities and the Reconstruction of Sickle Cell Anemia," in *Drawing Blood: Technology and Disease Identity in Twentieth-Century America* (Baltimore: Johns Hopkins University Press, 1997), 134–61. See also Tera Hunter, "Tuberculosis as the 'Negro Servant's Disease,'" in *To 'Joy My Freedom: Southern Black Women's Lives and Labors after the Civil War* (Cambridge, Mass.: Harvard University Press, 1997), 187–218; Katherine Ott, "Race-ing Illness at the Turn of the Century," in *Fevered Lives: Tuberculosis in American Culture since 1870* (Cambridge, Mass.: Harvard Univer-

sity Press, 1996), 100–110; Barbara Bates, "P.S. I Am Colored," in *Bargaining for Life: A Social History of Tuberculosis, 1876–1938* (Philadelphia: University of Pennsylvania Press, 1992), 288–310; and David McBride, *From TB to AIDS: Epidemics among Urban Blacks since 1900* (Albany: State University of New York Press, 1991). For more on Typhoid Mary, see Judith Walzer Leavitt, *Typhoid Mary: Captive of the Public Health* (Boston: Beacon Press, 1996). See also Alan Kraut, *Silent Travelers: Germs, Genes, and the "Immigrant Menace"* (New York: Basic Books, 1994).

3. C. Jeff Miller, "Special Problems of the Colored Woman," *Southern Medical Journal* 25 (1932): 734.

4. Syphilis, for example, was seen as a self-inflicted disease that had its roots in sexual vice throughout the region. See James Jones, *Bad Blood: The Tuskegee Syphilis Experiment* (New York: Free Press, 1981). See also Allan Brandt, *No Magic Bullet: The Social History of Venereal Diseases since 1880* (New York: Oxford University Press, 1985). In the pages of the *Southern Medical Journal*, one could also read about the disproportionate impact among black people of regional maladies such as hookworm anemia and pellagra. The African American was portrayed in southern public health discourse as both the victim of these diseases and a key vector of their transmission. See, for example, John Ettling, *The Germ of Laziness: Rockefeller Philanthropy and Public Health in the New South* (Cambridge, Mass.: Harvard University Press, 1981), and Elizabeth Etheridge, *The Butterfly Caste: A Social History of Pellagra in the South* (Westport, Conn.: Greenwood Press, 1972). See also Paul Preble, "A Review of Public Health Administration in Memphis, Tennessee," *Public Health Bulletin* 113 (Washington, D.C.: U.S. Government Printing Office, 1921).

5. Charles Spurgeon Johnson, *In the Shadow of the Plantation* (Chicago: University of Chicago Press, 1934), 195.

6. Ibid., 192. This view of the "fatalistic and ignorant Negro" was prevalent among many other popular and professional audiences, and such images had a long pedigree in American writing. See George Fredrickson, *Black Image in the White Mind: The Debate on Afro-American Character and Destiny, 1817–1914* (New York: Harper and Row, 1971), and John Haller, *Outcasts from Evolution: Scientific Attitudes of Racial Inferiority, 1859–1900* (Carbondale: Southern Illinois University Press, 1995). The image appeared in writings on syphilis, tuberculosis, typhoid, malaria, and numerous other disorders, alongside the literature of infant death. In some accounts, fatalism in the face of death could be portrayed as a religious virtue, as in the words of James Weldon Johnson's poem "Go Down Death": "Weep not, weep not, She is not dead; / She's resting in the bosom of Jesus. . . . / And Jesus took his own hand and wiped away her tears. / And he smoothed the furrows from her face." James Weldon Johnson, "Go Down Death," from *God's Trombones*, reprinted in *Trials, Tribulations, and Cele-*

brations: African-American Perspectives on Health, Illness, Aging, and Loss, ed. Marian Gray Secundy (Yarmouth, Maine: Intercultural Press, 1992), 171–73. But fatalism was seen by others as closely akin to ignorance and public health dangers. Writing in 1930, Morris Fishbein, editor of the *Journal of the American Medical Association*, described a young black man as ignorant, carefree, and proud of his "four-plus" score on a Wasserman test for syphilis. "Returning to his place of work," wrote Fishbein, the young man crowed, "Salute me, men, I'se a four plus niggah." Morris Fishbein, *Doctors and Specialists* (Indianapolis: Bobbs-Merrill, 1930), 92. Such images were widely broadcast. One 1932 Tennessee radio broadcast for Negro Health Week stated the conventional theme: "The Negro mother must learn that medical care is a necessity in [labor], that babies may not be raised on superstition; that the seeds of disease will as surely produce a crop as will the seed of cotton or corn." Radio broadcast, April 7, 1932, Records of the Tennessee Department of Public Health, Record Group 1, Box 11, Folder 2, Tennessee State Library and Archives, Nashville.

7. See Keith Wailoo, "A Disease 'sui generis': The Origins of Sickle Cell Anemia and the Emergence of Modern Clinical Research, 1904–1942," *Bulletin of the History of Medicine* 65 (1991): 185–208. Similar negotiations occurred for other diseases. In the case of syphilis, the motif of "bad blood" was only one among many poignant indicators of southern regional health attitudes. The difference between black and white definitions of that term is particularly telling. For Macon County, Alabama, blacks, "bad blood" signified only an amorphous collection of ills and fatigue. But for USPHS researchers, "bad blood" was equated with syphilis, and the casual use of the term by Alabama blacks stood as a clear indicator of rural ignorance, moral decay, and casual maleficence in the face of obvious health problems. See Jones, *Bad Blood*.

8. On visibility, invisibility, and social status, see Erving Goffman, *The Presentation of Self in Everyday Life* (Garden City, N.Y.: Doubleday, 1959), and Vance Packard, *The Status Seekers: An Exploration of Class Behavior in America and the Hidden Barriers That Affect You, Your Community, Your Future* (New York: McKay, 1959). Other observations on visibility and invisibility can be found in Maurice Merleau-Ponty, *The Visible and the Invisible*, ed. Claude Lefort, trans. Alphonso Lingis (Evanston: Northwestern University Press, 1968).

9. See Travis Winsor and George Burch, "Sickle Cell Anemia: 'A Great Masquerader,'" *Journal of the American Medical Association* 129 (November 17, 1945): 793–96.

10. See, for example, the speculations about the likely burdens and effects of sickle cell disease among blacks prior to its recognition as a clinical entity in Todd Savitt, "Sound Minds and Sound Bodies: The Diseases and Health Care of Blacks in Ante-bellum Virginia" (Ph.D. diss., University of Virginia, 1975); Peter Wood, *Black Majority: Negroes in Colonial South Carolina from 1670 through*

the Stono Rebellion (New York: Norton, 1974); and Kenneth Kiple and Virginia Himmelstein King, *Another Dimension to the Black Diaspora: Diet, Disease, and Racism* (New York: Cambridge University Press, 1981).

11. Elbridge Sibley, *Differential Mortality in Tennessee, 1917–1928* (Nashville: Fisk University, 1930). See also Dorothy Dickens, *A Nutritional Investigation of Tenants in the Yazoo-Mississippi Delta*, Mississippi Agricultural Experiment Station Bulletin 254 (A&M College, Mississippi, 1928), 1–28.

12. See Margaret Humphreys, *Yellow Fever and the South* (New Brunswick: Rutgers University Press, 1992).

13. Mortality figures are from Sibley, *Differential Mortality*, 96. See Daniel Drake, *Malaria in the Interior Valley of North America* (1850; reprint, Urbana: University of Illinois Press, 1964). Also see Erwin Ackerknecht, *Malaria in the Upper Mississippi Valley, 1760–1900* (New York: Arno Press, 1977), and, more recently, Conevery A. Bolton, "'The Health of the Country': Body and Environment in the Making of the American West, 1800–1860" (Ph.D. diss., Harvard University, 1998).

14. Ackerknecht, *Malaria in the Upper Mississippi*.

15. Sibley, *Differential Mortality*, 96.

16. Ackerknecht, *Malaria in the Upper Mississippi*, 5.

17. On the cultural meaning of pain in relation to medical notions of pain, see Martin Pernick, *A Calculus of Suffering: Pain, Professionalism, and Anesthesia in Nineteenth-Century America* (New York: Columbia University Press, 1985); see also Elaine Scarry, *The Body in Pain: The Making and Unmaking of the World* (New York: Oxford University Press, 1985).

18. On religion and healing in nineteenth- and twentieth-century America, see Ronald Numbers and Darrel Amundsen, eds., *Caring and Curing: Health and Medicine in the Western Religious Traditions* (New York: Macmillan, 1986).

19. For more on folk beliefs of the region and on the blues as an aspect of African American cultural expression, see N. N. Puckett, *Folk Beliefs of the Southern Negro* (Chapel Hill: University of North Carolina Press, 1926). See also Michael W. Harris, *The Rise of Gospel Blues: The Music of Thomas Andrew Dorsey in the Urban Church* (New York: Oxford University Press, 1992), and Clyde Woods, *Development Arrested: The Blues and Plantation Power in the Mississippi Delta* (New York: Verso, 1998). See especially Paul and Beth Garon, *Woman with Guitar: Memphis Minnie's Blues* (New York: Da Capo Press, 1992); Charles Keil, *Urban Blues* (Chicago: University of Chicago Press, 1966, 1991); and Daphne Duval Harrison, *Black Pearls: Blues Queens of the 1920s* (New Brunswick: Rutgers University Press, 1988).

20. See Hunter, "Tuberculosis as the 'Negro Servant's Disease.'" See also Ott, "Race-ing Illness," and Wailoo, "Detecting 'Negro Blood.'"

21. Lloyd M. Graves, "The Public Health Situation in Memphis," *Memphis Medical Journal* (March 1929): 56–59.

22. William D. Miller, *Memphis during the Progressive Era* (Memphis: Memphis State University Press, 1957).

23. J. F. Hamilton, "A Case of Sickle Cell Anemia," *Memphis Medical Journal* (November 1925): 253–55. See also editorial on sickle cell anemia in *Journal of the American Medical Association* 81 (December 15, 1923): 2036–37.

24. As historian Edwin Ayers has noted, even though black land owning had risen in the early twentieth century and peaked in 1910, "Blacks owned farms where land was cheap, where railroads had not arrived, and where stores were few: they got the 'backbone and spareribs' that white farmers did not value." There was little such land in the Memphis area. Edwin Ayers, *The Promise of the New South: Life after Reconstruction* (New York: Oxford University Press, 1992), 208.

25. Hamilton, "A Case of Sickle Cell Anemia," *Memphis Medical Journal* (November 1925): 254; also see J. F. Hamilton, "A Case of Sickle Cell Anemia," *U.S. Veteran's Medical Bulletin* 2 (1926): 497.

26. Hamilton, "A Case of Sickle Cell Anemia," *U.S. Veteran's Medical Bulletin* 2 (1926): 497.

27. Ibid.

28. Ibid.

29. Editorial, "The Spleen Rate as a Measure of Malaria Prevalence," *Memphis Medical Journal* (August 1927): 175.

30. Graves, "Public Health Situation in Memphis," 57. The blurring of the identity of sickle cell disease was not merely a Memphis phenomenon, nor was it related only to malaria. Abdominal and joint pains of sickle cell anemia were often taken for infected gallstones, appendicitis, or rheumatic fever. Because pneumonia and tuberculosis were widespread public health problems in every region and commonly affected sickle cell disease sufferers, people who might have been diagnosed in later years with sickle cell disease were largely indistinguishable from sufferers of tuberculosis, pneumonia, appendicitis, or just plain infant death. The obscurity of the malady, in Memphis and other locales, was linked to how physicians perceived the broader landscape and its distinctive disease context. Barbara Culliton, "Sickle Cell Anemia — The Path from Obscurity to Prominence," *Science* 177 (October 20, 1972); Todd Savitt, "Sickle Cell Anemia — Neglected Disease," *Journal of the National Medical Association* 64 (1976); and Todd Savitt, "The Invisible Malady — Sickle Cell Anemia in America, 1910–1970," *Journal of the National Medical Association* 73 (1981): 739–46. Most clinicians themselves found it difficult to diagnose cases of sickle cell anemia as they were presented, and many doctors, like Hamilton, found it hard to convince their peers that this was an authentic new category of pathological experience.

31. Graves, "Public Health Situation in Memphis," 57.

32. Ibid.

33. Patricia LaPointe, *From Saddlebags to Science: A Century of Health Care in Memphis, 1830–1930* (Memphis: The Foundation, 1984), 76.

34. Graves, "Public Health Situation in Memphis," 57.

35. Ibid.

36. See Michael Honey, *Southern Labor and Black Civil Rights: Organizing Memphis Workers* (Knoxville: University of Tennessee Press, 1993), 41–42.

37. Obituary, "L. M. Graves," *Memphis Commercial Appeal*, December 5, 1964. In his obituary Graves was credited with being "a leading advocate of slum clearance [who] made the arguments that convinced city officials of the need for the first housing project here."

38. Graves, "Public Health Situation in Memphis," 57.

39. Lemuel Diggs, "Practical Points in Blood Examination," *Memphis Medical Journal* (September 1935): 10.

40. Among the few to scrutinize these cases were pediatricians like Thomas Benton Cooley. See T. Cooley and P. Lee, "A Series of Cases of Splenomegaly in Children, with Anemia and Peculiar Bone Changes," *Transactions of the American Pediatric Society* 37 (1925): 29, and T. Cooley, E. Witwer, and P. Lee, "Anemia in Children," *American Journal of the Diseases of Children* 34 (1927): 347–63.

41. As one federal health inspector noted in 1921, even among the educated physicians, "Malaria infection has very frequently been returned as the cause of deaths and, it is believed, often without the support of laboratory diagnosis." Preble, "Public Health Administration," 84.

42. LaPointe, *From Saddlebags to Science*, 77.

43. See Molly Ladd-Taylor, ed., *Raising a Baby the Government Way: Mothers' Letters to the Children's Bureau, 1915–1935* (New Brunswick: Rutgers University Press, 1986).

44. See Thomas McKeown, *The Modern Rise of Population* (New York: Academic Press, 1976), and Samuel Preston and Michael Haines, *Fatal Years: Child Mortality in Late Nineteenth-Century America* (Princeton: Princeton University Press, 1991). See also "Demography and History around 1900: A Symposium on *Fatal Years*," *Bulletin of the History of Medicine* 68 (1994): 86–128. Some laboratory innovations, such as the diphtheria antitoxin, contributed to this decline, as would penicillin and other antibacterial agents in later decades. See also Judith Leavitt and Ron Numbers, "Sickness and Health in America," in *Sickness and Health in America: Essays in the History of Medicine and Public Health*, 3d ed., ed. Judith Leavitt and Ron Numbers (Madison: University of Wisconsin Press, 1997), 3–10. The reduction in infant mortality accounted for a gradual rise in overall life expectancy, as many more people survived childhood. See also C. E. A. Winslow, *The Conquest of Epidemic Disease: A Chapter in the History of Ideas* (Princeton: Princeton University Press, 1943).

45. See Jacqueline Dowd Hall, James Leloudis, Robert Korstad, Mary Murphy, Lu Ann Jones, and Christopher Daley, *Like a Family: The Making of a Cotton Mill World* (Chapel Hill: University of North Carolina Press, 1987).

46. Molly Ladd-Taylor, "'My Work Came Out of Agony and Grief': Mothers and

the Making of the Sheppard-Towner Act," in *Mothers of a New World: Maternalist Politics and the Origins of Welfare States*, ed. Seth Koven and Sonya Michel (New York: Routledge, 1993), 324. See also Viviana Zelizer, *Pricing the Priceless Child: The Changing Social Value of Children* (New York: Basic Books, 1985); Richard Meckel, *"Save the Babies": American Public Health Reform and the Prevention of Infant Mortality, 1850–1929* (Baltimore: Johns Hopkins University Press, 1990); Ladd-Taylor, *Raising a Baby the Government Way*; and Molly Ladd-Taylor, *Mother-Work: Women, Child Welfare, and the State, 1880–1930* (Urbana: University of Illinois Press, 1994).

47. Meckel, *"Save the Babies,"* 219.

48. See J. H. Mason Knox Jr., "The Health Problems of the Negro Child," *American Journal of Pediatric Health* 16 (August 1926): 805–9. See also *Journal of Negro Life* in the 1920s; John Kenney, "Health Problems of the Negroes," *Journal of the National Medical Association* 3 (1911): 127–35; Charles Garvin, "Negro Health — Discussion of Diseases," *Journal of Negro Life* 2 (November 1924): 341–42; "Racial Theory and Negro Mortality," *Opportunity* 2 (May 1924): 132; E. Franklin Frazier, "Three Scourges of the Negro Family," *Opportunity* 4 (July 1926): 210–13; W. Montague Cobb, "The Physical Constitution of the American Negro," *Journal of Negro Education* 3 (July 1934): 340–88; William Gannett, *Negro Life in Rural Virginia, 1865–1934* (Blacksburg, Va.: Virginia Polytechnic Institute, Virginia Agricultural Experiment Station, 1934); E. Franklin Frazier, "Family Disorganization among Negroes and the Effect upon Their Children," *Opportunity* 9 (July 1931): 204–7.

49. Sibley, *Differential Mortality*.

50. Consult Puckett, *Folk Beliefs of the Southern Negro*. John Dollard commented that blacks were "concerned with charms, fetishes, amulets, lucky and unlucky days, and the like." John Dollard, *Caste and Class in a Southern Town* (New Haven: Yale University Press, 1937), 264. See also William Reynolds Ferris Jr., "Black Folklore from the Mississippi Delta" (Ph.D. diss., University of Pennsylvania, 1969).

51. Mrs. M. M. Hubert Jackson, "Club Women's View of National Negro Health Week," *National Negro Health News* 3 (April–June 1935): 3.

52. Of course, there was an element of middle-class anxiety among such African Americans that their own ideals would be limited as long as these beliefs remained prevalent among working-class blacks. Historian Kevin Gaines has noted that "it was difficult for African Americans to ignore minstrelsy [since such images were] a major obstacle to the assertion of bourgeois black selfhood." Kevin Gaines, *Uplifting the Race: Black Leadership, Politics, and Culture in the Twentieth Century* (Chapel Hill: University of North Carolina Press, 1996), 68. To aspiring middle-class blacks, sickness was one of the many symbols of the gap in status, class, education, and culture between themselves and the black working class. The National Negro Health Week program, with its syphilis,

tuberculosis, and public health education campaigns, was one outgrowth of this attitude. As historian Susan Smith points out in her study of black women's health activism, this embarrassed sense of connection to rural, uneducated blacks brought elite black women into the Mississippi Delta on health missions. They commented from an educated distance on the strange charms worn around baby's necks to protect against illness, and on the curious paternalistic culture that shaped medical practices and beliefs in the hinterlands. Susan Smith, *Sick and Tired of Being Sick and Tired: Black Women's Health Activism in America, 1890–1950* (Philadelphia: University of Pennsylvania Press, 1995).

53. See Ira D. A. Reid, "Let Us Prey," *Opportunity* 4 (September 1926): 274–78.
54. Rev. M. W. Gilbert, "Baptism," in *The Negro Baptist Pulpit: A Collection of Sermons and Papers by Colored Baptist Ministers*, ed. Edward M. Brawley (Philadelphia: American Baptist Publication Society, 1890; reprint, Freeport, N.Y.: Books for Libraries Press, 1971), 130.
55. Dollard, *Caste and Class*, 238.
56. Ibid., 239.
57. Editorial, "Baby Shows," *Memphis Medical Journal* (October 1932): 192.
58. James R. Reinberger, "Modern Prenatal Supervision," *Memphis Medical Journal* (February 1932): 29.
59. See, for example, Sydney Halpern, *American Pediatrics: The Social Dynamics of Professionalism, 1880–1980* (Berkeley: University of California Press, 1988); Meckel, *"Save the Babies"*; and Rosemary Stevens, "Specialties and Specialty Boards: The Defining Process," in *American Medicine and the Public Interest* (New Haven: Yale University Press, 1971), 218–43.
60. Margaret Koenig, Narrative Report to Dr. Rude, Chief, Children's Bureau, September 23, 1922, p. 1, Box 47, Folder 20-24-5-5: "Correspondence with Bureau Agents," Records of the U.S. Department of Labor, Children's Bureau, Record Group 102, National Archives and Records Administration, College Park, Maryland. Elsewhere Koenig found no cases "of unbilical [*sic*] hernia," which she had expected to find, and "which is so prevalent among them" (p. 2). And in Gainesville she noted "a very nice class of colored people was present . . . of the children examined very little pathology was found" (p. 3). In a 1922 letter from Trenton, Tennessee, however, Koenig evaluated 500 African American children as "the most unsanitary of any examined, even though much public health work has been done among them. More pathology was found, many hernias and leutic infection . . . and much personal uncleanliness." Margaret Koenig to Dr. Oppenheimer, September 17, 1922, ibid.
61. Koenig to Rude, September 9, 1922, ibid.
62. Koenig to Rude, August 27, 1922, p. 4, ibid.
63. From the beginning, the Memphis Chamber of Commerce maintained close contact with the Children's Bureau. For example, E. C. Klaiber, president of the

Memphis Chamber of Commerce, wrote to Dr. Martha Eliot of the Children's Bureau on February 21, 1935: "Owing to the high infant mortality in Memphis, may I, as President of the Chamber of Commerce, invite you to make a survey." Box 132, Folder 20-159-6: "Correspondence with Outsiders," ibid.

64. Editorial, "Infant Mortality," *Memphis Commercial Appeal*, July 11, 1934.

65. "High Baby Mortality Laid to Two Causes — Indigent Outsiders and Negroes Held Responsible," *Memphis Commercial Appeal*, July 19, 1934.

66. "High Infant Mortality Rate Is Misleading Declare City's Obstetricians," *Memphis Commercial Appeal*, July 11, 1934.

67. Ibid.

68. "High Baby Mortality Laid to Two Causes," *Memphis Commercial Appeal*, July 19, 1934.

69. See Ladd-Taylor, *Raising a Baby the Government Way*; see also Kriste Lindenmeyer, *A Right to Childhood: The U.S. Children's Bureau and Child Welfare, 1912–1946* (Urbana: University of Illinois Press, 1997).

70. The 1930 White House Conference on Child Health and Protection had refocused attention on child welfare, as had the deepening Depression. See Katherine Glover and Evelyn Dewey, *Children of a New Day* (New York: Appleton-Century, 1934). See also *White House Conference on Child Health and Protection, Section I: Medical Service, Committee on Prenatal and Maternal Care, Fetal, Newborn, and Maternal Morbidity and Mortality* (New York: Appleton-Century, 1933). The South was well along the path to being labeled by the Roosevelt administration's 1938 report on economic conditions as the country's "number one economic problem." See David L. Carlton and Peter A. Coclanis, *Confronting Southern Poverty in the Great Depression: The Report on Economic Conditions of the South with Related Documents* (New York: Bedford Books, 1996), 1.

71. Lindenmeyer, *Right to Childhood*.

72. "Eleventh Ward Shoots Memphis Baby Death Record Up," *Memphis Commercial Appeal*, February 24, 1935.

73. "Expert Will Study Infant Mortality — Dr. Graves Instructed to Secure Authority," *Memphis Commercial Appeal*, January 5, 1935.

74. Dewey Grantham, *The South in Modern America: A Region at Odds* (New York: HarperCollins, 1994), 165.

75. Martha Eliot to Katharine Lenroot, February 26, 1935, Box 132, Folder 20-159-5: "Correspondence with Bureau Agents," Records of the U.S. Department of Labor, Children's Bureau.

76. See "Woman to Fight Infant Deaths," *Memphis Press-Scimitar*, January 15, 1935, an article on Martha Eliot. See also "Survey of Memphis Infant Deaths Begins — Dr. Oppenheimer Hints Mortality Study May Take Year," *Memphis Commercial Appeal*, April 23, 1935.

77. Martha Eliot to Edward Mitchell, July 24, 1935, and E. Mitchell to Martha

Eliot, July 30, 1935, Box 132, Folder 20-159-8: "Correspondence with Bureau Agents," Records of the U.S. Department of Labor, Children's Bureau.

78. Eliot sent a preliminary report to Mitchell. Only then did she tell him, "The opinion was expressed so often in Memphis that the infant mortality report was of sufficient general interest to be published, that we are planning to print it." Eliot to Mitchell, November 26, 1935, ibid. By the time of Oppenheimer's arrival, the city had already begun to address the problem. The *Commercial Appeal* noted that "new clinics and a full time pediatrician [were] installed" while the "report of the national expert was awaited." "City Acts to Lower Baby Fatality Rate," *Memphis Commercial Appeal*, August 23, 1935.

79. Eliot to Mitchell, January 24, 1936, Box 132, Folder 20-159-8: "Correspondence with Bureau Agents," Records of the U.S. Department of Labor, Children's Bureau.

80. Mrs. Hopkins to Miss Lenroot, July 24, 1936, ibid.

81. Sibley, *Differential Mortality*, 22.

82. John P. Kennedy, City Health Officer of the Department of Health, Atlanta, to Dr. Oppenheimer, November 21, 1935, and Oppenheimer to John Kennedy, November 18, 1935, Box 132, Folder 20-159-8: "Correspondence with Bureau Agents," Records of the U.S. Department of Labor, Children's Bureau.

83. U.S. Department of Labor, Children's Bureau, *Infant Mortality in Memphis*, Publication 233 (Washington, D.C.: U.S. Government Printing Office, 1937), 29.

84. Ibid., 26.

85. Ibid., 87. For a short analysis of Memphis's expansion and the politics of annexation, see Christopher Silver and John Moeser, *The Separate City: Black Communities in the Urban South, 1940–1980* (Lexington: University Press of Kentucky, 1995). See also Christopher Silver, "The Changing Face of Neighborhoods in Memphis and Richmond, 1940–1985," in *Shades of the Sunbelt: Essays on Ethnicity, Race, and the Urban South*, ed. Randall Miller and George Pozzetta (New York: Greenwood Press, 1988), 93–126.

86. "City Launches Drive to Curb Baby Deaths," *Memphis Press-Scimitar*, November 2, 1935. Graves later recalled, "In 1929, the limits of the city were extended to include almost twice the original area. This presented the problem of approximately forty thousand homes without sewers and water connections and other sanitary protection necessary in urban areas." L. M. Graves, "Symposium on Public Health: Public Health Progress in Memphis," *Memphis Medical Journal* (March 1941): 42–44. See also "Infant Mortality Rate in 1933 Shows Sharp Increase over 1932," *Memphis Commercial Appeal*, January 4, 1934.

87. Those with anti-immigrant sentiments had always used public health data to support their claims of the immigrant "threat." See Alan Kraut, *Silent Travelers: Germs, Genes, and the "Immigrant Menace"* (New York: Basic Books, 1994); Howard Markel, *Quarantine!: East European Jewish Immigrants and the New York Epidemics of 1892* (Baltimore: Johns Hopkins University Press, 1997); and Charles

Rosenberg, *The Cholera Years: The United States in 1832, 1849, and 1866* (Chicago: University of Chicago Press, 1962).

88. This thinking persisted well beyond the 1930s. See "Health Survey Proves Slum Areas Mankiller—Memphis Meets Menace with Decent Shelter," *Tri-State Defender*, September 27, 1952, 22.

89. Among other reasons given in city papers were these logical ones: "Depression Factor in Infant Mortality," *Memphis Commercial Appeal*, November 6, 1935; "Infant Death Figure Blamed on Epidemic, Non-Resident Cases," *Memphis Commercial Appeal*, October 30, 1935; "Education of Mothers, Biggest Need for Reducing Memphis' Infant Death Rate," *Memphis Press-Scimitar*, August 24, 1935; and "Baby Deaths Blamed on Strange Disease," *Memphis Commercial Appeal*, January 16, 1935.

90. S. L. Wadley, "The Present Meningitis Situation," *Memphis Medical Journal* (May 1930): 85–86.

91. Ibid., 85.

92. Ibid.

93. "Baby Clinics Launched to Curb Deaths," *Memphis Press-Scimitar*, August 22, 1935; "City Plans New Health Center," *Memphis Press-Scimitar*, June 23, 1937. On the new clinics, see David Goltman, "A Study of 137 Premature Babies Born during 1937 in Relation to the Present Infant Hygiene Setup in Memphis," *Memphis Medical Journal* (October 1938): 162.

94. Goltman, "Study of 137 Premature Babies," 161.

95. W. L. Rucks, quoted in Goltman, "Study of 137 Premature Babies," 162. Italics added for emphasis.

96. "Baby Death Battle Gains Ground Here," *Memphis Commercial Appeal*, May 22, 1936. Reports of progress in the "baby death battle" continued, even as officials also bemoaned the "Negro trend upward."

97. See Edward Beardsley, "The Federal Rescue of Southern Health Programs, 1933–1955," in *A History of Neglect: Health Care for Blacks and Mill Workers in the Twentieth-Century South* (Knoxville: University of Tennessee Press, 1987), 156–85.

98. Gilbert Levy, James Hughes, and S. R. Bruesch, "Pediatrics," in *History of Medicine in Memphis*, ed. Marcus Stewart and William T. Black (Jackson, Tenn.: McCowat-Mercer Press, 1971), 275.

99. For a discussion of this theme, see John S. Hughes, "Labeling and Treating Black Mental Illness in Alabama, 1861–1910," *Journal of Southern History* 59 (August 1993): 435–60. See also Albert Deutsch, "The First U.S. Census of the Insane (1840) and Its Use as Pro-Slavery Propaganda," *Bulletin of the History of Medicine* 15 (1944): 469–82, and Samuel Thielman, "Southern Madness: The Shape of Mental Health in the Old South," in *Science and Medicine in the Old South*, ed. Ronald Numbers and Todd Savitt (Baton Rouge: Louisiana State University Press, 1983).

100. See, for example, Thomas Mays, "Human Slavery as Prevention of Pulmo-

nary Consumption," *Transactions of the American Climatological Association* 20 (1904): 192–97.

101. For more on the discovery and unfolding national discourse of sickle cell anemia (and its relation to ideas of racial purity and intermarriage), see Wailoo, "Detecting 'Negro Blood.'"

102. See Frederick Hoffman, *Race Traits and Tendencies of the American Negro* (New York: Macmillan, 1896); Frederick Hoffman, *History of the Prudential Insurance Company of America, 1875–1900* (New York: Prudential Press, 1900); and Louis Dublin, "The Problem of Negro Health as Revealed by Vital Statistics," *Journal of Negro Education* 6 (1937): 268–75.

103. Sibley, *Differential Mortality*, 11. See also Elbridge Sibley, *Social Science Research Council: The First Fifty Years* (New York: The Council, 1974).

104. See M. O. Bousfield, "Major Health Problems of the Negro," *Hospital Social Service* 28 (1933): 543.

105. Diggs had trained at the Johns Hopkins School of Medicine, and two Hopkins researchers had produced early 1920s case reports on sickle cell anemia. See Verne Mason, "Sickle Cell Anemia," *Journal of the American Medical Association* 79 (October 14, 1922): 1318–19, and W. Taliaferro and J. Huck, "The Inheritance of Sickle Cell Anemia in Man," *Genetics* 8 (1923): 594–98. Mason and Huck were both at Hopkins at the time of these studies.

106. Lemuel Diggs, quoted in Thelma Tracy Mabry, *History of Medicine in Memphis: Interview with Dr. Lemuel Whitley Diggs* (Memphis: Oral History Research Office, Memphis State University, 1984), 2.

107. Ibid., 1–2.

108. Ibid., 14–15.

109. Ibid., 15.

110. Ibid. By the 1920s, specialists knew that splenic enlargement was common in sickle cell disease, but Diggs determined from this case that over years the spleen in the sickle cell anemia patient could wither away.

111. Lemuel Diggs, interview by author, Cordova, Tennessee, April 16–18, 1993.

112. Gibbs Milliken, "A Case of Sickle Cell Anemia," *Medical Records Annual* 22 (March 1928): 49.

113. W. C. Colbert, "The Classification and Therapeutic Indications of the Anemias," *Memphis Medical Journal* (June 1938): 99–101; Richard Ching, "Problems in the Diagnosis and Treatment of the Anemias," *Memphis Medical Journal* (August 1938): 130–33.

114. A. F. Cooper, "With the Editor: The Mid-South," *Memphis Medical Journal* (February 1941): 25.

115. Ibid.

116. For more on this diagnostic micropolitics, see Wailoo, "Detecting 'Negro Blood.'"

117. William Porter, quoted in James P. Baker, "Sickle Cell Anemia," *Virginia Medical Monthly* 69 (1942): 208–12.

118. Anthony C. Allison, "Protection Afforded by Sickle Cell Trait against Subtertian Malaria Infection," *British Medical Journal* 1 (1954): 290–94.

CHAPTER 3

1. See Robert Wiebe, *The Search for Order, 1877–1917* (New York: Hill and Wang, 1967).

2. See, for example, Vincent Franklin, *The Education of Black Philadelphia: The Social and Educational History of a Minority Community, 1900–1950* (Philadelphia: University of Pennsylvania Press, 1979), and, on education in the South, Jim Leloudis, *Schooling the New South: Pedagogy, Self, and Society in North Carolina, 1880–1920* (Chapel Hill: University of North Carolina Press, 1996). See also Laurence Veysey, *The Emergence of the American University* (Chicago: University of Chicago Press, 1965).

3. Owsei Temkin, "Health and Disease," in *The Double Face of Janus and Other Essays in the History of Medicine* (Baltimore: Johns Hopkins University Press, 1977), 419–40.

4. See Rosemary Stevens, *American Medicine and the Public Interest* (New Haven: Yale University Press, 1971) and *In Sickness and in Wealth: American Hospitals in the Twentieth Century* (New York: Basic Books, 1989). On the hospital in the early twentieth century, see David Rosner, *A Once Charitable Enterprise: Hospitals and Health Care in Brooklyn and New York, 1885–1915* (New York: Cambridge University Press, 1982).

5. Don Madison, "Paying for Health Care in America," in *The Social Medicine Reader*, ed. Gail Henderson, Nancy King, Ronald Strauss, Sue Estroff, and Larry Churchill (Durham, N.C.: Duke University Press, 1997), 415–46. According to one estimate, in 1940 there were only 12 million people in the United States with private health insurance. By 1950 the number had risen to 77 million, and by 1960 the number was 123 million—a fivefold increase in two decades. George Anders, *Health against Wealth: HMOs and the Breakdown of Medical Trust* (New York: Houghton Mifflin, 1996), 20. Anders uses figures from *Source Book of Health Insurance Data*, vol. 20 (New York: Health Insurance Association of America, 1994), xx.

6. Once Truman was elected, his proposal for national health insurance was successfully attacked by the American Medical Association as "socialized medicine."

7. On specialization after World War II, see Rosemary Stevens, *American Medicine*. See also W. Bruce Fye, *American Cardiology: The History of a Specialty and Its College* (Baltimore: Johns Hopkins University Press, 1996).

8. Lester Lamon, *Blacks in Tennessee, 1791–1970* (Knoxville: University of Tennessee Press, 1970). Fifty-five percent of the state's residents were urban.

9. John Lucius McGehee, "Report for the John Gaston Hospital for 1943," *Memphis Medical Journal* (February 1943): 27.

10. See Robert Watson Briggs Papers, Southern Historical Collection, Wilson Library, University of North Carolina at Chapel Hill.

11. Private Robert D. Van Dyke III to Mrs. R. D. Van Dyke Jr., October 9, 1943, MS #257, Box 4, Folder 120, Annie Pope Van Dyke Family Papers, Mississippi Valley Collection, McWherter Library, University of Memphis.

12. William D. Van Dyke to Mrs. R. D. Van Dyke Jr., August 27, 1943, p. 3, MS #257, Box 4, Folder 118, Van Dyke Family Papers.

13. L. M. Graves, "Emergency Maternity and Infant Care Program," *Memphis Medical Journal* (October 1943): 156.

14. Lemuel Diggs, quoted in Thelma Tracy Mabry, *History of Medicine in Memphis: Interview with Dr. Lemuel Whitley Diggs* (Memphis: Oral History Research Office, Memphis State University, 1984), 13.

15. Ibid.

16. Julius Bauer and Louis Fisher, "Sickle Cell Disease, with Special Reference to Its Nonanemic Variety," *Archives of Surgery* 47 (1943): 553–63.

17. It is unclear how the issue was resolved at the time. Diggs's opinions on the matter are not evident, nor is it clear that Bauer's article provoked any changes in policy. Indeed, it seems to have remained an obscure matter, dwarfed in significance by the American Red Cross blood segregation controversy. The published record suggests that the sickle cell question remained irrelevant to the debate on military integration or black participation in the armed forces. However, Diggs's subsequent position on military service by people with sickle cell trait (that is, his belief that people with the trait should not be admitted to the air force) suggests that he would have been willing to support Bauer's position, even if he disagreed with the inflammatory rhetoric of "biologic inferiority" or with the underlying assault on black participation in the military.

18. For more insight into this controversy, see Charles Hurd, *The Compact History of the American Red Cross* (New York: Hawthorn, 1959).

19. See, for example, "Aryan Blood Demand Handicaps Nazi Wounded," *New York Times*, March 1, 1942; "Blood and Prejudice — Segregation of White and Negro Blood Donations Brings a Protest," *New York Times*, June 14, 1942; and "Red Cross Plans Big Blood Supply — New Program for Country Stirs Row Over Supply from Various Races," *New York Times*, July 10, 1947.

20. Keith Wailoo, "Detecting 'Negro Blood': Black and White Identities and the Reconstruction of Sickle Cell Anemia," in *Drawing Blood: Technology and Disease Identity in Twentieth-Century America* (Baltimore: Johns Hopkins University Press, 1997), 134–61. An excellent study of these and other blood/race controversies is Spencie Love, *One Blood: The Death and Resurrection of Charles R. Drew* (Chapel Hill: University of North Carolina Press, 1997).

21. As historian Barbara Savage has observed, black migration transformed the

medium of radio, creating a larger audience and suggesting new marketing possibilities to advertisers. Moreover, "Television's emergence . . . transformed radio into a locally oriented medium with targeted markets." Savage notes that "by this time, the radio and advertising industry realized that many major urban areas had been transformed by the massive black migration of the war years." The black audience was seen as a valuable consumer, and out of this realization, WDIA in Memphis was born. Barbara Savage, *Broadcasting Freedom: Radio, War, and the Politics of Race, 1938–1948* (Chapel Hill: University of North Carolina Press, 1999), 260.

22. Quoted in Robert Gordon, *It Came from Memphis* (Boston: Faber and Faber, 1994), 11–12.

23. Ibid., 12.

24. Ibid.

25. In 1946 one Memphis columnist offered his readers a satirical view of the "typical" Delta black man named "the Reverend." "Up to dis pas' year," the man told his neighbor, "I been farming wid mules all my life . . . but . . . I mighty glad to Exchange mule farming for Boss' tractor working on de sheer crop. Mighty handy having tractors gittin up an' down de furrows." Ellen Orr, "De Rev'un an' De Mules," in Paul Flowers, *The Greenhouse* (Memphis: Paul Flowers, 1946).

26. "With the Editor: Amebiasis Research," *Memphis Medical Journal* (September 1947): 139.

27. Ibid.

28. David Rothman, *Strangers at the Bedside: How Law and Bioethics Transformed Medical Decision Making* (New York: Basic Books, 1991).

29. "Negro Body Racket at Gaston Hospital Disclosed by Tobey," *Memphis Commercial Appeal*, June 6, 1952.

30. See Virginia Van der Veer Hamilton, *Lister Hill: Statesman from the South* (Chapel Hill: University of North Carolina Press, 1987). See also David Barton Smith, *Health Care Divided: Race and Healing a Nation* (Ann Arbor: University of Michigan Press, 1999).

31. C. E. Thompson, "The Hospital Survey and Construction Act," *Memphis Medical Journal* (February 1946): 22.

32. L. M. Graves, "The Relation of Hospital Service to the Public Health," *Memphis Medical Journal* (May 1948): 93.

33. Thompson, "Hospital Survey and Construction Act," 22.

34. Edward Beardsley, *A History of Neglect: Health Care for Blacks and Mill Workers in the Twentieth-Century South* (Knoxville: University of Tennessee Press, 1987), 178.

35. Physicians were aware of their own migration problems, and many had begun to complain of the influx of refugee doctors — often German Jewish specialists. "With the Editor: The Refugee Physician," *Memphis Medical Journal* (February 1942): 17. See also the discussion of the role of a German Jewish refugee in the

founding of the American College of Cardiology in W. Bruce Fye, *American Cardiology: The History of a Specialty and Its College* (Baltimore: Johns Hopkins University Press, 1996).

36. "City to Use Old Carnes Home for Negro Clinic," *Memphis Press-Scimitar*, July 17, 1944.

37. C. E. Thompson, "The Hospital Survey and Construction Act," *Memphis Medical Journal* (February 1946): 21.

38. "Dr. L. M. Graves, Long-Time Health Director Is Dead," *Memphis Press-Scimitar*, December 4, 1964.

39. "LeBonheur to Keep Hospital Plan Alive," *Memphis Commercial Appeal*, July 30, 1949.

40. James G. Hughes, "Need for Hospital Facilities for Chronically Ill Children" [formal statement in support of LeBonheur Hospital, ca. 1949], 1, Records of the Tennessee Department of Public Health, Record Group 97, Series 3, Box 109, Folder 7, Tennessee State Library and Archives, Nashville.

41. Ibid., 2.

42. Ibid., 4.

43. "Lease Agreement," in Records of Tennessee Department of Public Health, ibid.

44. "Negro Memphis Asked to Give $15,000 to La Bonheur Effort," *Memphis World*, January 20, 1950.

45. Liz Conway, ed., *Memphis, 1948–1958* (Memphis: Memphis Brooks Museum of Art, 1986), 67.

46. Conservative black businessman J. E. Walker himself took a stand against segregation in support of integrated seating for a concert by Marian Anderson. Harry Holloway, "Memphis Tennessee: Independent Political Power," in *The Politics of the Southern Negro: From Exclusion to Big City Organization* (New York: Random House, 1969), 279.

47. In a 1929 book review, for example, one author noted that "they are not yet used to this class; they still regard an educated Negro much in the same way as we look upon a talking parrot. . . . When a white author writes about such a Negro he makes him out a fool, a pimp or a whiner." Aubrey Bowsen, "Superstition and Syphilis," review of Roark Bradford's *This Side of Jordan* (London: Harper and Brothers, 1929) in *New Amsterdam News*, March 1929, in *[L. S. Alexander] Gumby Collection of the American Negro, Scrapbooks* (New York: Columbia University Libraries, 1971–74), microfilm.

48. T. R. Montgomery, "Let Negroes Build Their Own Hospital," in Box 6, Folder 5: "Negro Hospital," Samuel Watkins Overton Papers, Mississippi Valley Collection, McWherter Library, University of Memphis.

49. "Negro Hospital Delay Explained by Overton," *Memphis Commercial Appeal*, May 19, 1949; see also "Mayor Invites Ideas for Negro Hospital," *Memphis Commercial Appeal*, July 22, 1949.

50. "Another Major Group Backs Negro Hospital," *Memphis Commercial Appeal*, July 24, 1949.

51. U.S. Representative Cliff Davis to Mayor Watkins Overton, July 27, 1949, Box 6, Folder 3, Overton Papers.

52. "Public Fund Drive for Negro Hospital Proposed by Mayor," *Memphis Commercial Appeal*, July 29, 1949; see also Editorial, "Planning Must Go On," *Memphis Commercial Appeal*, July 30, 1949.

53. Editorial, "Negro Hospital Need," *Memphis Commercial Appeal*, August 4, 1949.

54. Two excellent overviews of this new national politics in race and health are W. Montague Cobb, *Medical Care and the Plight of the Negro* (New York: National Association for the Advancement of Colored People, 1947), and W. Montague Cobb, *Progress and Portents for the Negro in Medicine* (New York: National Association for the Advancement of Colored People, 1948). See also the *Journal of Negro Education* 18 (Summer 1949), a special health issue.

55. "Sydenham Fight on Race Bias Cited," *New York Times*, February 11, 1948.

56. "Officials in Talks to Save Sydenham," *New York Times*, n.d., in *Gumby Collection*.

57. "Sydenham Becomes City Hospital; Funds Rushed for Medical Care," *New York Times*, March 4, 1949.

58. "Consultant Takes First Look at Negro Hospital Needs Here," *Memphis Commercial Appeal*, October 13, 1949.

59. Editorial, "Negro Hospital Progress," *Memphis Commercial Appeal*, October 30, 1949.

60. "Sydenham Fight on Race Bias Cited," *New York Times*, February 11, 1948. Quote by Dr. Peter Marshall Murray, staff member of Sydenham Hospital.

61. Basil MacLean, *The City of Memphis, Tennessee, 1949: A Study of Negro Hospital Needs* (Rochester, N.Y.: Basil C. MacLean, George William Graham and Lloyd Mussells, Associates, 1949), 43.

62. T. O. Fuller, *Bridging the Racial Chasms: A Brief Survey of Inter-racial Attitudes and Relations* (Memphis: T. O. Fuller, 1937), 70.

63. Graves, "Relation of Hospital Service to Public Health," 92.

64. "Higher Insurance Rates for Negroes," *Journal of the National Medical Association* 42 (1950): 184. In 1950 a New York state superintendent of insurance suggested that companies might be allowed to charge higher rates on African American lives in order to make such cases more economically appealing, thereby expanding insurance coverage for blacks. An official at the Atlanta Life Insurance Company responded sharply that segregation, not mortality, was the problem for blacks in America. "Negroes, as a race, are, if anything, stronger physically than whites. The fact that they have a higher death rate is not due to the physical structure of the race, but to the artificial barriers of all kinds and descriptions, enacted into laws by those who would keep us more or less enslaved." Ibid.

65. Robert Pharr, Assistant City Attorney to Mayor Overton, in a Meeting of the

Hospital Advisory Committee, Nashville, Tennessee, May 24, 1950, Box 6, Folder 1: "Negro Hospital," Overton Papers.

66. MacLean, *City of Memphis*, 45.

67. Ibid., 47.

68. "Bonheur Votes to Go Ahead on Hospital," *Memphis Press-Scimitar*, August 3, 1949.

69. The proposal was one focus of the General Conference of the CME Church in Kansas City, Missouri, in April 1950. For a short history of Collins Chapel, see Donald R. Harris, "A Hospital for the Negroes of Memphis: Collins Chapel Hospital, 1910–1970," Memphis and Shelby County Public Library, Memphis.

70. W. S. Martin to the Venerable Bishops, 22nd General Conference, CME Church, Kansas City, Missouri, [April 1950], in *Quadrennial Report of the Collins Chapel Connectional Hospital, CME Church, May 3, 1950* (Jackson, Tenn.: Publishing House, CME Church), Box 1, Folder 1: "Negro Hospital," Overton Papers. For local coverage, see "Two Negro Leaders Disapprove New Hospital Plan — So Far as Diverting Funds Is Concerned," *Memphis Press-Scimitar*, April 21, 1950.

71. Editorial, "Shortsighted Decision," *Memphis Commercial Appeal*, April 27, 1950.

72. Graves, "Relation of Hospital Service to Public Health," 93. This new Collins Chapel, Graves believed, would alleviate the lack of "adequate facilities for the training of Negro physicians and nurses or for the practice of Negro physicians located in the city."

73. As one newspaper article noted, the disparity between the rising "economic level of the negro here" and the structure of the private health care system was increasingly obvious. "Negro Hospital Seen as Spur for Doctors," *Memphis Commercial Appeal*, July 19, 1949.

74. Margaret McCulloch to Robert Hutcheson, March 3, 1951, Records of the Tennessee Department of Public Health, Record Group 97, Series 3, Box 104, Folder 13, Tennessee State Library and Archives.

75. "Bluff City Medical Society Backs City Hospital Plan," *Memphis World*, April 28, 1950; "Negro Doctors Back City Hospital Plan — Mayor Thanked, Cooperation of Group Pledged — Collins Program Stands," *Memphis Commercial Appeal*, April 26, 1950.

76. "Hospital Campaign Gets More Support," *Memphis Commercial Appeal*, May 6, 1950.

77. Editorial, "Negro Hospital Need," *Memphis Commercial Appeal*, August 4, 1949.

78. L. M. Graves, "Symposium on Public Health: Public Health Progress in Memphis," *Memphis Medical Journal* (March 1941): 42.

79. Ibid., 43.

80. Ibid., 44.

81. Ernst Boas, *The Unseen Plague; Chronic Disease* (New York: J. J. Augustin, 1940). See also the discussion of cardiac disease in Fye, *American Cardiology*.

82. Indeed, within a few years penicillin and other antibiotics would be produced

for wartime and then civilian use and would gradually push tuberculosis off this list. See David Adams, *The Greatest Good to the Greatest Number: Penicillin Rationing on the American Home Front, 1940–1945* (New York: P. Lang, 1991).

83. William Dameshek, "Is Leukemia Increasing?," *Blood* 1 (January 1947): 101. See also "The Leukemic Terror," *Newsweek*, March 7, 1949, 54.

84. S. L. Wadley, "Epidemiology of Poliomyelitis," *Memphis Medical Journal* (April 1950): 59.

85. Ibid.

86. Ibid.

87. Graves, "Relation of Hospital Service to Public Health," 92.

88. Ibid.

89. C. H. Sanford, "With the Editor: A Half Century of Progress," *Memphis Medical Journal* (September 1948): 154. Flood control in the 1930s had resulted in the dramatic decline of the threat of malaria. On malaria, see Harold C. Hofsommer, "Survey of Rural Problem Areas: Leflore County, Mississippi, Cotton Growing Area of the Old South," Bureau of Agricultural Economics Report, Record Group 83, National Archives, cited in James Cobb, *The Most Southern Place on Earth: The Mississippi Delta and the Roots of Regional Identity* (New York: Oxford University Press, 1992), 189.

90. See, for example, Russell Patterson, "The Surgical Implications of Sickle Cell Anemia," *Memphis Medical Journal* (August 1950): 120–22.

CHAPTER 4

1. "Herff Presents Grants for UT, Memphis State — $8,500 Set for Anemia Study," *Memphis Commercial Appeal*, February 4, 1953. See also Thelma Tracy Mabry, *History of Medicine in Memphis: Interview with Dr. Lemuel Whitley Diggs* (Memphis: Oral History Research Office, Memphis State University, 1984), 11.

2. "Grant Renewed to Trace Strange Malady's Secret," *Memphis Press-Scimitar*, May 22, 1954.

3. "LeBonheur Hospital Assured — Fund Over the Top by $50,000," *Memphis Press-Scimitar*, February 13, 1950; "Negro Memphis Asked to Give $15,000 to La Bonheur Drive," *Memphis World*, January 20, 1950. The LeBonheur activism in health matters was predated by the wartime activities of other women's groups, such as the Memphis chapters of the Daughters of the American Revolution, which raised money for blood plasma war projects. "Blood Plasma for the War, DARs Project," *Memphis Press-Scimitar*, October 14, 1942, Morgue Files, Folder 9981: "Blood Banks," Mississippi Valley Collection, McWherter Library, University of Memphis. See also Marsha Wedell, *Elite Women and the Reform Impulse in Memphis, 1875–1915* (Knoxville: University of Tennessee Press, 1991).

4. Robert Sigafoos, *From Cotton Row to Beale Street: A Business History of Memphis* (Memphis: Memphis State University Press, 1979), 259.

5. Indeed, the birth rate among Memphis's African American families was notably higher than that of their white counterparts.

6. Benjamin Spock, *The Common Sense Book of Baby and Child Care* (New York: Duell, Sloan, and Pearce, 1946). In the late 1940s, Spock's book sold record numbers of copies in its second and third editions. See Lynn Bloom, *Doctor Spock: Biography of a Conservative Radical* (Indianapolis: Bobbs-Merrill, 1972). On Salk, see Jane S. Smith, *Patenting the Sun: Polio and the Salk Vaccine* (New York: W. Morrow, 1990).

7. Paul Flowers, *The Greenhouse* (Memphis: Paul Flowers, 1955), 3.

8. Moreover, poor health in Memphis was no longer linked to the agricultural economy. Less and less of the regional economy revolved around cotton. Between 1953 and 1957, noted historian James Cobb, "the proportion of cropland devoted to cotton fell from 59 percent to 32 percent . . . [, and] the number of mechanized cotton pickers rose by 46 percent." James Cobb, *The Most Southern Place on Earth: The Mississippi Delta and the Roots of Regional Identity* (New York: Oxford University Press, 1992), 205.

9. "News Men and the Medical Profession," *Memphis Medical Journal* (September 1952): 129.

10. Ibid.

11. As Durham noted, "It probably is not the atom bomb so much as our production line that deters Joe Stalin and the men in the Kremlin." Ibid.

12. "With the Editor: Do You Know or Don't You?," *Memphis Medical Journal* (April 1958): 145.

13. Elaine Tyler May, "Baby Boom and Birth Control," in *Homeward Bound: American Families in the Cold War Era* (New York: Basic Books, 1988).

14. "Various 'Drives' to Be Studied," *Memphis Press-Scimitar*, June 26, 1959; "Criticism for 4 Voluntary Agencies," *Memphis Press-Scimitar*, January 6, 1960.

15. "Criticism for 4 Voluntary Agencies," *Memphis Press-Scimitar*, January 6, 1960. For more on the tension between physicians and the National Foundation, which was often accused of fear-mongering and publicity-grabbing in an effort to raise funds for polio, see Smith, *Patenting the Sun*.

16. See W. Bruce Fye, *American Cardiology: The History of a Specialty and Its College* (Baltimore: Johns Hopkins University Press, 1996), for a discussion of objections to voluntarism and the story of the creation of the American College of Cardiology as a response to the popular appeals of the American Heart Association.

17. Lloyd M. Graves and Alfred H. Fletcher, "Some Trends in Public Housing," *American Journal of Public Health* (January 1941): 70. For example, discussing the public housing construction at Lamar Terrace, Graves noted that "299 families (practically all colored) were displaced by 633 white families. . . . This involved a gradual replacement of a small poor class Negro business section with a new white business residential development to serve the 633 new white families moved in." With the construction of an additional public housing complex, a

small island of "46 colored families [was] allowed to remain" at one end of the neighborhood, but "this island was too noticeable to be forgotten." The resolution followed a pattern similar to that at Lauderdale Courts: "Through neighborhood agitation and with the aid of city officials . . . this area was purchased and will be converted into a park and playground." Ibid.

18. Christopher Silver, "The Changing Face of Neighborhoods in Memphis and Richmond, 1940–1985," in *Shades of the Sunbelt: Essays on Ethnicity, Race, and the Urban South*, ed. Randall Miller and George Pozzetta (New York: Greenwood Press, 1988), 112. As Silver has noted, city planner Harlan Bartholomew called for a strategy of slum clearance that would channel black housing in one direction.

19. Ibid., 115. By 1952 a confederation of twenty-four African American neighborhood groups formed the Bluff and Shelby County Council of Civic Clubs in order to lobby for their own interests. One of the most vocal was in the Eleventh Ward.

20. Harry Holloway, *The Politics of the Southern Negro: From Exclusion to Big City Organization* (New York: Random House, 1969), 280. As Holloway notes, whereas African Americans in cities like Houston and Atlanta "were either part of a coalition or in the early stages of developing one . . . , Memphis Negroes suddenly found themselves relatively independent" (ibid.).

21. "Ground Broken Here for Negro Hospital," *Memphis Commercial Appeal*, November 23, 1953.

22. See Steven Lawson, *Running for Freedom: Civil Rights and Black Politics in America since 1941* (New York: McGraw-Hill, 1991).

23. These years saw the creation of black radio in Memphis with WDIA, a station that would have a huge impact on black culture, consciousness, and activism. On other popular cultural shifts in black Memphis, see also Peter Marshall Ostenby, "Other Games, Other Glory: The Memphis Red Sox and the Trauma of Integration, 1948–1955" (master's thesis, University of North Carolina, 1989).

24. In cities across the nation, such media dramatized the plight of blacks in the South. In New York City, for example, WMCA began broadcasting a new program, *New World A'Coming*, in 1944. The program portrayed blacks as "daily victims of insult, violence, and discrimination in a nation talking loudly about expanding democracy." As historian Barbara Savage notes, "One program on [Memphis's] W. C. Handy concluded with a dramatization of an incident in which his wife was denied hospital emergency room care." Such dramatizations gained wider audiences in the 1950s. Barbara Savage, *Broadcasting Freedom: Radio, War, and the Politics of Race* (Chapel Hill: University of North Carolina Press, 1999), 254.

25. "50 Percent Increase in Bluff City Population Causes Many Headaches," *Tri-State Defender*, September 27, 1952. 17. Note also the city's attempts at self-

promotion in 1944–45, including *City of Memphis, Civic Progress, 1940–1945* (Memphis: City of Memphis, 1945) and Memphis Commissioners, *Benefits and Opportunities for Colored Citizens of Memphis* (Memphis: Memphis Commissioners, 1944). The transformation from tenant farming to sharecropping on the cotton plantations meant a dramatic mobility for rural Mid-South people — and a significant influx of rural citizens into Memphis. See James Cobb, *Most Southern Place*. See also Richard Day, "The Economics of Technological Change and the Demise of the Sharecropper," *American Economics Review* 57 (June 1967): 443.

26. Announcing a 1951 campaign for the Baptist Hospital, for example, the *Memphis Medical Journal* stated that "an extensive survey was made [of hospital conditions in the city,] and . . . the most alarming fact . . . was that of all the South (from Baltimore, Maryland to El Paso, Texas) of 100,000 population, Memphis has the lowest number of general beds per one thousand people." "With the Editor: Support the Baptist Building Fund," *Memphis Medical Journal* (March 1951): 31.

27. Silver, "Changing Face of Neighborhoods, 115.

28. Ibid. See also Christopher MacGregor Scribner, "Federal Funding, Urban Renewal, and Race Relations: Birmingham in Transition, 1945–1955," *Alabama Historical Quarterly* 57 (October 1995): 269–95, and Roger Biles, *Memphis in the Great Depression* (Knoxville: University of Tennessee Press, 1986).

29. "Doctors Set Aside Motion to Admit Negro Members — But Welcome Them to Scientific Sessions," *Memphis Press-Scimitar*, November 3, 1954.

30. Here was another vast system of discrimination in which (as in the Red Cross blood segregation controversy) no single organization would accept total blame.

31. "Doctors Set Aside Motion to Admit Negro Members," *Memphis Press-Scimitar*, November 3, 1954. See also "Medical Society Head to Try to Sell Plan — Admitting Negroes Is Topic Tonight," *Memphis Press-Scimitar*, November 2, 1954, Morgue Files, Mississippi Valley Collection, McWherter Library, University of Memphis.

32. The new policy noted that black doctors could apply for full membership, but "attendance at social functions would be by invitation only." "Medical Society Acts on Negroes — Membership Possible on Limited Basis," *Memphis Press-Scimitar*, July 6, 1955.

33. Russell H. Patterson, "The Surgical Implications of Sickle Cell Anemia," *Memphis Medical Journal* (August 1950): 120. See also Memphis authors Lemuel Diggs, "The Sickle Cell Crisis," *American Journal of Clinical Pathology* 26 (1956): 1109–18, and H. Rudner Jr. and H. Rudner Sr., "Abdominal Manifestations of Sickle Cell Anemia," *American Journal of Gastroenterology* 25 (1956): 11–21. For earlier writings along these lines by non-Memphis authors, see E. H. Campbell, "Acute Abdominal Pain in Sickle Cell Anemia," *Archives of Surgery* 31 (1935):

607, and A. Oschner and S. Murray, "Pitfalls in the Diagnosis of Acute Abdominal Conditions," *American Journal of Surgery* 41 (1938): 343–69.

34. Patterson, "Surgical Implications of Sickle Cell Anemia," 120.

35. "The most common complaint," Patterson noted, "was bone and joint pain." Ibid., 121.

36. Frank D. Smythe, "A Golden Opportunity for the University of Tennessee Medical College," *Memphis Medical Journal* (October 1924): 214–18.

37. Frankie Winchester, "The Path from Obscurity: Efforts to Gain Recognition for Sickle Cell Disease, Memphis, 1920–1975" (master's thesis, Memphis State University, 1991), 16.

38. Since the early 1920s, the University of Tennessee had held a contract with the city of Memphis to staff John Gaston Hospital. This arrangement was seen as a "golden opportunity for the University" because the wealth of clinical material brought students into intimate contact with a wide range of diseases. Smythe, "Golden Opportunity." This view of patients as "valuable clinical material" should not be surprising; it has always been part of medical education and research. See Kenneth Ludmerer, *Learning to Heal: The Development of American Medical Education* (New York: Basic Books, 1985).

39. See David Adams, *"The Greatest Good to the Greatest Number": Penicillin Rationing on the American Home Front, 1940–1945* (New York: Peter Lang, 1991).

40. See, for example, L. W. Diggs and Luis Barreras, "Pulmonary Emboli vs. Pneumonia in Patients with Sickle Cell Anemia," *Memphis and Mid-South Medical Journal* (October 1967): 375–80. Here the authors note that "patients with sickle cell disease also are susceptible to respiratory infections and pneumonia. In the past, practically all patients with chest symptoms and signs, fever, leukocytosis and infiltrative lesions as revealed by roentgenograms were diagnosed and treated as pneumonia" (379).

41. Clarence Taylor, "Sickle Cell Anemia in Pregnancy: Resume of Literature, with a Case Report," *Journal of the National Medical Association* 43 (1951): 168.

42. Mehdi Tavassoli to Maxwell Wintrobe, January 3, 1983, Box 25, Folder: "Tavassoli, Mehdi," Maxwell Myer Wintrobe Papers, Marriott Library Special Collections, University of Utah, Salt Lake City.

43. On the economy of laboratory science with its particular cycles of credit and exchange relations, see Bruno Latour and Stephen Woolgar, *Laboratory Life: The Construction of Scientific Facts* (Princeton: Princeton University Press, 1986).

44. "A Million Dollar Expansion for John Gaston—Three Vital Improvements Planned," *Memphis Press-Scimitar*, February 23, 1954.

45. They studied the disease from different perspectives (renal, cardiovascular, hemodynamic, and neurological). See, for example, F. S. Hill and B. C. Davis, "Electroencephalographic Studies of Sickle Cell Anemia," *American Journal of the Diseases of Children* 84 (1952): 214–18; F. S. Hill, "Neurological Manifestations in Sickle Cell Anemia," *Journal of the National Medical Association* 45

(1953): 421–24; J. Patterson, "Sickle Cell Anemia: A Surgical Problem," *Surgery* 28 (1950): 393–403; J. Patterson, "Sickle Cell Anemia: A Surgical Problem," *Surgery* 28 (1950): 641–51; James Etteldorf, "John Gaston Clinico-Pathological Clinic Sickle Cell Anemia," *Tennessee State Medical Journal* 27 (January 1951): 25–31; James Etteldorf, "Renal Function Studies in Pediatrics," *American Journal of the Diseases of Children* 83 (1952): 185–91; James Etteldorf et al., "Renal Hemodialysis in Adults with Sickle Cell Anemia," *American Journal of Medicine* (1955): 242–48; James Etteldorf et al., "Cardiovascular Dynamics in Sickle Cell Anemia," *Abstract from Combined Meeting of British Pediatric Association, Society for Pediatric Research, and Canadian Pediatric Society* (1955): 57–58; James Etteldorf et al., "Oxygen Disassociation in Sickle Cell Disease," *American Journal of the Diseases of Children* 90 (1955): 572; and James Etteldorf, Abstract, "Further Hemodynamic Observations in Children with Homozygous Hemoglobin S," *The Society for Pediatric Research Program and Abstracts* 34 (May 1959): 6.

46. This transformation was also occurring in other cities and regions in the 1950s.

47. Randall Miller, "The Development of the Modern Urban South: An Historical Overview," in Miller and Pozzetta, *Shades of the Sunbelt*, 6.

48. Scribner, "Federal Funding, Urban Renewal."

49. Suzanne Lebsock and Nancy Hewitt, eds., *Visible Women: New Essays on American Activism* (Urbana: University of Illinois Press, 1993); see also Wedell, *Elite Women*.

50. In 1954 Memphis pediatrician Fontaine S. Hill revealed the new status of research when he wrote, "Adequate service to sick makes mandatory the acquisition of . . . knowledge." F. S. Hill, *Practical Guide to Fluid Therapy in Pediatrics* (Philadelphia: W. B. Saunders, 1954), v. Hill also took an interest in sickle cell disease. On urban renewal, see Sigafoos, *Cotton Row to Beale Street*, 259.

51. One hematologist, Ernest Beutler, recalled initiating "investigations of the effect of methemoglobin forming drugs on red cell lifespan in patients with sickle cell anemia." "At that time," he noted, "it was quite possible to carry out such investigations after explaining the procedure to the patient and obtaining his consent. Nowadays, such studies would be virtually impossible. They would be mired in intramural and extramural committees which would question their propriety, morality, and safety." Ernest Beutler, biographical statement, Box 9, Folder: "Beutler," Wintrobe Papers,

52. David Rothman, *Strangers at the Bedside: A History of How Law and Bioethics Transformed Medical Decision Making* (New York: Basic Books, 1991). See also Susan Lederer, *Subjected to Science: Human Experimentation in America before World War II* (Baltimore: Johns Hopkins University Press, 1995).

53. Margaret Anderson, *The Children of the South* (New York: Farrar, Straus, Giroux, 1958). Written in the aftermath of the 1954 *Brown v. Board of Education* desegregation decision, Anderson's book was a schoolteacher's account of race relations in the public school. For popular psychoanalyst Erik Erikson, black identity itself

was shaped in childhood since "Negro babies often receive sensual satisfactions which provide them with enough oral and sensory surplus for a lifetime." For Erikson, this upbringing inevitably met disillusionment when black children became aware of the "master race." And here, in this tension, new identities emerged — "mammy's oral-sensual 'honey-child' . . . the evil identity of the dirty, anal-sadistic, phallic rapist 'nigger,' . . . and the clean anal-compulsive, restrained, friendly, but always sad 'white man's Negro.'" Erik Erikson, *Childhood and Society* (New York: W. W. Norton, 1950), 241–42. See also E. Franklin Frazier, *The Negro Family in the United States* (New York: Macmillan, 1949), and David Rosner and Gerald Markowitz, *Children, Race, and Power: Kenneth and Mamie Clark's Northside Center* (Charlottesville: University Press of Virginia, 1996).

54. Throughout America — in the 1940 White House Conference on Children in a Democracy, in Richard Wright's 1945 novel *Black Boy: A Record of Childhood and Youth* (New York: Harper and Row, 1945), and in the 1950 White House Conference on Children and Youth — the message was the same: the child was a product of a society in need of reform. See, for example, Charles Spurgeon Johnson, *Growing Up in the Black Belt: Negro Youth in the Rural South* (Washington, D.C.: American Council on Education, 1941). As Johnson wrote, "The racial position of Negroes in the South is a part of the institutional reorganization of the South and reflects a long history of racial conflicts and accommodations. . . . The situation is aggravated by the generally low economic condition of the area and the resulting inadequacy of provisions for education, housing, health. . . . The response of Negro youth to this situation is the objective of this study" (xviii).

55. See Kenneth and Mamie Clark, "The Development of Consciousness of Self and the Emergence of Racial Identity in Negro Preschool Children," *Journal of Social Psychology* 10 (1939): 591–99. For an astute analysis of the Clarks and their work, see Rosner and Markowitz, *Children, Race, and Power*, 23.

56. See Keith Wailoo, *Drawing Blood: Technology and Disease Identity in Twentieth-Century America* (Baltimore: Johns Hopkins University Press, 1997), 162–87.

57. "The Sickle Threat," *Time*, January 19, 1959, 42.

58. "Children's Hospital for Memphis — Began Over a Tea Cup Back in Flapper Era," *Memphis Press-Scimitar*, June 18, 1952.

59. "Le Bonheur Children's Hospital," *Memphis Medical Journal* (July 1952): 101.

60. "LeBonheur to Keep Hospital Plan Alive," *Memphis Commercial Appeal*, July 30, 1949; "Negro Memphis Asked to Give $15,000 to La Bonheur Drive," *Memphis World*, January 20, 1950; "LeBonheur Hospital Assured — Fund Over the Top by $50,000," *Memphis Press-Scimitar*, February 13, 1950. Newspapers marveled that well-off club women would undertake such a generous project: "What would a sleek, proud thorobred have to do with whether a sick child gets well? The answer: plenty." "Money Will Go to LeBonheur's New Hospital," *Memphis Press-Scimitar*, September 17, 1951.

61. "Putting Finishing Touches to LeBonheur Hospital," *Memphis Press-Scimitar*, February 5, 1952.

62. See "University of Tennessee News Notes," *Memphis and Mid-South Medical Journal* (June 1960): 255 and (February 1961): 77–78.

63. As I have written elsewhere, "Enamored of the new diagnostic tool, two clinicians reminded their peers in 1954 that 'it is no longer satisfactory to use the term sickle cell anemia without attempting to establish' the forms of hemoglobin responsible for the disease." John Moseley and John Manly, "Sickle Cell Disease: An Analysis of Recent Advances," *Journal of the National Medical Association* 46 (1954): 181, quoted in Wailoo, *Drawing Blood*, 157.

64. "University of Tennessee News," *Memphis Medical Journal* (July 1958): 293.

65. Frankie Winchester, *Sickle Cell Anemia Research in Memphis: Interview with Alfred P. Kraus, M.D.* (Memphis: Oral History Research Office, Memphis State University, 1989), 5.

66. In the early 1960s one biologist stated that "the study of sickle cell hemoglobin has not only provided much information about normal and abnormal hemoglobins but has opened an era of biochemical genetics." A. Atamer, "Hereditary Hemoglobinopathies," in *Blood Disease* (New York: Grune and Stratton, 1963), 175. As I have argued elsewhere, with the use of electrophoresis in many clinical settings a global cataloging of abnormal hemoglobins followed. Hemoglobin variations (with no evidence of clinical disorders) as well as clinically significant abnormalities turned up everywhere. See Wailoo, *Drawing Blood*, 157.

67. His wife, Lorraine Kraus, was equally prolific, if a bit more wide-ranging in her research interests.

68. See Robert Orsi, *Thank You, St. Jude: Women's Devotion to the Patron Saint of Hopeless Causes* (New Haven: Yale University Press, 1996).

69. Ibid., 14.

70. Winchester, *Interview with Kraus*, 6. Appropriately enough, Lemuel Diggs quickly became a key figure in the creation of St. Jude. "Pair of Herff Grants Made," *Memphis Press-Scimitar*, February 3, 1953.

71. See Leonard Dinnerstein and Mary Dale Pallson, *Jews in the South* (Baton Rouge: Louisiana State University Press, 1973).

72. For discussion of the gift relationship, see Marcel Mauss, *The Gift: Forms and Functions of Exchange in Archaic Societies* (New York: W. W. Norton, 1967), 69. For discussions of gift giving in the context of health care, see Richard Titmuss, *The Gift Relationship: From Human Blood to Social Policy* (New York: Pantheon, 1971); and see Renée Fox and Judith Swazey, *Spare Parts: Organ Replacement in American Society* (New York: Oxford University Press, 1992).

73. Norman Parks, "Tennessee Politics since Kefauver and Reece: A 'Generalist' View," *Journal of Politics* 28 (1966): 151–52.

74. Statement by Edmund Orgill, March 3, 1956, Box 16, Folder: "Negroes," Ed-

mund Orgill Papers, Mississippi Valley Collection, McWherter Library, University of Memphis. Italics added for emphasis.

75. Rev. Roy Love to Edmund Orgill, November 19, 1955, ibid.

76. Paul Vanderwood, "Council of Civic Clubs Roars Its Approval of a Pro-Segregation Resolution," *Memphis Press-Scimitar*, February 14, 1956, Morgue Files, Folder 51421, Mississippi Valley Collection, McWherter Library, University of Memphis. According to Memphian Paul Coppock, the powerful council got its start in the late 1920s by bringing white neighborhoods together to defend "custom" wherever boundaries of race relations seemed threatened. See Paul Coppock, "How the Civic Clubs Got Their Start," *Memphis Press-Scimitar*, May 24, 1981.

77. Vanderwood, "Council of Civic Clubs."

78. Dr. T. R. Montgomery to Mayor Edmund Orgill, February 27, 1956, Box 16, Folder: "Negroes — John Gaston," Orgill Papers.

79. Western Union telegram from Gordon Hollingsworth Sr. to Mayor Edmund Orgill, February 26, 1956, Box 16, Folder: "Negroes," Orgill Papers.

80. Paul Vanderwood, "Cool Reception to Speech Accusing Orgill of Creating Racial Hatred," *Memphis Press-Scimitar*, June 15, 1956.

81. In Box 16, Folder: "Negroes (hate)," Orgill Papers.

82. Black civic organizations and local radio personalities received increasing public attention and newspaper headlines. By the 1950s, physician A. L. Johnson had won local acclaim as a "prime mover of current efforts to establish a Negro hospital." The story of his receipt of an award from the Memphis chapter of Omega Psi Phi, a "national Negro fraternity, in a public ceremony at First Baptist Church (negro)," was carried in the *Commercial Appeal*, highlighting the widening public interest in such issues. "Negro Trophy Given to Dr. A. L. Johnson — Leader of Drive for Hospital Nurses' Training," *Memphis Commercial Appeal*, June 19, 1950.

83. Donald Young lists "visibility" of the African American, either physical or cultural, competition between whites and blacks, and the traditional low position of minority groups as key factors in race prejudice. Cited in John Dollard, *Caste and Class in a Southern Town* (New Haven: Yale University Press, 1937), 441. See Donald Young, *American Minority Peoples: A Study in Racial and Cultural Conflicts in the United States* (New York: Harper and Brothers, 1932), 589.

84. Mabry, *Interview with Diggs*, 10.

85. Ibid.

86. Ibid.

87. "The Memphis Medical Journal," *Memphis Medical Journal* (April 1958): 143.

88. For insight and contrast on this, see "Insurance Fees at John Gaston Hospital," *Memphis Medical Journal* (October 1958): 395.

89. To be sure, as historian Thomas Clark noted in 1961, there were still fundamen-

tal conflicts "between country and flourishing urban communities." But these conflicts had taken a turn in the post–World War II decades. To those in the hinterlands, urban growth now signaled a threat, an assault on tradition. As Clark noted, cities like "Atlanta, New Orleans, Norfolk-Newport News, Memphis, Louisville, Miami, and Charlotte form spreading metropolitan complexes which grasp old rural communities in their tentacles." "These places, and scores of others, have outgrown their bounds since 1940s," wrote Clark. "Every month the traditionally rural South is forced deeper into retreat." Thomas Clark, *The Emerging South* (New York: Oxford University Press, 1961), 273.

90. As an example of this new civic culture, see the description of a new council concerned with sickle cell anemia in the black community. "Pupils Visit Crump Hospital," *Memphis Commercial Appeal*, March 25, 1957. As one article noted, one "Negro Civic leader said the council would need the cooperation of other Negro groups in Memphis if it decided to tackle the anemia campaign." This was "a disease that killed thousands of Negroes each year." The following year, the papers pictured Diggs with the African American women of the Gentry Avenue Civic Club as they handed him a check for $200. *Memphis Commercial Appeal*, June 12, 1958. The new awareness of sickle cell disease was part of a larger liberal trend. As historian Joel Williamson has noted, "The New Liberals, the native white Southerners who participated in the breakup of the neo-Conservative order in the middle of the twentieth century, were, for the most part, decidedly not organized. Their rebellions against the rigid racial establishment were mainly individual, scattered, and evolved over the decades." Among this group were many academic liberals. Joel Williamson, *The Crucible of Race: Black-White Relations in the American South since Emancipation* (New York: Oxford University Press, 1984), 486.

CHAPTER 5

1. Psychiatrist/author Robert Coles traveled through the South in the early 1960s, for example, and saw both fear and hope in the faces of the region's children as a new, desegregated world appeared. "The first two years of desegregation in cities in the Deep South can hardly be easy for all," Coles reflected. "But young people in the South are growing up in a world which differs sharply from that of their parents." Robert Coles, "In the South These Children Prophesy," in *Farewell to the South* (Boston: Little, Brown, 1963), 59.

2. *Hearings before the United States Commission on Civil Rights: Hearing Held in Memphis, Tennessee, June 25–26, 1962* (Washington, D.C.: U.S. Government Printing Office, 1963). See also later Civil Rights Commission hearings: *Employment, Administration of Justice, and Health Services in Memphis–Shelby County, Tennessee* (Washington, D.C.: U.S. Government Printing Office, 1967); *Hearings before the United States Commission on Civil Rights: Hearing Held in Memphis, Tennessee, May 9, 1977* (Washington, D.C.: U.S. Commission on Civil Rights, 1978); and,

most recently, *Burning of African-American Churches in Tennessee and Perceptions of Race Relations: Transcripts of a Community Forum, Held July 10, 1996, Memphis, Tennessee* (Atlanta: U.S. Commission on Civil Rights, Southern Regional Office, 1996).

3. A 1963 U.S. Supreme Court decision in *Simkins v. Moses Cone Hospital* (in North Carolina) marked an eventful step in the fall of separate but equal hospital care. For further discussion, see David Barton Smith, *Health Care Divided: Race and Healing a Nation* (Ann Arbor: University of Michigan Press, 1999). On the 1960s, see David Steigerwald, *The Sixties and the End of Modern America* (New York: St. Martin's Press, 1995). The 1950s had established that the black consumer could be a force for change by withholding dollars from discriminating establishments. The 1960s established the black public protester as an additional agent of change—marches and public demonstrations undermined segregation in transportation, in education, in department stores, in hospital care, and at lunch counters. The new strategy had far-reaching effects. Many southerners, watching marches in Montgomery, Alabama, and Washington, D.C., saw their regional way of life in upheaval, their economy threatened, and their very identities being altered.

4. Richard Ely, "Bulletin No. 2: Memphis Citizens' Council, February 22, 1962," Box 13, Folder 1: "Memphis Committee on Community Relations, 1961–1964," Edward Meeman Papers, Mississippi Valley Collection, McWherter Library, University of Memphis.

5. Other health care cases also highlighted the inhumanity of racial exclusion. Consider, for example, the often-cited case of Charles Drew, the black surgeon and inventor of blood plasma transfusion who died after an automobile accident in North Carolina in 1950. According to legend, Drew was refused transfusion at a white-only hospital. While untrue in Drew's case, the situation did occur in many other instances—and the story of Drew's death resonated with African Americans for decades afterward. For an analysis, see Spencie Love, *One Blood: The Death and Resurrection of Charles R. Drew* (Chapel Hill: University of North Carolina Press, 1997).

6. This new politics of pain forced medicine to rethink its pain management practices and forced politicians and social activists to openly discuss remedies for the relief of suffering. The pain of sickle cell disease could be used to dramatize the blindness of mainstream culture to the experiences of marginal groups, and the disenfranchised could now embrace the illness experience as a vital, lived reality and a genesis of group identity. The rising focus on pain in sickle cell disease, in short, provides a keen insight into the new politics of patienthood and health care in the 1960s.

7. The rate had gone from 26 per 1145 in 1956 to 26.9 in 1958, and it was expected to increase yet again for 1959. "Increase in Infant Death Rate Puzzle," *Memphis Press-Scimitar*, January 5, 1960.

8. Roy Hamilton, "Same in Shelby: Infant Mortality Rate Is Up," *Memphis Press-Scimitar*, January 5, 1960.

9. Testimony of Dr. Nobel W. Guthrie, *Hearings before the United States Commission on Civil Rights, June 25–26, 1962*, 11.

10. Ibid., 12.

11. Ibid., 7.

12. Testimony of James W. Moore, Commissioner, City of Memphis, Accompanied by Oscar M. Marvin, Administrator, City of Memphis Hospitals, ibid., 33.

13. Testimony of M. K. Calleson, ibid., 43.

14. Testimony of G. W. Stanley Ish, ibid., 59.

15. Ibid., 60.

16. "Sickle Cell Fund Drive Launched," *Memphis Press-Scimitar*, April 5, 1963.

17. Moses Newsom, "Malady Afflicts Race," *Memphis Commercial Appeal* (1962), Folder: "Sickle Cell Anemia," Newspaper Clipping Files, Memphis and Shelby County Public Library.

18. For general insight into racial politics and the 1960s, see Stewart Burns, *Social Movements of the 1960s: Searching for Democracy* (Boston: Twayne Publishers, 1990), and Steigerwald, *The Sixties*.

19. "The Sickle Threat," *Time*, January 19, 1959, 42; "Incurable 'Negro Disease' Strikes Five in Family," *Ebony*, May 1966, 154–62.

20. Anthony C. Allison, "Sickle Cell and Evolution," *Scientific American* 195 (August 1956): 88.

21. As early as 1951, one author forecast that we "may be able to devise a small, innocuous molecule which will lock permanently on to the defective hemoglobin and prevent the abnormal molecule from misbehaving." George Gray, "Sickle Cell Anemia," *Scientific American* 185 (August 1951): 56–59. See a more extensive discussion of these ideals of molecular engineering in Keith Wailoo, *Drawing Blood: Technology and Disease Identity in Twentieth-Century America* (Baltimore: Johns Hopkins University Press, 1997).

22. Anthony C. Allison, "Protection Afforded by Sickle-Cell Trait against Subtertian Malariarial Infection," *British Medical Journal* 1 (1954): 290–94.

23. J. V. Neel, "Data Pertaining to Population Dynamics of Sickle Cell Disease," *American Journal of Human Genetics* 5 (1953): 154.

24. For a more detailed discussion, see Wailoo, *Drawing Blood*, 154–59. As Theodosius Dobzhansky wrote, "Race differences are compounds of individual differences; they are more often relative than absolute; races differ in frequencies of some genes more often than in that a certain gene is wholly absent in one race and present in every individual in another. This relativity, the lack of hard and fast dichotomies in race differences, is disappointing to the adherents of the old-fashioned typological concept of races. Curiously enough, it is also disappointing to some new-fashioned writers, who claim that since races are not airtight pigeonholes they do not exist." Theodosius Dobzhansky, "Biological Aspects of

Race in Man: Introduction," in *Science and the Concept of Race*, ed. Margaret Mead et al. (New York: Columbia University Press, 1968), 78.

25. "Pair of Herff Grants Made," *Memphis Press-Scimitar*, February 3, 1953.

26. Allison, "Sickle Cell and Evolution," 91.

27. Allison, "Protection Afforded by Sickle-Cell Trait," 291.

28. William Levin, "Editorial: 'Asymptomatic' Sickle Cell Trait," *Blood* 13 (1958): 905–6.

29. See A. P. Kraus, "Editorial: Genetics," *Memphis and Mid-South Medical Journal* 38 (May 1963): 201.

30. See, for example, discussions in postslavery America regarding the rise of mental illness and epidemic disease as a response to the new freedom of African Americans and their inability to cope with the burdens of individual responsibility. See John Haller, *Outcasts from Evolution: Scientific Attitudes of Racial Inferiority, 1859–1900* (Urbana: University of Illinois Press, 1971), and John Hughes, "Labeling and Treating Black Mental Illness in Alabama, 1861–1910," *Journal of Southern History* 59 (August 1993): 435–60.

31. See S. Weisenfeld, "Sickle Cell Trait in Human Biological and Cultural Evolution," *Science* 157 (September 8, 1967): 1134–40; R. Singer, "The Sickle Cell Trait in Africa," *American Anthropologist* 55 (1953): 634–48; L. Mednick and M. Orans, "The Sickle-Cell Gene: Migration versus Selection," *American Anthropologist* 58 (1958): 293–95; and F. Livingstone, "The Origins of the Sickle-Cell Gene," in *Reconstructing African Culture History*, ed. Creighton Gabel and Norman R. Bennett (Boston: Boston University Press, 1967), 139–66. For a more detailed discussion of these developments, see Wailoo, *Drawing Blood*, 180–86.

32. See Keith Wailoo, "Detecting 'Negro Blood': Black and White Identities and the Reconstruction of Sickle Cell Anemia," in *Drawing Blood*, 134–61.

33. Todd Lee Savitt, "Sound Minds and Sound Bodies: The Diseases and Health Care of Blacks in Ante-Bellum Virginia" (Ph.D. diss., University of Virginia, 1975); Peter Wood, *Black Majority: Negroes in Colonial South Carolina from 1670 through the Stono Rebellion* (New York: Norton, 1974).

34. "Incurable 'Negro Disease' Strikes Five in Family," *Ebony*, May 1966, 154–62.

35. Ibid., 160.

36. Ibid., 162.

37. "Abstracts and charts are also being made from case records of sc patients observed in the City of Memphis Hospitals during the last decades." *ALSAC News*, April 14, 1961, in Box 13, Folder: "Lemuel Diggs," Maxwell Myer Wintrobe Papers, Marriott Library Special Collections, University of Utah, Salt Lake City.

38. Mentioned in *ALSAC News*, April 14, 1961.

39. "University of Tennessee News Notes," *Memphis and Mid-South Medical Journal* (February 1961): 77.

40. "Medical News in Tennessee: University of Tennessee College of Medicine," *Journal of the Tennessee Medical Association* (September 1962): 383. Reference to

"availability of patients" appears in "Sickle Cell Center Added to UT," *University Center-Grams* 18 (February 1965): 1.

41. "Sickle Cell Fund Drive Launched; Negro Leaders Named," *Tri-State Defender*.

42. Lemuel Diggs, "Treatment of the Crisis," *Southern Medical Journal* 56 (1963): 472–74.

43. *Tri-State Defender*, June 13, 1964.

44. Public discussions about blood and blood transfusion had also begun to reshape attitudes toward race and segregation. In addition to my discussion above, see Love, *One Blood*.

45. "Policy Attacked of Segregating Blood Banks," *Memphis Press-Scimitar*, November 20, 1968, Morgue Files, Folder 9981: "Blood Banks," Mississippi Valley Collection, McWherter Library, University of Memphis.

46. Two official histories of St. Jude are Hazel Fath, *A Dream Come True: The Story of St. Jude Children's Research Hospital and ALSAC* (Memphis: St. Jude Children's Research Hospital, 1983), and Randall Bedwell, ed., *From His Promise: A History of ALSAC and St. Jude Children's Research Hospital* (Memphis: Guild Bindery Press, 1996).

47. Fath, *Dream Come True*, 33. While the acronym ALSAC remained the same throughout this period, the letters came to mean different things in different contexts. At first, the acronym drew attention to the Lebanese and Syrian origins of the group (American Lebanese and Syrian Associated Charities). Then, in some fund-raising contexts, perhaps reflecting the changing demographics of the organization, the name became American Lebanese Societies and Associated Charities. By 1961, Lemuel Diggs would state that the term ALSAC stood for "Aiding Leukemia Stricken American Children." This represented a dramatic shift in the identity of donors as well as in the purpose of the organization.

48. Ibid., 38.

49. "Chicago Chapter Proves There's a Santa," *ALSAC News*, April 14, 1961, 3.

50. See Robert Orsi, *Thank You, St. Jude: Women's Devotion to the Patron Saint of Hopeless Causes* (New Haven: Yale University Press, 1996).

51. Lemuel Diggs, "Organization of the St. Jude Children's Research Hospital," *ALSAC News*, April 14, 1961, 4.

52. As the official history of St. Jude presents it, "At the time, Danny's plan was to build a general pediatric hospital. [However, t]here did not seem to be much positive reaction to that idea in Memphis." Fath, *Dream Come True*. Memphis became a leading site because Thomas's close friend Cardinal Stitch, whose first parish had been in Memphis, suggested the Bluff City. Diggs Autobiographical Statement, [ca. 1984], 38, Wintrobe Papers.

53. Fath, *Dream Come True*, 19.

54. Diggs Autobiographical Statement, 39, Wintrobe Papers.

55. Lemuel Diggs, "St. Jude Hospital," *Memphis Medical Journal* (June 1960): 225.

56. Diggs, "Organization of St. Jude, 4.

57. Diggs, "St. Jude Hospital," 225.

58. Fath, *Dream Come True*, 68.

59. Diggs, "St. Jude Hospital," 225.

60. David Tucker, *Memphis since Crump: Bossism, Blacks, and Civic Reformers, 1948–1968* (Knoxville: University of Tennessee Press, 1980), 120.

61. Fath, *Dream Come True*, 69.

62. First quote from "1959–1960 Progress Report during First Year of Operation of ALSAC-St. Jude Research Grant," Box 13, Folder: "Lemuel Diggs," Wintrobe Papers. Second quote from "Sickle Cell Center Added to UT," *University Center-Grams* 18 (February 1965): 1.

63. Diggs, "Organization of St. Jude," 4.

64. Ibid. The effects of federal research financing were far-reaching, especially at the University of Tennessee, which also felt the economic pressure of patronage. In 1961–62 federal sources accounted for nearly $1.9 million of the total $2.2 million in contracts and awards for research. Foundations and voluntary health organizations contributed $111,000, an amount comparable to industry and individual contributions. Only $41,159 came from the city, county, and state. "News—University of Tennessee College of Medicine," *Journal of the Tennessee Medical Association* (December 1962): 489.

65. At the same time, authors like Robert Coles were exposing the poor health, economic deprivation, and debility of children in the rural South. Robert Coles, *Children of Crisis: A Study of Courage and Fear* (New York: Dell Publishing, 1964). Coles described his purpose as trying "to present five youths, not quite as I would at a clinical conference, but with the same purpose—to make them as individuals come alive." "Whatever illumination is supplied by these youths—and my acquaintance with them—has come," he noted, "from the success with which the truth of their experience is revealed" (224).

66. See James Cobb, *The Most Southern Place on Earth: The Mississippi Delta and the Roots of Regional Identity* (New York: Oxford University Press, 1992), 231–52.

67. Addison Scoville, "Editorial: Patient Care," *Journal of the Tennessee Medical Association* (July 1963): 298. See also Louis J. Vorhaus, "Sick People Need Care, Not Research," *Saturday Evening Post*, March 11, 1963. For more on how the proliferation of unregulated clinical research posed enormous problems in the ethics of human experimentation, see David Rothman, *Strangers at the Bedside: A History of How Law and Bioethics Transformed Medical Decision Making* (New York: Basic Books, 1991).

68. Scoville, "Editorial: Patient Care," 298.

69. Ibid.

70. John Herbers, "Integration Gains in Memphis; Biracial Leadership Takes Hold," *New York Times*, March 31, 1964.

71. Ibid.

72. Noted Vasco Smith to the ABC reporter, "Here in Memphis we have, I guess,

approximately a third of our restaurants that are now open, serving all individuals without regard to race, creed or color." Even one "militant" member of the committee conceded some progress, while also seeing much "tokenism," and a black banker from Beale Street noted that the city had yet to elect "a Negro to office." ABC News Broadcast, May 22, 1964, Morgue Files, Meeman Papers.

73. Herbers, "Integration Gains in Memphis."

74. Ibid.

75. ABC News Broadcast, May 22, 1964.

76. Many blacks, "despite their leaders' warnings, were impressed by Ingram's record as a city judge." Herbers, "Integration Gains in Memphis."

77. The project was financed, Diggs later noted, "by the wives of the colored doctors in Memphis, the Bluff City Medical Society, who helped me with the assembling of this material," demonstrating yet again the civic support for (and the conciliating social symbolism of) Diggs's work. Lemuel Diggs, quoted in Thelma Tracy Mabry, *History of Medicine in Memphis: Interview with Dr. Lemuel Whitley Diggs* (Memphis: Oral History Research Office, Memphis State University, 1984), 9.

78. Other authors also pursued these themes. See, for example, Samuel Charache and Stuart Richardson, "Prolonged Survival of a Patient with Sickle Cell Anemia," *Archives of Internal Medicine* 113 (1964): 844–49.

79. Lemuel Diggs, "With the Editor: The St. Jude Hospital, Memphis, Tennessee," *Memphis and Mid-South Medical Journal* (June 1961): 237.

80. See, for example, among many articles, L. W. Diggs, "The Vascular Lesions in Sickle Cell Disease," *Proceedings of the Eighth International Congress of Hematology* (Tokyo) (1960): 910–15; L. W. Diggs, "The Pathology of Hemoglobin S," *Proceedings of the Sixth International Congress on Tropical Medicine and Malaria* (Lisbon) (1958): 5–13; L. W. Diggs, "Pulmonary Emboli vs. Pneumonia in Patients with Sickle Cell Anemia," *Memphis and Mid-South Medical Journal* (October 1967): 375.

81. From its beginning, the Sickle Cell Anemia clinic was conceived as a central clearinghouse and a work site for the various specialists where "patients with sickle cell anemia and related hereditary anomalies [could be] studied from as many angles as possible. These include study of bone changes, under the direction of Dr. David S. Carroll; Coagulation, Dr. Marion Dugdale; Hemodynamic Studies, Dr. George Copeland; Phonocardiographic Studies, Dr. Nathan Salky; Vascular Changes, Miss Dorothy Williams, student, and Retinal Studies by Ophthalmology. Principle attention is being given to the changes taking place at the time of sickle cell crises." "University of Tennessee News Notes," *Memphis and Mid-South Medical Journal* (October 1961): 411. For later studies based on patients in the clinic, see, for example, H. Lemmi and R. Ang, "Sickle Cell Crisis in Adults' Electroencephalographic Findings," *Memphis and Mid-South Medical Journal* (May 1966): 131–33. See also Editorial, "Sickle Cell Disease and the

Nervous System," *Memphis and Mid-South Medical Journal* (May 1966): 147, and L. W. Diggs and Luis Barreras, "Pulmonary Emboli vs. Pneumonia in Patients with Sickle Cell Anemia," *Memphis and Mid-South Medical Journal* (October 1967): 376–80.

82. Congressman George Grider, "Memo for Files — Subject: The Sicle Cell Anemia Problem of the Negro People," November 25, 1964, Box 17, Folder 13, George Grider Papers, Mississippi Valley Collection, McWherter Library, University of Memphis.

83. Ibid.

84. E. L. Mason to George Grider, May 5, 1966, Box 7, Folder 28: "Hospital Desegregation," Grider Papers.

85. "Grider Blasted by Kuykendall," *Memphis Press-Scimitar*, December 3, 1965; "Kuykendall Tells about Plans," *Memphis Press-Scimitar*, October 11, 1965; "Shift to GOP Is Claimed," *Memphis Commercial Appeal*, August 10, 1966, all in Box 24, Folder 29, Grider Papers.

86. Grider, "Memo for Files." On Medicare, see Robert Johnson, "Citizens Speak Out on Medicare," *Memphis Press-Scimitar*, June 1, 1962. On HEW and the Civil Rights Act, see Ida Clemens, "Storm of Hospitals Brings No Yielding," *Memphis Commercial Appeal*, April 15, 1966: "Representative George Grider yesterday charged that Federal officials were not being candid in demanding Memphis hospitals comply with the Civil Rights Act without telling them how to achieve compliance." See also "Intent in Rights Compliance Is Decisive, Grider Says," *Memphis Commercial Appeal*, April 17, 1966. All in Box 30, Folder 18: "Memphis Hospitals," Grider Papers.

87. One excellent analysis of the Watts riots is Gerald Horne, *The Fire This Time: The Watts Uprising and the 1960s* (Charlottesville: University Press of Virginia, 1995).

88. Larry Haygood to Edward Meeman, September 10, 1965, 3, Morgue Files, Meeman Papers.

89. Ibid.

90. "No one should ever think of participating in a street demonstration without being thoroughly trained in the techniques of civility, good manners, and nonviolence," Haygood declared. Ibid., 4–5.

91. "One mark of the sea-change in the movement after the mid-1960s was the decline of freedom-talk and the emergence of the rhetoric of power." Richard King, *Civil Rights and the Idea of Freedom* (Athens: University of Georgia Press, 1996), 15.

92. Alfred P. Kraus, "Sickle Cell Disease," in *Current Therapy*, ed. Howard Conn (Philadelphia: W. B. Saunders, 1966), 199. After his arrival in Memphis in 1950, Kraus had pursued studies in (and promoted a wider awareness of) the relatively new medical field of genetics. See Kraus, "Editorial: Genetics," 201. On the changing relationship of genetics to medicine in this era, see Kenneth Lud-

merer, *Learning to Heal: The Development of American Medical Education* (New York: Basic Books, 1985), and Daniel Kevles, *In the Name of Eugenics: Genetics and the Uses of Human Heredity* (New York: Knopf, 1985; Cambridge, Mass.: Harvard University Press, 1995). In the mid-1950s, Kraus became interested in the new field of hemoglobin variants, an area that was full of excitement after Linus Pauling's 1949 work on the role of hemoglobin molecules in sickle cell anemia. See, for example, K. Singer, A. P. Kraus, et al., "Studies of Abnormal Hemoglobins: X. A New Syndrome: Hemoglobin C–Thalassemia Disease," *Blood* 9 (1954): 1172, and L. M. Kraus, D. B. Morrison, and A. P. Kraus, "Abnormal Human Hemoglobins. I. Biosynthesis in Vitro of Fe-59 Labeled Hemoglobin A and Hemoglobin S," *Blood* 14 (1959): 1103. Kraus's intense interest in genetics is revealed by his attendance at a 1961 course at the Rockefeller Institute, sponsored by the American Eugenics Society and the Population Council, after which he offered his own course on medical genetics in Memphis in 1962–63. See Kraus's curriculum vitae (1975) in Morgue Files, Mississippi Valley Collection, McWherter Library, University of Memphis.

93. William H. Bullock, "Sickle Cell Disease," in Conn, *Current Therapy* (1965), 196.

94. For example, in 1966 Kraus wrote, "Sickle cell–hemoglobin C disease (hemoglobin C plus hemoglobin S) occurs once in every 100 sickle cell disease patients . . . [and] occasionally hemoglobin S is found together with one of the other abnormal hemoglobins (D, G, etc.)." A. P. Kraus, "Sickle Cell Disease," in Conn, *Current Therapy* (1966), 199.

95. In 1963 a University of Tennessee master's thesis chronicled the features of this new rare form of hemoglobin. See E. Yeaglin, "Characterization of Hemoglobin N Memphis" (master's thesis, University of Tennessee, 1963). On *Hemoglobin Memphis*, see also A. P. Kraus et al., "Hemoglobin Memphis/S: A New Variant of Sickle Cell Anemia," *Transactions of the Association of American Physicians* 80 (1967): 297–304. See also L. Kraus, T. Miyami, I. Iuchi, and A. P. Kraus, "Characterization of alpha 23 Glu NH2 in Hemoglobin Memphis Hemoglobin/S, a New Variant of the Molecular Disease," *Biochemistry* 5 (1966): 3701–8; A. P. Kraus and L. M. Kraus, "Biosynthesis in Vitro of Hemoglobin Labeled with Iron-59 in Sickle Cell-Hemoglobin C Disease," *Federal Proceedings* 19 (1960): 78; A. P. Kraus, B. Koch, and L. C. Burckett, "Two Families Showing Interaction of Hemoglobin C or Thalassaemia with High Fetal Hemoglobin in Adults," *British Medical Journal* 1 (1961): 1434; R. J. Hill and A. P. Kraus, "Studies on Amino Acid Sequence of Hemoglobin A2," *Federal Proceedings* 22 (1963): 597; and T. Imamura and A. Riggs, "Identification of H Oak Ridge with Hemo D. Punjab (Los Angeles)," *Biochemical Genetics* 7 (October 1963): 127–30. See also A. P. Kraus, "Editorial: Genetics," 201; A. P. Kraus et al., "A New Variety of Sickle Cell Anemia with Clinically Mild Symptoms Due to an Alpha Chain Variant of Hemoglobin a23gluNH2," Abstract, *Journal of Labora-*

tory and Clinical Medicine 66 (1965): 66; A. P. Kraus and L. M. Kraus, "Hemoglobin Defect Found in Sickle Cell Anemia," *Journal of the American Medical Association* 201 (September 18, 1967): 23; T. Wajima and A. P. Kraus, "Low Leukocyte Alkaline Phosphatase Activity in Sickle Cell Anemia," *Journal of Laboratory and Clinical Medicine* 72 (1968): 980; M. R. Cooper, A. P. Kraus, W. L. Ramseur, J. H. Felts, and C. L. Spurr, "Characterization of a New Hemoglobinopathy: Hemoglobin Memphis/Sickle Cell Disease," *Clinical Research* 17 (1969): 322; C. L. Neely, T. Wajima, A. P. Kraus, L. Diggs, and L. Barreras, "Lactic Acid Dehydrogenase Activity and Plasma Hemoglobin in Sickle Cell Disease," *American Journal of Clinical Pathology* 52 (1969): 167–69.

96. "The alleviation of the classical symptoms of sickle cell anemia and the behavior of cells and hemoglobin under low-oxygen tension indicate that [*Hemoglobin Memphis*] does not follow the same molecular behavior as [*Hemoglobin S*]." Kraus, Miyami, Iuchi, and Kraus, "Characterization of alpha 23 Glu NH2 in Hemoglobin Memphis," 3701.

97. Ibid., 3707.

98. Ibid., 3703.

99. A. P. Kraus and L. M. Kraus, "Hemoglobin Defect Found in Sickle Cell Anemia," 23.

100. As Alfred Kraus explained to the readers of the *Memphis and Mid-South Medical Journal* in late 1964, close scrutiny of the hemoglobin was also a valuable tool for doctors. In the case of a hypothetical patient, Mrs. Jones, he explained, a finding of abnormal hemoglobin could lead in many different therapeutic directions depending on the type of hemoglobin abnormality. "If her maiden name had been Vivaldi . . . the possibility of thalassemia minor would likely have been considered earlier. . . . Should she be Negro, hemoglobin C disease or one of its variants would have to be considered. . . . Having established the correct diagnosis, we are now in the position of handling Mrs. Jones's problem intelligently." Alfred P. Kraus, "Yes, It's Not Tired Blood," *Memphis and Mid-South Medical Journal* (November 1964): 418–19.

101. Commenting on the role of sympathy in the modern doctor-patient relationship, two astute British authors noted in 1966 that "two modern trends have both acted to reduce the traditional display of sympathy between doctor and patient. The first trend results from the growth of scientific medicine. The therapeutic revolution we have witnessed in the last thirty years makes it possible for so much to be done for the patient which was hitherto impossible that doctors are conditioned to think in terms of cure of symptoms by pharmacy and surgery. . . . The other trend is the growth of insurance schemes and in this country [the United Kingdom] the capitation system of payment. . . . In such a system . . . the less [the doctor] sees the patient for the same illness the easier he is earning his money, and sympathy, which may encourage a more intimate and perhaps a more dependent relationship between patient and doctor, becomes

rationed." Kevin Browne and Paul Freeling, "The Doctor-Patient Relationship III: The Role of Sympathy (Part I)," *Practitioner* 196 (March 1966): 454. See also Browne and Freeling, "The Doctor-Patient Relationship IV: The Role of Sympathy," *Practitioner* 196 (April 1966): 593–96. In the fields of clinical psychology and nursing, "empathy" emerged as a therapeutic factor in later years. See, for example, C. B. Traux, "Length of Therapist Response, Accurate Empathy and Patient Improvement," *Journal of Clinical Psychology* 26 (1970): 539–41, and L. Zderad, "Empathy—From Cliché to Construct (with Reflections on Synthesis)," *Nursing Theory Conferences* 3 (January 1970): 46–75. For assessments of new pain management techniques in sickle cell disease, see, for example, P. M. Barnes, R. Hendrickse, and E. J. Watson-Williams, "Low-Molecular Weight Dextran in Treatment of Bone Pain Crises in Sickle-Cell Disease," *Lancet* 2 (1965): 1271, and P. M. Barnes, "Treatment of Painful Sickle Cell Crises: Assessment of New Methods," *Clinical Pediatrics* 5 (November 1966): 650–51.

102. This warning appears in Paul Switzer, "Sickle Cell Anemia," in Conn, *Current Therapy* (1964), 191; Bullock, "Sickle Cell Disease," in Conn, *Current Therapy* (1965), 196; A. P. Kraus, "Sickle Cell Disease," in Conn, *Current Therapy* (1966), 200; and A. P. Kraus, "Sickle Cell Disease: Method of A. P. Kraus," in Conn, *Current Therapy* (1967), 210.

103. Lemuel Diggs, "Sickle Cell Diseases," in Conn, *Current Therapy* (1968), 224.

104. Howard Pearson, "Sickle Cell Anemia," in Conn, *Current Therapy* (1969), 240–42. "Therapy of painful crises is directed at correcting dehydration and acidosis, as well as symptomatically controlling pain . . . Propoxyphene (Darvon) (32 to 65 mg.) and if necessary small doses of codeine (30 to 60 mg.) are used for analgesia" (241).

105. "Sickle Cell Fight Encourages Unity," *Memphis Commercial Appeal*, September 4, 1967. See also "Worse Than Polio—Strange Sickle Cell Anemia Neglected," *Tri-State Defender*, March 26, 1968.

106. Dane Boggs Autobiographical Statement, November 17, 1982, Box 9, Folder: "Dane Boggs," Wintrobe Papers. See also D. R. Boggs, "The Frequency of Heterozygosity for Abnormal Hemoglobins in Western Pennsylvania," *Blood* 44 (1974): 699.

107. "Sickle Cell Fight Encourages Unity," *Memphis Commercial Appeal*, September 4, 1967.

108. Frankie Winchester, *Sickle Cell Anemia Research in Memphis: Interview with Alfred P. Kraus, M.D.* (Memphis: Oral History Research Office, Memphis State University, 1989), 8. See A. P. Kraus et al., "Hemoglobin Memphis/S."

109. Thus, while a 1965 USPHS public information pamphlet on sickle cell anemia spoke impersonally about the *disease* and "people with sickle cell anemia," the 1969 edition spoke directly to the *patient*, explaining "How It Makes You Sick" and "How You Get It." The 1965 pamphlet asked, "How is it recognized?" and

answered, "People with sickle cell anemia show the usual symptoms of severe anemia. They are often poorly developed, having a short trunk with long arms and legs." The 1969 booklet addressed specific concerns of patients, counseling them to "be careful about staying outside and getting wet in cold rainy and snowy weather. Do not go to visit friends who are sick with colds, measles, flu and other diseases that are catching." "Sickle Cell Anemia," Public Service Publication No. 1341, Health Information Series No. 119, U.S. Department of Health, Education, and Welfare, Public Health Service, FS2.50:119, November 23, 1965; "Sickle Cell Anemia," U.S. Department of Health, Education, and Welfare, Public Health Service, National Institutes of Health, FS2.22 An3-2, December 15, 1969.

110. Mitchell noted that Tennessee's implementation of Medicaid, the federal health insurance program for the poor, was just on the horizon: "In addition to the impact of Medicare and the regional medical program we shall experience in 1969 the implementation of Medicaid." Labor unrest in the now vast health care industry had also emerged, and Mitchell reported that Memphis "experienced in 1968 a heretofore unheard of strike of hospital employees at the City of Memphis Hospitals which has seriously curtailed the activities of that institution." B. G. Mitchell, "Mid-South Medicine — 1968," *Memphis and Mid-South Medical Journal* (December 1968): 98. These upheavals — health insurance for the poor and hospital workers striking for higher wages — were by-products of uneven economic growth in the 1960s. See Leon Fink and Brian Greenberg, *Upheaval in the Quiet Zone: A History of Hospital Workers' Union, Local 1199* (Urbana: University of Illinois, 1989).

111. J. Edwin Stanfield, *In Memphis: Mirror to America?* (Atlanta: Southern Regional Council, 1968), 28.

112. A useful collection elaborating on this theme of public pain and suffering is Arthur Kleinman, Veena Das, and Margaret Lock, *Social Suffering* (Berkeley: University of California Press, 1997). In the introduction the authors note, "From the perspective of theories of social suffering, such a preoccupation with individual certainty and doubt simply seems a less interesting, less important question to ask than that of how such suffering is produced in societies and how acknowledgment of pain, as a cultural process, is given or withheld" (xii).

113. Mabry, *Interview with Diggs*, 6–7.

114. David Vincent, "Research Revs Up Here on Disabling Sickle Cell Disease," *Memphis Commercial Appeal*, April 19, 1970. Ernestine Flowers, a retired teacher who worked with Lemuel Diggs, added, "We have been documenting the economic burden of the disease and its psychological effects. . . . Simply speaking, it causes poverty because it is so disabling." "Also," Flowers continued, "sickle cell children tend to achieve at lower levels educationally than their peers. It is not that they have lower intelligence but because they're so tired they can't listen and learn" (ibid.).

115. "University of Tennessee News Notes: New Procedure for Detection of Sickle Hemoglobin," *Memphis and Mid-South Medical Journal* (January 1969): 20; Lemuel Diggs, Lillian Barreras, and Ronald Joyner, "The Test Tube Turbidity Method as a Screening Procedure for the Detection of Sickle Cell Hemoglobin," *Memphis and Mid-South Medical Journal* (November 1969): 313–15; "Research and Writing Now for Our Dr. Diggs," *Memphis and Mid-South Medical Journal* (May 1969): 151.

CHAPTER 6

1. The Sidney Poitier movie was entitled *A Warm December*; the Bill Cosby movie was entitled *To All My Friends on Shore*.

2. Richard Nixon, "Health Message," February 18, 1971, *Congressional Quarterly Almanac* 27 (February 1971): 37A–38A.

3. See Stephen Skowronek, *The Politics Presidents Make: Leadership from John Adams to George Bush* (Cambridge, Mass.: Harvard University Press, 1993), and Leon Friedman and William F. Levantrosser, eds., *Richard M. Nixon: Politician, President, Administrator* (New York: Greenwood Press, 1991).

4. A. James Reichley, *Conservatives in a Age of Change: The Nixon and Ford Administrations* (Washington, D.C.: Brookings Institution, 1981). Another historian has noted that Nixon "pleaded for unity, but his appeals to the silent majority deepened cleavages between the races and generations." David Steigerwald, *The Sixties and the End of Modern America* (New York: St. Martin's Press, 1995). See also *Presidential Studies Quarterly* 26 (Winter 1996), an issue devoted to Nixon, especially H. D. Graham, "Richard Nixon and Civil Rights: Explaining an Enigma," 93–106; John Whitaker, "Nixon's Domestic Policy: Both Liberal and Bold in Retrospect," 131–53; and Dwight Ink, "Nixon's Version of Reinventing Government," 57–69.

5. For example, see "Concern with Urban Problems Spurs Interest in Sickle Cell Anemia," *New York Times*, July 25, 1971.

6. For a discussion of cardiology, cardiovascular disease, and the debate over political lobbying, see W. Bruce Fye, *American Cardiology: The History of a Specialty and Its College* (Baltimore: Johns Hopkins University Press, 1996).

7. Eugene Fowinkle, "The Health Industry," in *Memphis in the Seventies: Action Leaders Look at Urban Development*, ed. Bergen S. Merrill (Memphis: Memphis State University, 1970).

8. Felix I. D. Konotey-Ahulu, "Chwechweechwe: The African Rheumatic Syndrome That Came to Be Known as Sickle Cell Disease — A Personal Testimony," 5, Box 18, Folder: "Konotey-Ahulu," Maxwell Myer Wintrobe Papers, Marriott Library Special Collections, University of Utah, Salt Lake City. See also Stuart B. Edelstein, *The Sickled Cell: From Myths to Molecules* (Cambridge, Mass.: Harvard University Press, 1986).

9. Konotey-Ahulu, "Chwechweechwe," 5.

10. Ibid.

11. Ibid., 6.

12. Ibid., and see Chinua Achebe, *Things Fall Apart* (London: Heinemann, 1958), which has references throughout to childhood symptoms that echo those of sickle cell disease. See also Edelstein, *Sickle Cell Anemia*, and Paul Ramsey, *The Patient as Person: Explorations in Medical Ethics* (New Haven: Yale University Press, 1970).

13. Alfred Kraus, Oral History, Mississippi Valley Collection, McWherter Library, University of Memphis.

14. Lemuel Diggs and Alfred Kraus had received numerous federal grants in the early 1960s to run the University of Tennessee clinic and to pursue research.

15. "Health Industry Probably Largest in Memphis," *Memphis and Mid-South Medical Journal* (November 1969): 336.

16. Ibid.; Timothy Richard Campbell, "Agriculture's Second Great Depression of the Twentieth Century: Federal Policy and the Agricultural Economy of the 82-County Primary Memphis Trade Region (PMTR) between 1969 and 1987" (Ph.D. diss., University of Memphis, 1995).

17. Editorial, "Spotlight on a Killer," *Memphis Press-Scimitar*, March 4, 1971.

18. Jane S. Smith, *Patenting the Sun: Polio and the Salk Vaccine* (New York: W. Morrow, 1990), 73.

19. "Sickle Cell Anemia — Research and Treatment," broadcast on WRC-TV, Washington, D.C., August 1971, transcript in *Congressional Record*, October 8, 1971, S16089.

20. Ibid.

21. Other new organizations included the American Sickle Cell Anemia Association, Cleveland, Ohio (1972); the Sickle Cell Disease Association of America, California (1971); the National Association for Sickle Cell Disease; the Sickle Cell Research Foundation of Los Angeles; the National Sickle Cell Disease Foundation; and the National Sickle Cell Anemia Foundation, based in Memphis.

22. With the cost of medical care, Medicare, and Medicaid growing rapidly, politicians had drawn attention to a burgeoning health care crisis. One political response to the crisis, by Senator Edward Kennedy, called for a national health insurance plan, which would control costs more strictly than Medicare. Nixon had countered with his own proposal, an employer mandate for private insurance. At the same time, both Congress and Nixon embraced the Health Maintenance Organization Act of 1972 as a further step along the road to controlling costs. For a discussion of these and other trends, see Don Madison, "Paying for Health Care in America," in *The Social Medicine Reader*, ed. Gail Henderson et al. (Durham, N.C.: Duke University Press, 1997), 415–46.

23. Dr. Marvin Sipperstein, "Presidential Address," Southern Society of Clinical

Investigation, sent March 10, 1971, to D. Kuykendall via Vanderbilt University professor, in Folder HEW, Dan Kuykendall Papers, Mississippi Valley Collection, McWherter Library, University of Memphis.

24. For insight into this controversy, see "Problems Seen in Genetic Tests: Mass Screenings Are Called Psychological Danger," *New York Times*, May 25, 1972, 1; "Sickle Cell: Resentment Complicates the Case," *New York Times*, November 5, 1972; Tabitha Powledge, "The New Ghetto Hustle," *Saturday Review of the Sciences* 1 (February 1973): 38–40; and "The Row over Sickle-Cell," *Newsweek*, February 12, 1973, 63–65.

25. Kathleen Cleaver, "Position of the Black Panther Party on the 7th Congressional District Election in Alameda County," January 31, 1968, Social Protest Collection, Carton 18, Folder: "Black Panther Party," Bancroft Library, University of California at Berkeley.

26. See "The Ethnic Diseases: Going After Two Killers," *New York Post*, February 20, 1971.

27. See "House Steps Up Fight on Sickle Cell Anemia," *Memphis Press-Scimitar*, October 8, 1971.

28. Graham, "Richard Nixon and Civil Rights," 93.

29. Skowronek, *The Politics Presidents Make*.

30. Whitaker, "Nixon's Domestic Policy." One characteristic urban assault on Nixon was Joann Rogers, "Nixon Hit for Ghetto Health Failures," *San Francisco Sunday Examiner and Chronicle*, June 22, 1969, A21.

31. David Tucker, *Memphis since Crump*.

32. Other than this strong success in Tennessee, however, the Republicans enjoyed little success in the South. Dewey Grantham, *The South in Modern America: A Region at Odds* (New York: HarperCollins, 1994), 284.

33. Kuykendall was an organizer of Nixon's congressional team. See, for example, the memo from Clark MacGregor to the President, February 22, 1971, regarding "Meeting with 'Captains' of Congressional Teams." MacGregor writes, "At the request of Congressman Dan Kuykendall (R. Tennessee) a meeting has been arranged to discuss strategies which might be used to gather support for the 'Big Five' Legislative programs ... Revenue Sharing, Executive Reorganization, Welfare Reform, Environment, and Health." Box 19, Folder: "EX LE legislation," White House Central Files, Subject Files, Nixon Presidential Materials Project, National Archives and Records Administration, College Park, Maryland.

34. When Tennessee's Republican senators Brock and Baker ended their support of Nixon in 1974, Kuykendall publicly berated them for disloyalty. Only at the last minute did Kuykendall announce his withdrawal of support for Nixon. See David Flynn, "Kuykendall Hits GOP Disloyalty," *Memphis Press-Scimitar*, January 19, 1974; "Kuykendall Admits 'Closed Mind' on Question of Impeachment," *Memphis Press-Scimitar*, February 13, 1974; "Kuykendall in 'Toughest' Contest,"

Memphis Commercial Appeal, May 1, 1974; "8th District Repub. Poll: Kuykendall Finds Change in Opinions on Nixon," *Memphis Press-Scimitar*, August 8, 1974; "Nixon Quizzes Kuykendall: Do They Want to Pick Carcass?" *Memphis Press-Scimitar*, August 27, 1974.

35. *Congressional Record*, October 8, 1971, S16080.

36. Ibid., S16082.

37. Included in the *Congressional Record*, October 8, 1971, were Robert Scott, "Health Care Priorities and Sickle Cell Anemia," *Journal of the American Medical Association* 214 (October 26, 1970): 731–34; "Sickle Cell Cure — The Promise, the Peril: Urea Combats Crisis of Disease but Can Cause Dehydration," *Medical World News*, January 8, 1971; "Sickle Cell Disease — Progress Amidst Chaos," *Medical World News*, May 28, 1971; "Detecting an Old Killer," *Time*, October 4, 1971, 57; and "Sickle Cell Anemia — Research and Treatment," WRC-TV transcript, August 1971. See also Richard Goldsby, *Race and Races* (New York: Macmillan, 1971), which calls for premarital screening for sickle cell anemia.

38. *Congressional Record*, October 8, 1971, S16080, Tunney quoting Scott, "Health Care Priorities and Sickle Cell Anemia."

39. See Peter Kihss, " 'Benign Neglect' on Race Is Proposed by Moynihan," *New York Times*, March 1, 1970, 1; "Text of the Moynihan Memorandum on the Status of Negroes," *New York Times*, March 1, 1970, 69; and Max Frankel, "Is 'Benign Neglect' the Real Nixon Approach?" *New York Times*, March 8, 1970, sec. 4, p. 1.

40. It was in 1964, only seven years earlier, that Democratic congressman George Grider, upon learning of the existence of research on sickle cell anemia, had commented, "This seems like a very attractive and necessary activity and one that we ought to keep in our minds." See Chapter 5.

41. Harry Bloomfield to Dan Kuykendall, April 24, 1969, Series 3, Box 51, Folder 24, Henry Loeb III Papers, Cossitt Branch Library, Memphis.

42. "Gardner Makes It Clear Funds Will Be Halted," *Memphis Commercial Appeal*, April 15, 1966, and "Eight Hospitals Accused in Racial Complaints," *Memphis Press-Scimitar*, April 29, 1965, in Box 7, Folder 28, George Grider Papers, Mississippi Valley Collection, McWherter Library, University of Memphis. The caption of a photo with four men arguing read, "THE ARGUMENT over whether Memphis hospitals are complying with the Civil Rights Act spilled over into the corridors as Dr. Charles L. Dinkins, president of Owen College, tried to make a point with William Page, regional director of the Department of Health, Education, and Welfare. Representative George Grider got in some words of his own with Dr. Leo Gehrig of the United States Surgeon General's Office" (*Memphis Press-Scimitar*, April 29, 1965).

43. "How to Hew to HEW Line Is Our Hospitals' Dilemma," *Memphis Press-Scimitar*, April 15, 1966, in Box 7, Folder 28, Grider Papers. The Department of

Health, Education, and Welfare needed to see a rise in white patients at the E. H. Crump Hospital, which had been created as a black hospital in the 1950s, and a rise in black patients at Baptist Memorial Hospital, Methodist Hospital, and St. Joseph Hospital. Oscar Marvin, Administrator, Memphis City Hospitals, to Robert Nash, Chief of the HEW Office of Equal Health Opportunity, May 20, 1966, ibid.

44. Writing to a supporter, Grider noted, "I did feel . . . that the folks from Atlanta and Washington were unrealistic. They gave me the impression that they intended to withhold approval until goals which can't possibly be reached for many years have been attained. I can assure you that I have already begun efforts up here to cause a reappraisal in this position. . . . At the same time, there are some things in Memphis that need correcting. I gather that steps are being taken now by the hospitals, by the city of Memphis hospital group, and by the private practicing physicians to move in good faith toward desegregation." George Grider to A. Roy Tyrer, April 20, 1966, ibid.

45. On the black vote, Kuykendall stated, "We have recognized that Negroes are voting in a bloc [for the Democrats]," but he predicted that "[as blacks] become better informed, better educated, and the emotion of the moment dies, the Negro will rejoin the Republican Party." "Gore Ignores People, Kuykendall Says," *Knoxville News Sentinel*, August 13, 1964. See also Dale Enoch, "Kuykendall Launches Drive, Says Gore 'Deserted' State," *Memphis Commercial Appeal*, September 1, 1964; "GOP Candidates Criss-Cross City—Kuykendall, Baker Hammer at 'Galloping Federalism,' Lawlessness on Streets," *Memphis Commercial Appeal*, September 8, 1964, in Box 24, Folder 29, Grider Papers.

46. "Beaming GOP Finds Power in Redrawn Ninth District," *Memphis Commercial Appeal*, August 10, 1966. "A check of how precincts in the new Ninth District voted in the 1964 November election bears out the GOP contentions that the new district is more favorable." See also Null Adams, "Kuykendall To Seek Grider's Seat," *Memphis Press-Scimitar*, May 25, 1966, and Jack Martin, "Confident Kuykendall Says, 'This Is Republican Year,'" *Memphis Commercial Appeal*, June 29, 1966, in Box 24, Folder 29, Grider Papers.

47. Transcript of WHBQ Press Conference with Dan Kuykendall, April 3, 1966, p. 6, Box 24, Folder 29, Grider Papers.

48. *Memphis Commercial Appeal*, March 23, 1969.

49. "Loeb Threat on Hospitals Renewed," *Memphis Press-Scimitar*, January 30, 1969.

50. "Hospital Fund Moves Closer," *Memphis Commercial Appeal*, May 29, 1969. It was clear, however, that some citizens in Mississippi had little sympathy for Memphis. One radio station editorialized that Memphis was always complaining, but that "for too many years, over a hundred, in fact, Mississippi dollars have helped build large metropolitan centers . . . just beyond our state boundaries." WKOR Editorial, August 15, 1969, Box 42, Folder 4, Loeb Papers.

51. From Norman Casey, Mid-South Medical Center Council, February 13, 1970,

after conversation with Alton Cobb, M.D., Administrator of Mississippi Medicaid Program, Box 43, Folder 4, Loeb Papers.

52. Lee Stillwell, "Kuykendall, Quillen Feud about New Medical School," *Memphis Press-Scimitar*, September 29, 1971.

53. In early 1972 one Memphian noted that "sickle cell disease, largely ignored as 'just a Negro blood disorder in the South,' [had] gained a national place among diseases to be destroyed." Charles Thornton, "Science Unlocking Sickle Cell," *Memphis Press-Scimitar*, January 11, 1972. In his testimony before Congress, Kuykendall "told a Senate subcommittee that progress is being made in Memphis in research on sickle cell anemia." "Sickle Cell Progress Reported," *Memphis Press-Scimitar*, November 9, 1971.

54. See Leon Panetta, *Bringing Us Together: The Nixon Team and the Civil Rights Retreat* (Philadelphia: Lippincott, 1971). See also the essays on Nixon in *Presidential Studies Quarterly* 26 (Winter 1996).

55. "New Crisis Plagues St. Jude," *Memphis Press-Scimitar*, February 11, 1971; Editorial, "St. Jude in Need," *Memphis Commercial Appeal*, February 12, 1971; Lee Stillwell, "HEW Gives Aid Pledge to St. Jude," *Memphis Press-Scimitar*, February 20, 1971; Lee Stillwell, "Leukemia Patients, Parents Say 'Thank You' to 3 Legislators," *Memphis Press-Scimitar*, April 7, 1971, 1. For the statement on St. Jude's dependence on federal funds, see letter to Elliot Richardson from Dan Kuykendall and Senators Baker and Brock, February 19, 1971, Box 41, Folder: "St. Jude Hospital," Kuykendall Papers.

56. "Backdrop — Pennies from Heaven," *Memphis Commercial Appeal*, May 21, 1972; see also "St. Jude Hospital to Receive 5 Million Dollar Federal Grant," *Memphis Commercial Appeal*, May 18, 1972; Brown Alan Flynn, "St. Jude Supporters Jubilant Over $5 Million U.S. Grant," *Memphis Press-Scimitar*, May 18, 1972.

57. Morris Cunningham, "Administration's Racial Policy Changes Often," *Memphis Commercial Appeal*, July 11, 1971.

58. As early as May 1971, Kuykendall saw that his district would change, contending "that the population makeup of the proposed [new] district makes it virtually certain that a black candidate would win the Democratic nomination and that this would polarize the situation even further." See William Street, "Some Aspects on Remap Plan Seem at Variance with Facts," *Memphis Press-Scimitar*, May 7, 1971.

59. "Politics This Morning — GOP-Negro Democrat Negotiations Set Political Ripples to Swirling," *Memphis Commercial Appeal*, January 15, 1971; see also Null Adams, "Democrats Warned by Rep. Kuykendall," *Memphis Press-Scimitar*, February 9, 1972, and Johnnie Vaughn, "Kuykendall in Squeeze," *Memphis Press-Scimitar*, April 13, 1972.

60. Dan Kuykendall to A. M. Scruggs, July 20, 1971, Box 54, Folder: "Dan Kuykendall Office," Kuykendall Papers. Scruggs had criticized Kuykendall for engaging in "an out and out case of . . . trying to buy black votes." As Kuykendall later

noted in the newspapers, "I failed to get black votes last time but I intend to get black votes this time." "Kuykendall Drops Redistricting Lawsuit," *Memphis Press-Scimitar*, April 18, 1972.

61. Dan Kuykendall to James Culbertson, Program Coordinator and Director of Memphis Regional Medical Program for Heart Disease, Cancer, Stroke, and Kidney Disease, [ca. August 10, 1971], Box 54, Folder: "Dan Kuykendall Office," Kuykendall Papers; "Redditt to Return to Former Beat as Liaison for GOP Lawmakers," *Memphis Commercial Appeal*, July 7, 1971. See also Frankie Winchester, *Sickle Cell Anemia Research in Memphis: Interview with Alfred P. Kraus, M.D.* (Memphis: Oral History Research Office, Memphis State University, 1989), 29. For Redditt's defense of Nixon, see "Black GOPs Not Together," *Tri-State Defender*, May 20, 1972, 1.

62. This group could claim Robert Church as their early-twentieth-century predecessor in the Republican Party, the party of Lincoln and emancipation. The majority of African Americans had, of course, long supported the Republican Party, but the FDR era had seen a sea change in African American affiliation. The *Memphis World*, a significant newspaper in the 1930s and 1940s, represented a holdover from these earlier days. For more on African American political affiliation, see Nancy J. Weiss, *Farewell to the Party of Lincoln: Black Politics in the Age of FDR* (Princeton: Princeton University Press, 1983).

63. An interesting analysis of these two papers is found in Hugh Davis Graham, *Crisis in Print: Desegregation and the Press in Tennessee* (Nashville: Vanderbilt University Press, 1967). On the newspapers and print media of Memphis, see also Thomas Harrison Baker, *The Memphis Commercial Appeal: The History of a Southern Newspaper* (Baton Rouge: Louisiana State University Press, 1971).

64. For coverage on Nixon, see Editorial, "President Nixon Replies," *Memphis World*, June 19, 1971, and Editorial, "The Doctors Agree," *Memphis World*, June 19, 1971 (this article supports Nixon's drug abuse policy); see also "The Black Nixon and Community," *Memphis World*, October 30 1971, 2. The two sickle cell articles are "Sickle Cell Gets Boost," *Memphis World*, July 5, 1971, and "VA Joins Sickle Cell Fight," *Memphis World*, March 25, 1972, 2.

65. "Black Officials Battle for Sickle Cell Funding," *Tri-State Defender*, December 18, 1971.

66. "Factors in Heart Disease," *Memphis World*, February 19, 1972, 4; "Sickle Cell Benefit," *Tri-State Defender*, February 19, 1972, 10. See also a similar parallel in "Dr. Jackson to Head MD Sickle Cell Team," *Tri-State Defender*, April 1, 1972, 1, and "Heart Disease and Cancer Leading Causes of Death," *Memphis World*, April 1, 1972, 5.

67. "Tri-State's Endorsements. . . . It's Patterson, Anderson," *Tri-State Defender*, October 28, 1972, 1. These sentiments are also echoed in Powledge, "The New Ghetto Hustle."

68. "Sickle Cell Cure," *Medical World News*, January 8, 1971.

69. Ibid.

70. "Black Perspective Aires Sickle Cell Anemia," *Tri-State Defender*, July 31, 1971, 2.

71. Winchester, *Interview with Kraus*, 14.

72. Ibid., 17.

73. See Kuykendall testimony in Senate Committee on Labor and Public Welfare, Subcommittee on Health, *National Sickle Cell Anemia Prevention Act: Hearings before the Subcommittee on Health of the Committee on Labor and Public Welfare, U.S. Senate*, 92d Cong., 1st sess., November 11–12, 1971 (Washington, D.C.: U.S. Government Printing Office, 1972). See also "Kuykendall Urges Sickle Cell Funds," *Memphis Commercial Appeal*, November 12, 1971, and House Committee on Interstate and Foreign Commerce, Subcommittee on Public Health and Environment, *Hearings on Research, Treatment, and Prevention of Sickle Cell Anemia*, 92d Cong., 1st sess., November 12, 1971 (Washington, D.C.: U.S. Government Printing Office, 1972).

74. "HEW Sees: Drug Abuse Challenge of Nation," *Memphis World*, January 22, 1972, 5; Norman Kempster, "Nixon Vows No Sympathy for Drug Pushers Now," *Memphis World*, March 25, 1972, 2.

75. "Saving Addicts on Channel 10," *Tri-State Defender*, December 25, 1971, 15.

76. Kraus, Oral History.

77. Editorial, "Spotlight on a Killer," *Memphis Press-Scimitar*, March 4, 1972.

78. "Sickle Shows Draw Protest," *Tri-State Defender*, May 20, 1972.

79. "Black Med Students Give Sickle Cell Tests," *Tri-State Defender*, February 5, 1972, 4; "G.G.'s Eye Sickle Cell Benefit," *Tri-State Defender*, February 15, 1972; "Sickle Cell Benefit Set," *Tri-State Defender*, February 19, 1972, 10; "Black Stars Join in Sickle Cell Fight," *Tri-State Defender*, April 22, 1972, 14; "Sickle Cell Benefit May 20," *Tri-State Defender*, May 20, 1972, 1; "Stars Help Raise Nearly $800,000 on Telethon," *Tri-State Defender*, December 30, 1972, 11.

80. Earl Caldwell, "The Panthers: Dead or Regrouping?," *New York Times*, March 1, 1971, 1; Earl Caldwell, "Panthers Must Merge with the People," *Los Angeles Free Press*, September 13, 1968; David Anderson, "Panthers: More Symbol Than Substance," *Wall Street Journal*, June 7, 1971, 12. See also Alan Althshuler, *Community Control: The Black Demand for Participation in Large Cities* (New York: Pegasus, 1970), and Black Panther Party, *All Power to the People* (Oakland, Calif.: People's Press, 1970). For a discussion of health initiatives by the Black Panthers, see G. Louis Heath, ed., *Off the Pigs! The History and Literature of the Black Panther Party* (Metuchen, N.J.: Scarecrow Press, 1976). Heath notes that "although no appointment was ever announced to a national 'Ministry of Health,' a number of chapters announced in the party's newspaper the opening or imminent opening of free medical clinics. . . . HCIS witnesses testified that clinics were actually operative in Seattle and Philadelphia. . . . A 'People's Free Health Clinic' was serving citizens in Brooklyn, New York, in November 1969 under the auspices of the local Panther Party branch" (98–99).

81. "Black Panther Survival Conference Successful," *Tri-State Defender*, June 22, 1972, 3. See also Dick Hallgren, "Black Panthers Draw Big Crowd: 'Survival' Rally," *San Francisco Chronicle*, March 30, 1972, 4.

82. "Black Panther Survival Conference Successful," *Tri-State Defender*, June 22, 1972.

83. "Dr. Jackson's War on the Sickle Cell," *Smithsonian*, June 1972, 70.

84. "Busing Creates Sickle Cell Problem," *Memphis Press-Scimitar*, February 1, 1973.

85. "500 at Ossining Prison Tested for SCA: All but 10 Are Cleared," *New York Times*, August 30, 1972 (the story implies wrongdoing on the part of those not cleared); Rita Delfiner, "Close Up: Fighting Disease and Stigma," *New York Post*, September 1972; Wendell Rose, Chief, Immunology-Hematology Section, Duke Medical Center, "Sickle Cell Anemia . . . Curse of the Black Man," *The Health Bulletin* (Duke Medical Center) (1972).

86. Robert Wilson, "Medical Units Get Sickle Cell Grant," *Memphis Press-Scimitar*, June 30, 1972. Washington, D.C., was also a research center. In the North, Boston, New York, and Philadelphia received funding, and in the Midwest, Cincinnati, Chicago, and Indianapolis received grants. Los Angeles was the only western state receiving funds.

87. Charles Thornton, "$3 Million Allotted for Sickle Cell Fight," *Memphis Press-Scimitar*, May 31, 1972.

88. "Sickle Cell Center Gets $457,000," *Tri-State Defender*, June 10, 1972, 1.

89. "Dr. Jackson to Head MD Sickle Cell Team," *Tri-State Defender*, April 1, 1972, 1.

90. See, for example, Goldsby, *Race and Races*. Goldsby argued for mandatory screening for sickle cell trait on marriage licenses.

91. Numerous experts stepped into the debate, noting that the price of stigma was high and that screening children who were not old enough to be making reproductive decisions or to make use of the information served no obvious function. See, for example, Doris Wilkinson, "Politics and Sickle Cell Anemia," *Black Scholar* 5 (May 1974): 26; Helen Ranney et al., "Why Do Sickle Screening in Children? The Trait Is the Issue," *Pediatrics* 51 (April 1973): 742–45; J. Bowman, "Ethical, Legal, and Humanistic Implications of Sickle Cell Programs," *INSERM* 44 (1975): 353–78; and Philip Reilly, "State Supported Mass Genetic Screening Programs," in *Genetics and the Law*, ed. Aubrey Milunsky and George Annas (New York: Plenum, 1976), 159–94.

92. "Sickle Cell Law Attacked," *Memphis Press-Scimitar*, June 29, 1972.

93. For a discussion of these debates in the early 1970s, see Daniel Kevles, "Varieties of Presumptuousness," in *In the Name of Eugenics: Genetics and the Uses of Heredity* (New York: Knopf, 1985; Cambridge, Mass.: Harvard University Press, 1995), 269–90. The debate began in 1969 but continued through 1972 and 1973. See, for example, Duston Harvey, "Controversy over White Black Intelligence Rages," *Pittsburgh Courier*, June 24, 1972, 16.

94. "Spotlight on a Killer," *Memphis Commercial Appeal*, March 4, 1972.

95. Statement by Dan Kuykendall in House Committee, *Hearings*, 45.

96. Linus Pauling, "Reflections on a New Biology: Foreword," *UCLA Law Review* 15 (1968): 269.

97. Ibid.

98. Lemuel Diggs, "Genetic Counseling for Sickle Cell Disease Carriers," *New England Journal of Medicine* 285 (November 25, 1971): 1266.

99. "Science Unlocking Sickle Cell," *Memphis Press-Scimitar*, January 11, 1972.

100. David Vincent, "Research Revs Up Here on Disabling Sickle Cell Disease," *Memphis Commercial Appeal*, April 19, 1970. See also Lois Gilbert, "Intelligence Impairment in Children with Sickle Cell Disease" (Ph.D. diss., Memphis State University, 1970).

101. See, for example, Lois Gilbert and A. P. Kraus, "Intelligence and Mental Capacity of Patients with Sickle Cell Disease," *Proceedings of the Thirteenth International Congress of Hematology* (Munich) (August 1970), and Gilbert, "Intelligence Impairment in Children."

102. See "Sickle Cell Study Disputes Defects," *Memphis Press-Scimitar*, September 29, 1973. The story discusses an article in the September 29, 1973, issue of the *New England Journal of Medicine* and the last four years of controversy over the mental status of people with sickle cell trait.

103. Kuykendall testimony in House Committee, *Hearings*, 45.

104. Kuykendall testimony in Senate Committee, *Hearings*.

105. Barbara Culliton, "Sickle Cell Anemia: National Program Raises Problems as Well as Hopes," *Science* 177 (October 20, 1972): 284.

106. Ibid.

107. "Banquet to Honor Dr. L. W. Diggs," *Tri-State Defender*, April 22, 1972. Diggs was among twenty-eight honorees presented for special distinction.

108. "Whites Have Sickle Cell," *Tri-State Defender*, May 20, 1972, 15; Robert Wilson, "Expert Explains Blood Disease," *Memphis Press-Scimitar*, May 11, 1972.

109. Wilson, "Expert Explains Blood Disease."

110. Frank Gardner, quoted in "Sickle Cell Cure—The Promise, the Peril," *Medical World News*, January 8, 1971, reprinted in *Congressional Record*, October 8, 1971, S16086.

111. Walter Seegers, quoted in "Sickle Cell Cure—The Promise, the Peril," reprinted in ibid., S16093.

112. Public following of the urea story was intense. See, for example, R. M. Nalbandian et al., "Sickle Cell Crises Terminated by Intravenous Urea in Sugar Solutions—A Preliminary Report," *American Journal of Medical Science* 261 (1971): 309–24, and "Sickle Cell Cure Found?," *Pittsburgh Courier*, May 6, 1972, 2. By October 1971, *Time* magazine reported that "Nalbandian's treatment, tested on 25 patients at 4 hospitals, has thus far proved safe and effective." "Detecting an Old Killer," *Time*, October 4, 1971, 57, reprinted in *Congressional Record*, October 8, 1971, S16094. By December 1972, the *Mem-*

phis Press-Scimitar reported, "Although the treatment is not a cure, its developers deserve praise and gratitude for providing a method of control and relief from pain." "Sickle Cell Control," *Memphis Press-Scimitar*, December 30, 1971.

113. Charles Thornton, "Science Unlocking Sickle Cell," *Memphis Press-Scimitar*, January 11, 1972.

114. Paul McCurdy, letter, "Sickle Cell Crisis and Urea," *Journal of the American Medical Association* 230 (December 9, 1974): 1386.

115. Kraus's writings in the 1970s (many written with Lorraine Kraus) included A. P. Kraus and L. Kraus, "Carbamyl Phosphate Mediated Inhibition of the Sickling of Erythrocytes from Sickle Cell Anemia Patients in Whole Blood *In Vitro*," *Biochemical and Biophysical Research Communications* 44 (1971): 1381–87; A. P. Kraus, "Observations on an Automated Solubility Test for the Identification of Sickle Cell Disease," Abstract, *Technicon International Congress Symposium* (1972); A. P. Kraus and L. Kraus, "Alteration of Structure of the Sickling Phenomenon Resulting from Carbamyl Phosphates Modification of Hemoglobins," Abstract, *Federal Proceedings* 31 (1972): 484 (#1523); A. P. Kraus (3rd author), "Carbamyl Phosphate Modification of Hb S Structure Resulting in Altered Sickling," in *Proceedings of the Second International Conference on Red Blood Cell Metabolism and Function*, ed. George Brewer (New York: Plenum Publishing, 1972); A. P. Kraus and L. Kraus, "Sickle Cell Anemia — Prolonged Red Cell Survival and Altered Sickling Mediated by Carbamyl Phosphate," presented at meetings of Central Society for Clinical Research, Chicago, November 1972, Abstract in *Clinical Research* 20 (1972): 788; A. P. Kraus (6th author), "Sickle Cell Anemia: Carbamyl Phosphate and Affinity Labeling Agent Prolongs Red Cell Survival," presented at Fifteenth Annual Meeting of American Society of Hematology, Hollywood, Florida, December 1972, Abstract in *Blood* 40 (1972): 928; A. P. Kraus (5th author), "Mechanism of Action of Carbamyl Phosphate Modification of the Sickling Phenomenon," presented at annual meeting of the Federation of the American Society for Experimental Biology and Medicine, Atlantic City, New Jersey, April 1972; A. P. Kraus (2nd author), "A Third Case of Hemoglobin Memphis/Sickle Cell Disease: Whole Blood Viscosity Used as a Screening Test," *American Journal of Medicine* 55 (1973): 535–41; A. P. Kraus (6th author), "Prolongation of *In Vivo* Survival of Sickle Cell Erythrocytes by Carbamyl Phosphate (CP)," submitted to annual meeting of Association of American Physicians, Atlantic City, New Jersey, May 1973; A. P. Kraus, "Hemoglobinopathies That Interact with Hb-S," and "Other Therapeutic Approaches in Sickle Cell Anemia," both presented at "Recent Advances in Sickle Cell Anemia" conference, Medical College of Georgia, Augusta, April 1973; A. P. Kraus, review of M. Murayama and R. Nalbandian, *Sickle Cell Hemoglobin: Molecule to Man*, in *Journal of the American Medical Association* 227 (February 18, 1974): 805–6; "Clinical Trials of Therapy

for Sickle Cell Vaso-Occlusive Crisis: A Cooperative Study," *Journal of the American Medical Association* 228 (May 27, 1974): 1120–24; A. P. Kraus (5th author), "Carbamyl Phosphate Effects on Human and Dog Hemoglobin Structure-Function Relationships," presented at meeting of International Society of Hematology, Israel, September 1974; A. P. Kraus (2nd author), "Leukocyte Alkaline Phosphatase Scores in Sickle Cell Anemia," submitted to Central Society for Clinical Research for presentation in Chicago, October 1974; A. P. Kraus, "Nomenclature of Abnormal Human Hemoglobins," in *The Detection of Hemoglobinopathies*, ed. R. M. Schmidt, T. H. J. Huisman, and H. Lehmann (Cleveland: CRC Press, 1974); A. P. Kraus and T. Wajima, "Leukocyte Alkaline Phosphatase Scores in Sickle Cell Anemia," *New England Journal of Medicine* 293 (October 30, 1974): 918–19; A. P. Kraus (4th author), "*In Vivo* Effects of Carbamyl Phosphate in Dogs," in *International Conference on Red Cell Metabolism*, ed. G. F. Brewer and Alan Liss (Ann Arbor, Mich.: University of Michigan, 1974); A. P. Kraus (3rd author), "Carbamyl Phosphate, an Antisickling Agent, Mechanism of Action *In Vitro* and *In Vivo*," in *Sixteenth International Congress of Hematology* (Kyoto) (September 1976); J. C. Morrison, A. P. Kraus, W. D. Whybrew, E. T. Bucovaz, and W. L. Wiser, "Fluctuation of Fetal Hemoglobin in Sickle Cell Anemia," *American Journal of Obstetrics and Gynecology* 125 (1976): 1945–48; A. P. Kraus (4th author), "Anion and Cation Effects of the Anti-Sickling Agents Disodium Carbamyl Phosphate (NaCP), Sodium Cyanate (NaNCO), or Dilithium Carbamyl Phosphate (LiCP)," *Clinical Research* 25, no. 4 (October 1977): 612; A. P. Kraus (4th author), "Antisickling Agents: *In Vivo* Differences Due to the Anions Carbamyl Phosphate (CP) or Cyanate (NCO) and the Cations Sodium or Lithium," *Blood* 50, suppl. 1 (1977): 110; A. P. Kraus (4th author), "Disodium Carbamyl Phosphate and Sodium Cyanate: Comparative Toxicity and Detoxification in Mice," submitted to *Toxicology and Applied Pharmacology* (March 1978); A. P. Kraus, "Sickle Cell Anemia," presented at Max Planck Institute, Munich, August 1978; A. P. Kraus (3rd author), "Zinc Metabolism in Sickle Cell Anemia," *Journal of the American Medical Association* 242 (December 14, 1979): 2686; A. P. Kraus (4th author), "Antisickling Effects of Carbamyl Phosphate or Cyanate on Survival, Erythrocytes, and Leukocytes in the Mouse," *American Journal of Hematology* 6 (1979): 343–51; A. P. Kraus (3rd author), "The Prevalence of Diabetes Mellitus among Pregnant Patients with Sickle Cell Hemoglobinopathies," *Journal of Clinical Endocrinology and Metabolism* 48 (1979): 192–95; A. P. Kraus (4th author), "Carbamyl Phosphate, an Antisickling Agent," in *Meeting on the Development and Therapeutic Agents for Sickle Cell Disease*, ed. J. Rosa, Y. Beuzard, and J. Hercules (Paris: INSERM, 1978), 205–16.

116. "Insurance Denials to Blacks Topic of Probe," *Memphis Press-Scimitar*, November 13, 1972.

117. Winchester, *Interview with Kraus*, 28.

118. See "Accomplishments of Congressman Dan Kuykendall of Particular Interest to the Black Community," Box 1, Folder: "Kuykendall Office, Baker, Brock, Kuykendall Community Service," Kuykendall Papers. The statement noted, "As a member of the powerful House Commerce Committee which writes health legislation Congressman Kuykendall was very influential in seeing enactment of legislation which will provide over $100 million during the next 3 years for various sickle cell programs. . . . A considerable portion of this money will be coming back to us in Memphis to fund the Sickle Cell program at the University of Tennessee."

119. Annual Report, St. Jude 1971, Box 41, Folder: "General, St. Jude Hospital," Kuykendall Papers.

120. "Sickle Cell Anemia will be an exclusive disease for the Black child and his brothers and sisters," the caucus wrote. "Whether or not he has it or its trait will depend upon chance. And chance will also determine whether or not he dies from it, because not enough is known about Sickle Cell Anemia to offer him a cure." Congressional Black Caucus, U.S. House of Representatives, *A Position on Health in the Black Community* (Washington, D.C.: Congressional Black Caucus, April 1972), 1–2, 8.

121. Ibid., 15. Meharry Medical College did receive funding to organize a conference on this theme in June 1972, and a Sickle Cell Center was created there the same year.

122. Winchester, *Interview with Kraus*, 27.

123. Ibid.

124. William Hines, "Sickle Cell Anemia: A Stylish Disease," *Memphis Commercial Appeal*, November 11, 1971.

125. Ibid.

126. Letter in *Memphis Commercial Appeal*, December 22, 1971.

127. Barbara Culliton, "Cooley's Anemia: Special Treatment for Another Ethnic Disease," *Science* 178 (November 10, 1972): 590–93.

128. Ibid. Congressman Giaimo drew a contrast between the expansion of sickle cell anemia research funding and the nonexistent funding for Cooley's anemia. The issue had obvious political resonance in local New Haven politics.

129. The formation of a Cooley's support group in Memphis in August 1971 attracted local press attention. See "Chapter Sets Up to Help Victims of Fatal Anemia," *Memphis Press-Scimitar*, August 16, 1971, Morgue Files, Folder 9981: "Blood Banks," Mississippi Valley Collection, McWherter Library, University of Memphis.

130. Culliton, "Cooley's Anemia," 592.

131. Richard Rettig, "Origins of the Medicare Kidney Disease Entitlement: The Social Security Amendments of 1972," in *Biomedical Politics*, ed. Kathi Hanna (Washington, D.C.: National Academy Press, 1991), 187–89.

132. For more discussion of the social, political, intellectual, and economic context

of kidney dialysis, see Alonzo Plough, *Borrowed Time: Artificial Organs and the Politics of Extending Lives* (Philadelphia: Temple University Press, 1986); see also Stephen Peitzman, "From Bright's Disease to ESRD," in *Framing Disease: Studies in Cultural History*, ed. Charles Rosenberg and Janet Golden (New Brunswick: Rutgers University Press, 1992).

133. On May 18, 1972, sickle cell legislation became law. P.L. 92-294, 92d Cong., 1st sess., *An Act to Amend the Public Health Service Act to Provide for the Control of Sickle Cell Anemia.* The law set aside $115 million for three years of funding for sickle cell disease. On August 29, 1972, the Cooley's anemia act was passed. P.L. 92-414, 92d Cong., 1st sess., *National Cooley's Anemia Control Act.*

134. "Sickle Cell Myths," *Tri-State Defender*, October 21, 1972, 6.

135. Ibid.

136. Editorial, "Planned Neglect Caused VD Deaths," *Tri-State Defender*, August 19, 1972, 6. A full history of the experiment appears in James Jones, *Bad Blood: The Tuskegee Syphilis Experiment* (New York: Free Press, 1984). As U.S. Representative Ralph Metcalfe noted on the floor of Congress, it was shocking that "a group of syphilitic victims were denied proper treatment for the disease in order that autopsies could be performed . . . to determine what effect the disease had on the human body if left untreated. . . . My question now is 'How many more of these human sacrifices are being made elsewhere in the country?'" "Text of Metcalfe Speech," *Pittsburgh Courier*, August 5, 1972, 1.

CHAPTER 7

1. Francis Davis, *The History of the Blues: The Roots, the Music, the People from Charley Patton to Robert Cray* (New York: Hyperion, 1995), 130.

2. See, for example, Michael Honey, *Southern Labor and Black Civil Rights: Organizing Memphis Workers* (Urbana: University of Illinois Press, 1993); Davis, *History of the Blues*, 129.

3. Pete Daniel, *Standing at the Crossroads: Southern Life in the Twentieth Century* (New York: Hill and Wang, 1986); Marcus Pohlman and Michael Kirby, *Racial Politics at the Crossroads: Memphis Elects Dr. W. W. Herenton* (Knoxville: University of Tennessee Press, 1996).

4. Serina K. Gilbert, "The Health Insurance Plight of Patients with Sickle Cell Disease," *Journal of the National Medical Association* 78 (1986): 663–65.

5. As Robert Petersdorf and Kathleen Turner have noted, "The major sources of support for [academic medical centers] have changed in the last several decades, reflecting significant changes in these institutions' external environments. Most dramatic has been the decline in the proportion of medical school revenues received from the federal government for activities other than the provision of medical services. . . . The rate of increase for funding though the National Institutes of Health has declined in recent years, limiting the availability of research grants." Petersdorf and Turner, "Are Academic Medical Centers in Trou-

ble?" in *The Metropolitan Academic Medical Center: Its Role in an Era of Tight Money and Changing Expectations*, ed. David E. Rogers and Eli Ginzburg (San Francisco: Westview Press, 1995), 31–32.

6. "Concern with Urban Problems Spurs Interest in Sickle Cell Anemia," *New York Times*, July 25, 1971.

7. "Counterattack on a Killer—Blacks Fight to End Tragic Toll of Sickle Cell Anemia," *Ebony*, October 1971, 85.

8. Ibid.

9. Ibid.

10. Samuel Charache, "The Treatment of Sickle Cell Anemia," *Archives of Internal Medicine* 133 (April 1974): 699.

11. Elisabeth Rosenthal, "The Pain Game," *Discover* (November 1993): 56.

12. This question paraphrases one of the main questions addressed in Arthur Kleinman, Veena Das, and Margaret Lock, eds., "Introduction," *Social Suffering* (Berkeley: University of California Press, 1997), xiii.

13. A useful discussion of this ambivalence about popular movements in medicine can be found in W. Bruce Fye, *American Cardiology: The History of a Specialty and Its College* (Baltimore: Johns Hopkins University Press, 1996).

14. For a discussion of AIDS politics, see Randy Shilts, *And the Band Played On: Politics, People, and the AIDS Epidemic* (New York: St. Martin's Press, 1987), and Stephen Epstein, *Impure Science: AIDS, Activism, and the Politics of Knowledge* (Berkeley: University of California Press, 1996). For a discussion of cancer politics in the 1970s, see Ralph Moss, *The Cancer Industry: The Classic Exposé on the Cancer Establishment* (Brooklyn, N.Y.: Equinox, 1980).

15. After the failure of Senator Kennedy's national health insurance legislation, the Health Maintenance Organization Act was a conservative answer to increased access to health care.

16. Rosenthal, "The Pain Game," 56.

17. See, for example, Loch Adamson, "Sickle-Cell Patients Seek Respect," *Bronx Beat Online*, November 6, 1995, http://www.columbia.edu/cu/bb/sickle.html. See also K. Gorman, "Sickle Cell Disease: Do You Doubt Your Patient's Pain?" *American Journal of Nursing* 3 (March 1999): 38–43. On Reagan's anecdotes on "welfare queens," see Dan Miller, "The Chutzpa Queen: Favorite Reagan Target as Welfare Cheat Remains Unflappable at Trial in Chicago," *Washington Post*, March 17, 1977, A3, and also Mary McGrory, "Legal Board Members Avoid Joining 'Em by Representing 'Em," *Washington Post*, December 21, 1982, A3.

18. Adamson, "Sickle-Cell Patients Seek Respect.".

19. Ibid.

20. Kathryn Kramer and Kermit Nash article.

21. K. H. Todd et al., "Ethnicity and Analgesic Practice," *Annals of Emergency Medicine* 35 (January 2000): 11–16. In a study of patients with long-bone fractures,

the authors found that "white patients were significantly more likely than black patients to receive ED analgesics . . . despite similar records of pain complaints in the medical record. The risk of receiving no analgesic while in the ED was 66 percent greater for black patients than for white patients."

22. See Peter T. Kilborn, "Memphis Blacks Find Cycle of Poverty Difficult to Break," *New York Times*, October 5, 1999.

23. Frankie Winchester, *Sickle Cell Anemia Research in Memphis: Interview with Alfred P. Kraus, M.D.* (Memphis: Oral History Research Office, Memphis State University, 1989), 33.

24. See discussion of narcotics in Memphis in Chapter 6, especially Kraus's comparison of therapeutic decision making in Oakland as compared with Memphis.

25. Thelma Tracy Mabry, *History of Medicine in Memphis: Interview with Dr. Lemuel Whitley Diggs* (Memphis: Oral History Research Office, Memphis State University, 1984), 7.

26. For interpretations of the significance of pain discourse in medicine and culture, see Kleinman, Das, and Lock, *Social Suffering*; Mary S. Sheridan, *Pain in America* (Tuscaloosa: University of Alabama Press, 1992); Elaine Scarry, *The Body in Pain: The Making and Unmaking of the World* (New York: Oxford University Press, 1985); Roselyne Rey, *The History of Pain* (Cambridge, Mass.: Harvard University Press, 1993); and David Morris, *The Culture of Pain* (Berkeley: University of California Press, 1991).

27. S. Charache and M. Moyer, "Treatment of Patients with Sickle Cell Anemia—Another View," *Progress in Clinical and Biological Research* 98 (1982): 81.

28. Randall Holcombe and Jason Griffin, "Effect of Insurance Status on Pain Medication Prescriptions in a Hem/Onc Practice," *Southern Medical Journal* 86 (February 1993): 151–56.

29. Richard Payne, "Pain Management in Sickle Cell Disease: Rationale and Techniques," in *Sickle Cell Disease*, ed. Charles Whitten and John Bertles (New York: New York Academy of Sciences, 1989), 189–206.

30. "Pain becomes a harbinger of potential catastrophe; tissues die from lack of oxygen. Patients sometimes suffer strokes, but the most deadly manifestation of sickle-cell disease in adults is 'acute chest syndrome,' in which blood vessels in the lungs become clogged, dramatically increasing the danger of infection." Adamson, "Sickle-Cell Patients Seek Respect."

31. Orah Platt, "Easing the Suffering Caused by Sickle Cell Disease," *New England Journal of Medicine* 330 (March 17, 1994): 783.

32. See Todd, "Ethnicity and Analgesic Practice." See also Adamson, "Sickle-Cell Patients Seek Respect." Notes Adamson, quoting Charles Pollack in *Emergency Medical Clinics of North America*: "There have been studies that demonstrate that sicklers display no more of a propensity for narcotic dependence and drug seeking than any other patient with chronic pain."

33. See, for example, Robert Aronowitz, "From Myalgic Encephalitis to Yuppie Flu: A History of Chronic Fatigue Syndromes," in *Making Sense of Illness: Science, Society, and Disease* (New York: Cambridge University Press, 1998).

34. Platt, "Easing the Suffering." See also Orah Platt, "Pain in Sickle Cell Disease: Rates and Risk Factors," *New England Journal of Medicine* 325 (July 4, 1991): 11–16, and Elliot Vichinsky et al., "Multidisciplinary Approach to Pain Management in Sickle Cell Disease," *American Journal of Pediatric Hematology-Oncology* 4 (Fall 1982): 328–33.

35. Bruce Jancin, "Gatekeeper Model Dangerous in Sickle Cell Disease," *Pediatric News* 32 (1998): 26.

36. Ibid. The author cited a survey done by physician Peter A. Lane, director of the Colorado Sickle Cell Treatment and Research Center at the University of Colorado, Denver.

37. Thomas Maugh II, "Sickle Cell (II): Many Agents Near Trials," *Science* 211 (January 30, 1981): 468–70.

38. Larry Churchill, *Rationing Health Care in America: Perceptions and Principles of Justice* (Notre Dame: University of Notre Dame Press, 1987).

39. "Switch on Genes," *Newsweek*, December 20, 1982, 85. See also T. J. Ley, J. DeSimone, N. Anagnou, G. Keller, K. Humphries, P. Turner, N. Young, P. Heller, and A. Nienhuis, "5-azacytidine Selectively Increases Gamma-Globin Synthesis in a Patient with Beta-Thalassemia," *New England Journal of Medicine* 307 (December 9, 1982): 1469–75; P. Heller and J. DeSimone, "5-azacytidine and Fetal Hemoglobin," *American Journal of Hematology* 17 (1984): 439–47; O. S. Platt, "Chemotherapy to Increase Fetal Hemoglobin in Patients with Sickle Cell Anemia," *American Journal of Pediatric Hematology-Oncology* 7 (Fall 1985): 258–60; and G. J. Dover et al., "Progress toward Increasing Fetal Hemoglobin Production in Man: Experience with 5-azacytidine and Hydroxyurea," *Annals of the New York Academy of Science* 445 (1985): 218–24.

40. "Genetic Fix: Turning on Fetal DNA," *Time*, December 20, 1982, 72.

41. Ibid.

42. See, for example, discussion in Howard A. Pearson, "Pharmacologic Manipulation of Fetal Hemoglobin Levels in Sickle Cell Diseases and Thalassemia: Promise and Reality," *Advances in Pediatrics* 43 (1996): 309–34.

43. A. Bank, D. Markowitz, and N. Lerner, "Gene Transfer: A Potential Approach to Gene Therapy for Sickle Cell Disease," *Annals of the New York Academy of Science* 565 (1989): 42.

44. Marian Segal, "New Hope for Children with Sickle Cell Disease," *FDA Consumer* 23 (March 1989): 14–19. Charles Whitten called gene therapy "the ultimate therapy."

45. Ron Winslow, "Sickle Cell Anemia Pain Curbed Dramatically by Drug, Study Says," *Wall Street Journal*, January 31, 1995, B6.

46. Charles Marwick, "Sickle Cell Problems Continue to Challenge Medical Sci-

ence, But Some Progress Is Noted," *Journal of the American Medical Association* 263 (January 26, 1990): 492.

47. Rodgers quoted in "A Switch for Sickle Cells," *U.S. News and World Report*, April 23, 1990. See also "Sickle Cell Breakthrough — New Drugs Quell Symptoms," *American Health* 9 (May 1990): 16, and "Waking Up Genes: A Flavor Enhancer May Provide the First Treatment for Sickle-Cell Anemia," *Time*, January 25, 1993, 23.

48. Pearson, "Pharmacologic Manipulation," 330.

49. Griffin Rodgers, "Recent Approaches to the Treatment of Sickle Cell Anemia," *Journal of the American Medical Association* 265 (April 24, 1991): 2100. Italics added for emphasis.

50. E. Vichinsky and B. Lubin, "A Cautionary Note Regarding Hydroxyurea in Sickle Cell Disease," *Blood* 83 (February 15, 1994): 1124–28.

51. Samuel Charache, "Experimental Therapy on Sickle Cell Disease: Use of Hydroxyurea," *American Journal of Pediatric Hematology-Oncology* 16 (1994): 62–66.

52. Warren Leary, "Sickle Cell Trial Called Success, Halted Early," *New York Times*, January 31, 1995, C1, C7.

53. Ibid. Italics added for emphasis.

54. Ibid.

55. Ibid.

56. As George Annas has written, the 1980s produced strange bedfellows, for "the antiregulation Reagan/Bush administrations and the gay community probably had only one interest in common: deregulating the drug approval process." George Annas, "Faith (Healing), Hope, and Charity at the FDA: The Politics of AIDS Drug Trials," in *Standard of Care: The Law of American Bioethics* (New York: Oxford University Press, 1993), 136. The trend continued into the 1990s. Increasingly, pharmaceutical companies themselves realized the value of allying with aggressive patient advocacy groups in bringing pressure on the FDA. This mixture of disease activism and free market ideologies sped new drugs, and some measure of relief, to the consumer.

57. This description appears on the National Cancer Institute Web site, http://cancertrials.nci.nih.gov/understanding/indepth/fda/history.html.

58. Ron Winslow, "Technology and Health: Sickle Cell Anemia Pain Curbed Dramatically by Drug, Study Says," *Wall Street Journal*, January 31, 1995, B6.

59. Ibid. See also Warren Leary, "Sickle Cell Trial Called Success, Halted Early," *New York Times*, January 31, 1995, C1, C7.

60. G. Rodgers and A. Schechter, "Sickle Cell Anemia — Basic Research Reaches the Clinic," *New England Journal of Medicine* 332 (May 18, 1995): 1372–73.

61. Samuel Charache, "Experimental Therapy," *Hematology/Oncology Clinics of North America* 10 (December 1996): 1376.

62. Gina Kolata and Kurt Eichenwald, "Health Business Thrives on Unproven

Treatment, Leaving Science Behind," *New York Times*, October 3, 1999. As Kolata and Eichenwald noted, more recent studies showed that BMT was not an effective alternative to chemotherapy and radiation in the treatment of breast and ovarian cancer, but even these findings did not dent the popularity of these centers.

63. "Marrow Transplant Found To Be a Cure in Sickle Cell Case," *New York Times*, September 20, 1984.

64. F. L. Johnson, "Bone Marrow Transplantation in the Treatment of Sickle Cell Anemia," *American Journal of Pediatric Hematology-Oncology* 7 (Fall 1985): 254–57. Johnson, chief of the Bone Marrow Transplantation Division of St. Jude and an associate professor of pediatrics at the University of Tennessee School of Medicine at Memphis, first presented this paper at a Washington, D.C., conference in October 1984. He warned that "the patient's course illustrates both the promise and problems of bone marrow transplantation in the treatment of sickle cell anemia."

65. "Marrow Transplant Found to Be a Cure in Sickle Cell Case," *New York Times*, September 20, 1984. See also Johnson, "Bone Marrow Transplantation."

66. E. Hardy and E. V. Ikpeazu, "Bone Marrow Transplantation: A Review," *Journal of the National Medical Association* 81 (1989): 523.

67. Ibid.

68. R. B. Scott, "Advances in the Treatment of Sickle Cell Disease in Children," *American Journal of the Diseases of Children* 139 (1985): 1219–22.

69. F. T. Billings III, "Treatment of Sickle Cell Anemia with Bone Marrow Transplantation — Pros and Cons," *Transactions of the American Clinical and Climatological Association* 101 (1989): 8–19; Ronald Nagel, "The Dilemma of Marrow Transplantation in Sickle Cell Anemia," *Seminars in Hematology* 28 (July 1991): 233–34; and E. Donnall Thomas, "The Pros and Cons of Bone Marrow Transplantation for Sickle Cell Anemia," *Seminars in Hematology* 28 (July 1991): 260–62.

70. Sergio Piomelli, "Sickle Cell Disease in the 1990s: The Need for Active and Preventive Intervention," *Seminars in Hematology* 28 (July 1991): 227–31.

71. Nagel, "Dilemma of Marrow Transplantation," 234.

72. Ernest Beutler, "Bone Marrow Transplantation for Sickle Cell Anemia: Summarizing Comments," *Seminars in Hematology* 28 (July 1991): 263–67.

73. Thomas, "Pros and Cons," 261.

74. Nagel, "Dilemma of Marrow Transplantation," 234.

75. Ibid.

76. Renée Fox and Judith Swazey, *Spare Parts: Organ Replacement in American Society* (New York: Oxford University Press, 1992).

77. Eric Kodish et al., "Bone Marrow Transplantation for Sickle Cell Disease," *New England Journal of Medicine* 325 (November 7, 1991): 1353.

78. As the authors noted, "Parents who had graduated from high school were

significantly more likely to accept some risk in exchange for cure than those who were not high-school graduates. . . . Parents who were employed or in school were more likely to accept some risk than those who were not occupied outside the home. . . . Finally, parents were more likely to consent to bone marrow transplantation for girls than for boys." Ibid., 1351.

79. Orah Platt and E. C. Guinan, "Bone Marrow Transplantation in Sickle Cell Anemia—The Dilemma of Choice," *New England Journal of Medicine* 335 (August 8, 1996): 426.

80. Ibid.

81. In the national discussion over sickle cell anemia therapies, some researchers believed that the BMT evidence suggested strongly that "the search for other therapies not based on marrow transplantation should be continued." Mentzer et al., "Availability of Related Donors." Others sought to avoid the complex ethical problems associated with BMT by passing the difficult decisions on to the consumers and their families, by redefining the therapeutic status of BMT, and by changing the regulatory status of the modality. "Although some knowledge may be gained from offering transplantation to patients with sickle cell disease," noted one study, "we suggest that the use of transplantation for patients with sickle cell disease is not primarily a matter of research." Kodish et al., "Bone Marrow Transplantation," 1353.

82. Susan Miller, "A Cure for Sickle Cell?" *Newsweek*, August 19, 1996, 64. See also Curtis Rist and Cindy Dampier, "A Life Now Worth Living," *People*, November 11, 1996, 201–2.

83. Samuel Charache, "Experimental Therapy," *Hematology/Oncology Clinics of North America* 10 (December 1996): 1375 (special issue on sickle cell anemia).

84. "In the United States," reported Charache, "only about 18% of [sickle cell anemia] patients would be expected to have HLA-identical full siblings." Ibid.

85. Ibid.

86. Richard Carter, "Insurance Coverage for Bone Marrow Transplants," reprinted from *BMT Newsletter*, May 1994. See also M. C. Walters et al., "Barriers to Bone Marrow Transplantation for Sickle Cell Anemia," *Biology of Blood and Marrow Transplantation* 2 (May 1996): 100–104. Here the authors point out that "among 4848 patients less than 16 years of age . . . 315 (6.5 percent) patients were reported to meet protocol entry criteria for transplantation . . . [and in this eligibility there was] wide variation among the [22] institutions. . . . [Among the 315 eligible,] 128 (41 percent) had HLA typing performed, and of these 44 (14 percent of those meeting the criteria) had an HLA-identical sibling." See, additionally, W. C. Mentzer et al., "Availability of Related Donors for Bone Marrow Transplantation in Sickle Cell Anemia," *American Journal of Pediatric Hematology-Oncology* 16 (February 1994): 27–29.

87. In the 1950s, for example, men like Mayor Edmund Orgill were such reformers. Orgill embraced social change and wider African American participation in

municipal life, but he was careful to do so not in the name of "integration" but in the name of democracy, fair representation, and (ironically) the preservation of the racial status quo. What was true in Memphis was also true statewide. In the 1960s Tennessee Democrats like Albert Gore Sr. found themselves forced into the position of supporting liberalization of racial attitudes, but opposing the Civil Rights Act of 1964. See Speech by Albert Gore Sr., April 1964, Governor Frank Clement Papers, Tennessee State Library and Archives, Nashville.

88. "Science Unlocking Sickle Cell," *Memphis Commercial Appeal*, January 11, 1972. One author in the same local newspaper noted that "it was probably considered a 'racial disease' and, in some quarters, a mark of inferiority." "Spotlight on a Killer," *Memphis Commercial Appeal*, March 5, 1972.

89. L. Diggs and D. Brookoff, Commentary, "Multiple Cerebral Aneurysms in Patients with Sickle Cell Disease," *Southern Medical Journal* 86 (April 1993): 377–79.

90. Julius Bauer and Louis Fisher, "Sickle Cell Disease, with Special Regard to Its Nonanemic Variety," *Archives of Surgery* 47 (1943): 558.

91. Robert Wilson, "Medical Units Get Sickle Cell Grant," *Memphis Commercial Appeal*, June 30, 1972, Morgue Files, Folder 80145, Mississippi Valley Collection, McWherter Library, University of Memphis.

92. Lemuel Diggs and Ernestine Flowers, "High School Athletes with Sickle Cell Trait (Hb A/S)," *Journal of the National Medical Association* 68 (1976): 492–93.

93. See discussion of "Doc" Ellis in Chapter 6.

94. Lemuel Diggs, "The Sickle Cell Trait in Relation to the Training and Assignment of Duties in the Armed Forces — IV. Consideration and Recommendation," *Aviation Space and Environmental Medicine* 55 (June 1984): 487–92; see also Lemuel Diggs, "The Sickle Cell Trait in Relation to the Training and Assignment of Duties in the Armed Forces — I. Policies, Observations, and Studies," *Aviation Space and Environmental Medicine* 55 (March 1984): 180–84; Lemuel Diggs, "The Sickle Cell Trait in Relation to the Training and Assignment of Duties in the Armed Forces — II. Aseptic Splenic Necrosis," *Aviation Space and Environmental Medicine* 55 (April 1984): 271–76; Lemuel Diggs, "The Sickle Cell Trait in Relation to the Training and Assignment of Duties in the Armed Forces — III. Hyposthenuria, Hematuria, Sudden Death, Rhabdomyolosis, and Acute Tubular Necrosis," *Aviation Space and Environmental Medicine* 55 (May 1984): 358–64; and Lemuel Diggs, "Opinions Related to Vascular Occlusive Lesions in Individuals with Sickle Cell Trait," *Military Medicine* 148 (September 1983): 757–58.

95. Diggs, "Sickle Cell Trait — I," 82.

96. I. M. Weisman, R. J. Zeballos, T. W. Martin, and B. D. Johnson, "Effect of Army Basic Training in Sickle-Cell Trait," *Archives of Internal Medicine* 148 (November 1988): 2420.

97. A. T. Fort, J. C. Morrison, L. W. Diggs, S. A. Fish, and L. Barreras, "Counseling

the Patient with Sickle Cell Disease about Reproduction: Pregnancy Outcome Does Not Justify the Maternal Risk," *American Journal of Obstetrics and Gynecology* 111 (October 1, 1971): 324–27.

98. Richard Severo, "Genetic Screening at DuPont: Blacks Only Need Apply," *The Nation*, September 20, 1980, 243–45.

99. Jeff Levine, "As Gene Technology Improves, So Does Prospect for Discrimination," *CNN Interactive*, October 24, 1996. "A case in point is Larry Allen," the report noted, "who said he lost his job and therefore his insurance partly because of medical bills associated with his children's sickle-cell disease."

100. Carter, "Insurance Coverage for Bone Marrow Transplants."

101. Diggs, conversation with the author, April 1993; Celeste Williams, "Penicillin Found Helpful for Victims of Sickle Cell — Memphis Doctor Is in Study Group," *Memphis Commercial Appeal*, June 12, 1986, B1.

102. Gregg Meyer and David Blumenthal, "The Initial Effects of TennCare on Academic Health Centers," *Commonwealth Fund Report*, November 1996, on Commonwealth Fund Web site, http://www.commonwealthfund.org/programs/taskforc/tenncare.asp.

103. David Manning, vice president of Columbia/HCA Healthcare Corporation declared in January 1995, "To suggest that [health care] problems will be solved by government intervention in the market, ignores the important lessons of history in this important area. Their only solution rests with market forces." David Manning, "TennCare: Market Based Medicaid Reform," January 1995, Columbia Center for Medicaid and the Uninsured Web site.

104. Jackson Baker, "Don Sundquist: Do We Really Have a Friend in Nashville?" *The Memphis Flyer*, March 20–26, 1997.

105. Ibid.

106. Deborah Gesensway, "How Internists in One Southern City Integrated Rather Than Faded Away," *American College of Physicians Observer*, November 1996, 1.

107. Pohlmann and Kirby, *Racial Politics at the Crossroads*.

108. G. Meyer and D. Blumenthal, "Initial Effects of TennCare." See also Gregg Meyer and David Blumenthal, "TennCare and Academic Medical Centers: The Lessons from Tennessee," *Journal of the American Medical Association* 278 (September 4, 1996): 672–76.

109. David Mirvis and Cyril Chang, "Grading TennCare," *TMA Medwire*, March 1998, http://www.medwire.org/html/news/mar98-grdingtnc.html. See also D. Mirvis, C. Chang, C. J. Hall, G. T. Zaar, and W. B. Applegate, "Tenncare: Health Care Reform for Tennessee," *Journal of the American Medical Association* 274 (October 18, 1995): 1274.

110. Meyer and Blumenthal, "Initial Effects of TennCare."

111. Ibid.

112. "The MED [medical center] faces special problems because of its location at

the border of Arkansas and Mississippi. The poor of these two states account for 25 percent of the deliveries at the MED. Tennessee DSH [the state program] once subsidized care for Mississippi and Arkansas (the MED is among the top five providers for both states), but with [DSH's] elimination the MED is now trying to cover these costs from operations. This geographically-based adverse selection could be repeated by other 'border' AHCs." Ibid.

113. Jon Hamilton, "TennCare Revitalized," *Physician's Weekly* 13 (June 17, 1996): 1–3.

114. "In a survey by the University of Tennessee, the percentage of uninsured who indicated receiving poor care increased from 13 percent in 1993 to 25 percent in 1994, i.e., an increase of over 90 percent from before to after initiation of TennCare." Mirvis and Chang, "Grading TennCare."

115. Hamilton, "TennCare Revitalized."

116. Baker, "Don Sundquist."

117. Ibid.

118. "Columbia Fraud 'Systemic': FBI, in Affidavit, Charges Health Giant with Scheme to Swindle Government," *CNNfn Interactive*, October 7, 1997. See also "Consumers Confront Managed-Care Revolution," *CNN Interactive*, September 6, 1996; "Columbia/HCA Profits Dim—Troubled Health-Care Giant Slashes Earnings Projections Amid Fraud Probe," *CNNfn Interactive*, September 9, 1997.

119. Increasingly, the future of specialties like hematology-oncology was weighed against the new political and economic climate. See T. P. Duffy, "Rationing Health Care: Its Impact and Implications for Hematology-Oncology," *Yale Journal of Biology and Medicine* 65 (March–April 1992): 75–82; J. van Eys, "The Impact of Medicaid on Research-Based Care in Pediatric Hematology-Oncology," *American Journal of Pediatric Hematology-Oncology* 13 (1991): 91–96.

120. Elliot Vichinsky, lecture at the 1997 national meetings of the Sickle Cell Disease Association of America, November 1997, Washington, D.C.

121. Ibid.

122. Ibid. In response to these trends, at least one author insisted that hematologist-oncologists should be classified as primary care practitioners because of the nature of the diseases they treat. S. W. Rypkema and R. F. Holcombe, "The Role of Hematologist/Oncologist as a Primary Care Provider," *American Journal of Medical Sciences* 308 (December 1994): 360–64.

123. Bob Herbert, "Hidden Agenda," *New York Times*, July 15, 1996, A13.

124. J. A. Wilimas, "A Randomized Study of Outpatient Treatment with Ceftiaxone for Selected Febrile Children with Sickle Cell Disease," *New England Journal of Medicine* 329 (August 12, 1993): 472–76. See comments on this paper as well in *New England Journal of Medicine* 329 (August 12, 1993): 501–2 and 330 (January 20, 1994): 219, 220.

CONCLUSION

1. One sees similar symbolism in discussions of Tay-Sachs disease among Askenazi Jews. See, for example, Jared Diamond, "Curse and Blessing of the Ghetto," *Discover* 12 (March 1991): 60–65.

2. Other historians and historian-epidemiologists have used the case of other diseases, such as hypertension, to explore similar themes in African American history. There are those, for example, like Clarence Grim who have argued that the Middle Passage experience selected for particular traits and encouraged the high prevalence of hypertension in African American men. See, for example, T. W. Wilson and C. E. Grim, "Biohistory of Slavery and Blood Pressure Differences in Blacks Today: A Hypothesis," *Hypertension* 17 (1991): 1122–1128. For commentaries and critiques of this biohistorical argument, see Philip Curtin, "The Slavery Hypothesis for Hypertension among African-Americans: The Historical Evidence," *American Journal of Public Health* 82 (December 1992): 1681–86, and K. A. Fackelmann, "The African Gene? Searching through History for the Roots of Black Hypertension," *Science News* 140 (1991): 254–55.

3. See Charles Bosk, *All God's Mistakes: Genetic Counseling in a Pediatric Hospital* (Chicago: University of Chicago Press, 1992).

4. See Ruth Hubbard and Elijah Wald, *Exploding the Gene Myth: How Genetic Information Is Produced and Manipulated by Scientists, Physicians, Employers, Insurance Companies, Educators, and Law Enforcers* (Boston: Beacon Press, 1993); Philip Kitcher, *The Lives to Come: The Genetic Revolution and Human Possibilities* (New York: Simon and Schuster, 1996); Daniel Kevles and Leroy Hood, eds., *The Code of Codes: Scientific and Social Issues in the Human Genome Project* (Cambridge, Mass.: Harvard University Press, 1992); and Susan Lindee and Dorothy Nelkin, *The DNA Mystique: The Gene as a Cultural Icon* (New York: Freeman Press, 1995).

5. "Discriminating Disease," *Time*, December 21, 1970, 41.

6. Rodgers and Schechter, "Sickle Cell Anemia — Basic Research Reaches the Clinic," *New England Journal of Medicine* 332 (May 18, 1995): 1372–73.

7. P. David Marshall, *Celebrity and Power: Fame in Contemporary Culture* (Minneapolis: University of Minnesota Press, 1997), x. See, particularly, the introduction and chapter 3, "Tools for the Analysis of the Celebrity as a Form of Cultural Power."

8. Ibid., xi. As Marshall also notes, "The celebrity sign effectively contains this tension between authentic and false cultural value."

9. This debate — about the role of government in enforcing health care equality, and the relationship of popular disease constituencies to biomedical research — still manifests itself today in the politics of AIDS and breast cancer. The case of sickle cell disease signaled an important stage in these relationships, for it highlighted that patients' experiences were now significant forces in American biomedical research.

10. James Grossman, *Land of Hope: Chicago, Black Southerners, and the Great Migration* (Chicago: University of Chicago Press, 1989); Allan Spear, *Black Chicago: The Making of a Negro Ghetto, 1890–1920* (Chicago: University of Chicago Press, 1967); Nicholas Lemann, *The Promised Land: The Great Black Migration and How It Changed America* (New York: Knopf, 1991).

11. Charles Rosenberg and Janet Golden, eds., *Framing Disease: Studies in Cultural History* (New Brunswick: Rutgers University Press, 1992).

12. Skeptics wondered at the time why preferential attention was given to this particular form of pain and suffering. Was this not a kind of "irrational" ethnic disease politics influencing medical research funding? In the wake of sickle cell disease legislation came calls for research funding for other diseases prevalent in other ethnic groups, as discussed in Chapter 6. See Barbara Culliton, "Cooley's Anemia: Special Treatment for Another Ethnic Disease," *Science* 178 (November 10, 1972): 590–93. On the politics of pain, see Mary-Jo Delvecchio Good et al., *Pain as Human Experience: An Anthropological Perspective* (Berkeley: University of California Press, 1992), and David Morris, *The Culture of Pain* (Berkeley: University of California Press, 1991).

13. In the early 1970s, for example, gay rights activists disrupted meetings of the American Psychiatric Association, calling for changes in the *Diagnostic and Statistical Manual*'s inclusion of homosexuality as a disease. At the same time, passage of legislation ensured that sufferers from kidney failure would have federally financed access to kidney dialysis. See Ronald Bayer, *Homosexuality and American Psychiatry* (Princeton: Princeton University Press, 1987). See also Abraham Bergman, *The "Discovery" of Sudden Infant Death Syndrome: Lessons in the Practice of Political Medicine* (Seattle: University of Washington Press, 1986), and Richard Rettig, "Origins of the Medicare Kidney Disease Entitlement: The Social Security Amendment of 1972," in *Biomedical Politics*, ed. Kathi Hanna (Washington, D.C.: National Academy Press, 1991), 176–208. On AIDS in the 1980s, see Steven Epstein, *Impure Science: AIDS, Activism, and the Politics of Knowledge* (Berkeley: University of California, 1996).

14. George Anders, *Health against Wealth: HMOs and the Breakdown of Medical Trust* (New York: Houghton Mifflin, 1996), 90. See, in particular, Bruce Jancin, "Gatekeeper Model Dangerous in Sickle Cell Disease," *Pediatric News* 32 (1998): 26.

15. Ralph Ellison, *Invisible Man* (New York: Random House, 1952), 433.

16. Ibid., 433.

17. Here my comments on pain are informed by Good et al., *Pain as Human Experience*, and Pierre Bourdieu, *Language and Symbolic Power* (Cambridge, Mass.: Harvard University Press, 1982).

18. Historians too have become skeptical of arguments from experience. As historian Joan Scott has noted, "Experience is not a word we can do without, although given its usage to essentialize identity and reify the subject, it is tempting

to abandon it altogether. . . . It serves as a way of talking about what happened, of establishing difference and similarity, of claiming knowledge that is 'unassailable.'" But as Scott also notes, "Given the ubiquity of the term, it seems to me more useful to work with it, to analyze its operations and to redefine its meaning. This entails focusing on processes of identity production, insisting on the discursive nature of 'experience' and on the politics of its construction." This describes the process I have pursued throughout this book. Joan W. Scott, "The Evidence of Experience," *Critical Inquiry* 17 (Summer 1991): 4.

Primary Sources

MANUSCRIPT COLLECTIONS
Bancroft Library, University of California, Berkeley
   Social Protest Collection
Columbia University, New York
   L. S. Alexander Gumby Collection of the American Negro, Scrapbook
Cossitt Branch Library, Memphis
   Henry Loeb III Papers
Marriott Library Special Collections, University of Utah, Salt Lake City
   Maxwell Myer Wintrobe Papers
Memphis and Shelby County Public Library, Memphis
   George Washington Lee Collection
   Newspaper Clipping Files
Mississippi Valley Collection, McWherter Library, University of Memphis
   George Grider Papers
   Dan Kuykendall Papers
   Edward Meeman Papers
   Morgue Files of the *Memphis Press-Scimitar*
   Edmund Orgill Papers
   Samuel Watkins Overton Papers
   Annie Pope Van Dyke Family Papers
Moreland-Spingarn Research Centers, Howard University, Washington, D.C.
   Louis T. Wright Papers
National Archives and Records Administration, College Park, Maryland
   Richard Nixon Presidential Materials Project
   Records of the U.S. Department of Labor, Children's Bureau
   Records of the U.S. Public Health Service
Regenstein Library, University of Chicago
   Julius Rosenwald Papers

Southern Historical Collection, University of North Carolina, Chapel Hill
  James Robinson Papers
Tennessee State Library and Archives, Nashville
  Hill McAllister Papers
  Malcolm Rice Patterson Papers
  Records of the Tennessee Department of Public Health

JOURNALS

ALSAC News
American Journal of the Diseases of
  Children
American Journal of Pediatric
  Hematology-Oncology
American Journal of Public Health
American Journal of Surgery
Archives of Internal Medicine
Atlantic
Aviation Space and Environmental
  Medicine
Black Scholar
Blood
British Medical Journal
Congressional Quarterly
Congressional Record
Crisis
Discover
Ebony
FDA Consumer
Hematology/Oncology Clinics of North
  America
Journal of the American Medical
  Association
Journal of Laboratory and Clinical
  Medicine
Journal of the National Medical Association

Journal of Negro Education
Journal of Negro Life
Journal of Social Psychology
Memphis and Mid-South Medical Journal
Memphis Flyer
Memphis Medical Journal
Nation
New England Journal of Medicine
New-Orleans Medical and Surgical
  Journal
Newsweek
Opportunity
Phylon
Planters Journal
Public Health Bulletin
Saturday Evening Post
Saturday Review of the Sciences
Science
Scientific American
Smithsonian
Southern Medical Journal
Tennessee State Medical Journal
Time
Transactions of the American Pediatric
  Society
U.S. News and World Report
Veteran's Medical Bulletin

NEWSPAPERS

Memphis Commercial Appeal
Memphis Press-Scimitar
Memphis World
New York Times
Pittsburgh Courier

San Francisco Chronicle
San Francisco Examiner
Tri-State Defender
Wall Street Journal
Washington Post

Index

Health, 16–17, 32, 38, 62, 70. *See also* Graves, Lloyd; Wadley, S. L.

Memphis General Hospital (MGH), 17, 32, 36–37, 38, 45, 50–51, 79, 80, 96, 106. *See also* John Gaston Hospital

Memphis Medical Journal, 38, 62, 68, 91, 106, 110, 120

Memphis Minnie. *See* Douglas, Lizzie

"Memphis Minnie-jitis Blues," 1–3, 25, 54, 55

Memphis Press-Scimitar, 51, 72, 138, 157, 182

Memphis Sickle Cell Anemia Council, 178

Memphis State University, 157

Memphis World, 95, 103, 112, 179

Mencken, H. L., 19

Meningitis, 2, 40, 65, 76, 78

Metropolitan Life Insurance Co., 100

Meyer, Gregg, 221

Miller, Randall, 117

Miller, William, 41

Mississippi, 10, 19, 44, 50, 53, 54, 72, 176–77, 181, 220, 221

Mississippi Delta, 2, 11, 156

Mississippi River, 11, 19, 47, 60, 63, 77

Mitchell, B. G., 162

Mitchell, Edward Clay, 72–74

Moore, Gatemouth, 90–91

Mortality, infant, 10, 32, 38, 55–59, 65–77, 103, 234

Moynihan, Daniel Patrick, 174

Murrell, Thomas, 14–15

Nagel, Ronald, 202, 213–14, 216

Nalbandian, Robert, 190–91, 228

Nashville, Tenn., 16, 50, 57, 101, 119, 220, 232

Nation, 136

National Association for the Advancement of Colored People (NAACP), 89, 90, 138, 171, 180

National Association of Patients on Hemodialysis, 195–96

National Institutes of Health (NIH), 8, 9, 148–49, 166, 170, 172, 183, 185, 193, 313

National Medical Association, 49

National Negro Health Week, 66

New England Journal of Medicine, 187, 188

New Orleans, La., 26, 27, 54, 100

Newsom, Moses, 143

Newsweek, 206

New York, N.Y., 2, 21, 28, 58, 98, 100, 119, 151, 180, 181, 220, 230; health care in, 39, 43, 101, 202

New York Age, 42

New York Times, 156, 223

Nixon, Richard M., 7, 12, 22–23, 165, 170–75, 181, 184, 192–93, 195

Oakland, Calif., 73, 181–83, 223

Obstetricians, 38–39, 70

Oppenheimer, Ella, 72–76, 98, 127

Orgill, Edmund, 111–13, 123–25, 127, 135, 157, 319–20

Orsi, Robert, 122

Our Bodies, Our Selves, 185

Overton, Watkins, 71, 97–98

Pain: African Americans and, 15–16, 55, 82, 107–9, 118, 128, 139, 150; experience of, 10, 13, 55, 57, 59, 161–64, 233–34; interpretations of, 59–65, 204–5, 299. *See also* Sickle cell disease: and narcotics; Sickle cell disease: and pain

Patients, 1, 6, 14–17, 33, 37, 46–47, 56, 104, 147–50, 155; activism by, 9, 110–11, 166–67; illness experiences of, 4–5, 9–10, 24, 160–64, 167–68, 169, 196, 227, 230, 233–34 (*see also* Sickle cell disease: experiences of patients with); as research subjects, 80, 82, 91–92, 95, 114–18, 120–22, 125–28, 148, 152, 155, 208, 211–16, 221, 230; used in medical education, 17, 29, 36–38, 79–81, 95, 106, 221, 249–50. *See also* Disease

Patterson, Russell, 114–15

Pauling, Linus, 5–6, 12, 106, 114, 116, 167, 186–87, 206, 228, 231, 234

Pearson, Howard, 161, 189, 208

Pediatricians, 68, 70, 72, 73, 77, 82, 95, 116–17, 126

Pediatrics, 117

Pellagra, 57, 60, 61, 254–55

Penicillin, 84, 86, 115–16

Perkins, Frances, 71

Pharmaceutical industry, 85, 206–11, 224, 227. *See also* Plough, Abe

Philanthropists, 30, 36, 45, 47–52. *See also* American Lebanese and Syrian Associated Charities; Herff, Herbert; Plough, Abe; Thomas, Danny

Phillips, Ulrich, 15

Physicians, 33, 34, 52, 61, 70–71, 75, 79–82, 93, 96, 113–14, 116–17. *See also* African Americans: as physicians

Pinkel, Don, 154

Platt, Orah, 204, 216

Plessy v. Ferguson, 26

Plough, Abe, 34, 122, 123

Pneumonia, 10, 55, 59, 65, 99, 104, 116

Poe, Clarence, 19

Poitier, Sidney, 165, 169–70, 182, 199

Polio, 94, 104–5, 110–11, 119, 168, 169

Preble, Paul, 47

Presley, Elvis, 11, 197

Price, Hollis, 157

Race. *See* African Americans; Memphis, Tenn.: white citizens of

Ray, James Earl, 162

Reagan, Ronald, 202, 209

Redditt, Edward, 178

Republican Party, 42, 168, 171–73, 175; in Tennessee, 42–44, 172–73, 176, 178, 179, 220, 231–32

Rheumatism, 10, 167

Richardson, Elliot, 172, 173

Richmond, Va., 82, 100

Robinson, James H., 19

Rockefeller, John D., 48, 50

Rodgers, Griffin, 208

Roe v. Wade, 185

Rosenthal, Elisabeth, 200, 201–2

Rosenwald, Julius, 48–50, 52, 238, 256

Rothman, David, 117

Royal Circle Hospital, 44

St. Jude Children's Research Hospital, 11, 21, 105, 121–22, 125, 127, 148, 150–56, 163, 169, 177, 180, 183, 192, 211, 223, 230

St. Louis, Mo., 58, 116

Salk, Jonas, 108

Science, 106, 194

Scoville, Addison, 155

Segregation, 97, 140–42. *See also* African Americans: and segregation; Hospitals, and desegregation; Memphis, Tenn.: segregation in

Selma, Ala., 156

Severo, Richard, 136

Sheppard-Towner Maternity and Infancy Protection Act, 65–66

Shockley, William, 186

Sibley, Elbridge, 60

Sickle Cell Anemia Control Act, 7, 169–96, 201

Sickle cell disease: and Africa, 144–47, 167–68, 182, 188–89, 204, 233; and African-American identity, 4–5, 78–79, 83, 139, 145–47; and Black Panther Party, 22, 164, 182–83; and

cardiovascular disease, 193–94; in
cinema and television, 165, 168, 169–
70, 180, 181–82; and Cooley's Anemia, 194, 195, 201, 212; and discrimination, 182, 191, 195–96; economic
aspects of, 12, 23, 138–39, 143–44,
147–49, 213–16, 222–23; and evolution, 5–7, 145–47, 186–87, 225–26,
233; experiences of patients with, 4–
5, 10, 21, 55, 59, 116, 119, 121, 134,
147–48, 161–64, 167–68, 169, 183–
84, 191, 199–200, 202, 204, 217, 227,
229, 233–34, 298–99; and hemoglobin, 116, 120–21, 206; *Hemoglobin Memphis*, 156–62; and heredity, 22, 78–79, 199, 231; and HMOs,
211; and inferiority debates, 185–90,
191, 199, 231; and malaria, 6, 22, 59–
65, 144–47, 188–89, 225–26, 233;
and malpractice, 205; and managed
care, 23, 198, 201, 216–24, 231; and
medical specialists, 80–83, 116–18,
120–23, 126–28; and Memphis
clinic, 3, 10, 21, 79–82, 107–9, 118–
23, 126–28, 156–62, 184, 191–92,
219, 294; and mental health, 187–88,
191; and molecular biologists, 5–6, 8,
114–18, 144–47, 186–87, 228, 230;
and narcotics, 23, 135, 160–62, 164,
181–82, 191, 199–205, 210, 215, 216,
231; neglect of, 23, 166, 174, 230,
231; obscurity and invisibility of, 8,
55–83, 184; and pain, 107–9, 114–
15, 121–22, 125–28, 158–64, 191,
192, 198–205, 208–10, 230–31, 233;
political significance of, 7–8, 22–23,
165–96; and popular culture, 7, 9, 22,
16; scientific significance of, 3, 79–
83, 106, 114–18, 120–21, 122–23,
125–28, 144–47, 158, 160–62, 196;
social meaning of, 3, 82–83, 125–28,
138–39, 155–56, 160–62, 165–96,

288; and soldiers, 88–89, 146, 180,
216–18
— treatment of, 23, 135, 158, 160–62,
164, 190, 205–16, 222–23; antibiotics in, 9, 84, 86, 115–16; blood
transfusion in, 119, 134, 223; bone
marrow transplantation in, 205, 211–
16, 220, 319; carbamyl phosphate in,
191; desickling agents in, 190–91;
5-azacytidine in, 206–7; gene therapy
in, 206–7, 227; hydroxyurea in, 207–
11, 212, 215, 220, 228; urea in, 190–
91, 228; zinc in, 191. *See also* Sickle
cell disease: and narcotics
Sickle cell trait: genetic screening for
and counseling controversies involving, 7, 174, 180–96, 226–27, 308; and
employment restrictions, 8, 136, 146,
180, 188–89, 216–19; and reproductive rights, 7–8, 171, 185–90, 191,
218, 227; theories about carriers of,
6, 144–47, 180, 188–89, 195, 225–26
Silver, Christopher, 113
Simkins v. Moses Cone Hospital, 289
Sipperstein, Marvin, 170
Smith, Vasco, 157
Southern Christian Leadership Con-
ference, 171
Spock, Benjamin, 94, 108
Stanfield, J. Edwin, 162
Stargell, Willie, 169
Sundquist, Don, 220, 222
Swazey, Judith, 214
Sydenham Hospital, 98
Syphilis, 13, 22, 56, 61, 65, 78, 79, 83,
103, 109, 196, 229

Tay-Sachs Disease, 8, 195
TennCare, 197–98, 201, 219–24, 232
Tennessee Hospital Association, 93
Tennessee State Medical Journal, 117
Terrell Memorial Hospital, 35, 44, 49

Thomas, Danny, 121–22, 150–52, 169, 177. *See also* American Lebanese and Syrian Associated Charities; St. Jude Children's Research Hospital

Thomas, E. Donnall, 213

Thompson, C. E., 93

Time, 119, 143

Tobey, Frank, 112

Tomes, Nancy, 31

Tri-State Defender, 95, 108, 112, 150, 179, 182, 184

Truman, Harry S., 85, 93

Tuberculosis, 2, 10, 16, 32, 38, 55, 56, 57, 59, 60, 61, 62, 65, 78, 79, 81, 83, 99, 104, 106, 109, 116, 144, 229

Tucker, David, 27

Tunney, John, 171–74

Tuskegee Institute, 16, 46, 49, 50; and Veterans Hospital controversy, 46–48

"Tuskegee Syphilis Experiment," 13, 22, 48–49, 166, 196

Typhoid fever, 16, 32, 47, 55, 60, 62–63, 106

UCLA Law Review, 186

United States, federal government of, 44–48, 51–52, 65–66, 84, 85, 137, 165, 176. *See also* Armed forces; Civil Rights Act; Funding, health care and research; Hill-Burton Hospital Survey and Construction Act; Medicaid; Medicare; Sickle Cell Anemia Control Act

U.S. Agricultural Adjustment Administration, 52

U.S. Children's Bureau, 59, 68, 69–77, 138

U.S. Civil Rights Commission, 138, 140–43, 150

U.S. Congress, 7, 88, 156, 185, 194, 195

U.S. Department of Health, Education, and Welfare (HEW), 158–59, 172, 177

U.S. Department of Justice, 222

U.S. Food and Drug Administration (FDA), 208–11, 213, 317

U.S. Health Care Financing Administration, 222

U.S. Public Health Service, 13, 41, 47, 48, 69–70, 71, 138, 148, 154, 196

U.S. Public Works Administration (PWA), 51–52, 76, 77

U.S. Supreme Court, 26, 112, 113, 118–19, 123, 185, 289

U.S. Veterans Hospitals, 44–48, 61, 120

Universal Life Insurance Co., 33, 39, 53, 123

University of Chicago, 214

University of Mississippi, 157

University of Pittsburgh, 162

University of Rochester, 50, 79

University of Tennessee Medical School, Memphis, 17, 21, 29, 36, 51, 53, 87, 177, 183, 189, 219–21; research at, 37, 79–82, 91–92, 108–9, 114–28, 148–49, 155, 162, 184, 191–92, 230; segregation at, 97, 140–42. *See also* Sickle cell disease: and Memphis clinic

Van Dyke, Annie Pope, 87–88

Van Dyke, Robert, 87

Van Dyke, William, 87–88, 93

Venereal Disease, 2, 144

Vichinsky, Elliot, 216, 223

Vocational School for Negro Girls, 43

Voting Rights Act, 137, 165, 176

Wadley, S. L., 76, 104–5

Walker, Joseph E., 25–26, 27, 30, 33, 34, 42, 44, 52, 53, 123–24, 127, 242

Wallace, George, 172

STUDIES IN SOCIAL MEDICINE